Cambridge Studies in Social and Emotional Development

General editor: Martin L. Hoffman

Social cognitive development

D0729955

Social cognitive development

Frontiers and possible futures

Based on seminars sponsored by the
Committee on Social and Affective Development During Childhood
of the Social Science Research Council

Edited by

JOHN H. FLAVELL *and* LEE ROSS

CAMBRIDGE UNIVERSITY PRESS

Cambridge
London   New York   New Rochelle
Melbourne   Sydney

Published by the Press Syndicate of the University of Cambridge
The Pitt Building, Trumpington Street, Cambridge CB2 1RP
32 East 57th Street, New York, NY 10022, USA
296 Beaconsfield Parade, Middle Park, Melbourne 3206, Australia

First published 1981

Printed in the United States of America
Typeset by Huron Valley Graphics, Inc., Ann Arbor, Michigan
Printed and bound by Vail-Ballou Press, Inc., Binghamton, New York

Library of Congress Cataloging in Publication Data

Main entry under title:

Social cognitive development.

(Cambridge studies in social and emotional development)

Includes index.

1. Social perception in children.
I. Flavell, John H. II. Ross, Lee.
III. Social Science Research Council. Committee on Social and Affective
Development During Childhood. IV. Series.
BF723.S6S63   155.4′18   80-25706
ISBN 0 521 23687 8 hard covers
ISBN 0 521 28156 3 paperback

Contents

List of contributors   *page* vi

Editorial preface   vii

1 The "intuitive scientist" formulation and its developmental
   implications *Lee Ross*   1

2 The development of thoughts about animate and inanimate
   objects: implications for research on social cognition *Rochel
   Gelman and Elizabeth Spelke*   43

3 Perspectives on the difference between understanding people
   and understanding things: the role of affect *Martin L.
   Hoffman*   67

4 "Concrete thinking" and the development of social
   cognition *Stephen M. Kosslyn and Jerome Kagan*   82

5 Social cognition in a script framework *Katherine Nelson*   97

6 Role taking and social judgment: alternative developmental
   perspectives and processes *E. Tory Higgins*   119

7 Exploring children's social cognition on two fronts *William
   Damon*   154

8 Relations between social cognition, nonsocial cognition, and
   social behavior: the case of friendship *Thomas J. Berndt*   176

9 Self-referent thought: a developmental analysis of
   self-efficacy *Albert Bandura*   200

10 Metacognition and the rules of delay *Water Mischel*   240

11 Monitoring social cognitive enterprises: something else that
    may develop in the area of social cognition *John H. Flavell*   272

12 The moral intuitions of the child *Richard A. Shweder, Elliot
    Turiel, and Nancy C. Much*   288

13 Concluding remarks *John H. Flavell and Lee Ross*   306

    Index   317

Contributors

Albert Bandura
Department of Psychology
Stanford University

Thomas J. Berndt
Department of Psychology
Yale University

William Damon
Department of Psychology
Clark University

John H. Flavell
Department of Psychology
Stanford University

Rochel Gelman
Department of Psychology
University of Pennsylvania

E. Tory Higgins
Department of Psychology
University of Western Ontario

Martin L. Hoffman
Department of Psychology
City University of New York
Graduate Center

Jerome Kagan
Department of Psychology and
Social Relations
Harvard University

Stephen M. Kosslyn
Department of Psychology and
Social Relations
Harvard University

Walter Mischel
Department of Psychology
Stanford University

Nancy C. Much
Committee on Human
Development
University of Chicago

Katherine Nelson
Department of Psychology
City University of New York
Graduate Center

Lee Ross
Department of Psychology
Stanford University

Richard A. Shweder
Committee on Human
Development
University of Chicago

Elizabeth Spelke
Department of Psychology
University of Pennsylvania

Elliot Turiel
Department of Education
University of California, Berkeley

Editorial preface

This book offers a collection of invited essays on social cognition and its development. These essays, as the title suggests, constitute less a comprehensive survey of current terrain than a prospectus for future exploration. The roster of contributors includes several researchers whose work on social cognitive development is probably familiar to the reader, but it also includes others who are best known for research that lies outside this area. Fairness both to the prospective reader and to our contributors thus demands that we clearly indicate the origins and goals of this volume.

During 1977–78, a series of small and informal conferences were held under the sponsorship of the Social Science Research Council's Committee on Social and Affective Development During Childhood. The intent of these conferences was to forge closer intellectual links between investigators long concerned with the field of social cognitive development and other investigators whose work in related disciplines – principally social anthropology, social psychology, cognitive psychology, and nonsocial cognitive development – seemed to offer potentially rich implications for that field. At each conference, several guests were invited to discuss their work, and the developmental issues it explicitly or implicitly raised, with the SSRC panelists. A number of these guests and most of the panelists then further volunteered (in some cases with a little gentle coercion) to prepare individually authored or jointly authored essays on topics that had figured heavily during our conference discussions. To those of the invited contributors who pleaded that they had only questions and speculations to offer, and to those who expressed qualms about venturing outside their accustomed scholarly realms, we insisted that the volume was to be more concerned with new ideas and perspectives than with detailed research reports or literature reviews. We thank them for their willingness to accept our challenge. We would also remark that some of the contributors turned out to be "closet" social cognitive developmentalists who "just happened" to have some relevant data lying around after all.

A few of the distinguished panelists and guests were unable to accept our invitation to set pen to paper. Nevertheless, the reader will find their ideas and influence apparent in the essays ultimately prepared by the rest of us. In this regard we gratefully acknowledge the stimulating contributions to the conferences made by Robert Abelson, Roy D'Andrade, Eleanor Rosch, Theodore Schwartz, and Amos Tversky. We also thank Janet Dafoe and Barbara Abrahams Everett for their assistance in transcribing the conference proceedings.

The strategy of inviting colleagues first to ponder and discuss, and ultimately to write about developmental topics that had previously not been the focus of their research programs was a deliberate one. Not only do we believe that the topics of greatest concern to the social and cognitive psychologist today are likely to be the "hot" developmental topics of tomorrow, but we also believe that the differing perspectives of the developmentalist and the nondevelopmentalist can be mutually enlightening (a theme to which we return in the concluding essay). The nondevelopmentalists were thus urged to give free rein to their imaginations and intuitions. They were invited to raise developmental questions and explore conceptual, methodological, or empirical issues without worrying about the need for conventional literature reviews, extensive documentation, or customary nods to colleagues who might have considered similar related issues before them. Essayists who were already veteran researchers and contributors to the social cognitive literature similarly were invited to speculate freely and relatively uncritically, to go further beyond their data than might normally be deemed appropriate for the conservative scientist.

Inevitably, our invitation to be wildly speculative and undisciplined has been inconsistently honored. Many of the contributors have supplemented their flights of fancy and speculation with a good deal of solid scholarship. Most have endeavored to show the relationship between their own ideas and those of earlier investigators, and some have favored us with provocative previously unpublished data.

The result, both of our choice of contributors and of the promptings and processes that culminated in their essays, is a collection that varies on a great many dimensions. Some of the essays offer primarily conceptual analysis or synthesis, others feature proposals for (or even descriptions of) seminal research, and still others focus on novel research tactics and techniques. Some of the essays deal primarily with classic topics and issues (for instance, the relationship between social cognitive development and nonsocial cognitive development, or the nature and origins of perspective-taking ability in children), whereas others deal with issues that are decidedly less classic (for instance, the child's intuitive appreciation of various principles of twentieth-century psychological theory and research, or the potential applications of concrete visualization tasks in exploring the child's developing social perceptions). Finally, essays differ widely in the explicitness with which they focus on specifically developmental issues. Thus, although some of the essays offer virtual battle plans for attacking particular developmental phenomena, others are less concerned with specific research proposals than with new perspectives on exactly what it is that ultimately develops in social cognition. Because each essay contains its own summary or conclusion, there is no need for us to abstract them here.

Our task as editors has benefited from the wisdom and efforts of many whose names do not appear here as authors. Themes for the book emerged from stimulating discussions in the Social Science Research Council's newly formed Committee on Social and Affective Development During Childhood. A complete list of the Committee's membership at that time appears facing the title page of this volume. The articles contained here reflect the Council's continuing mandate to advance social science research. This project and other committee efforts would not have been possible without the generous support of the Bush Foundation and the Foundation for Child Development. Peter B. Read, as Council staff to the committee, managed the myriad details required to obtain and sustain the involvement of keenly interested but overcommitted scholars. Susan Milmoe's editorial initiative at Cambridge University Press has allowed us to assemble and publish this distinctly nontraditional set of essays in an appropriately inviting format.

Like the compilers of any invited collection of papers, we hope that the collection's total contribution will be more than the sum of its separate parts. More specifically, we hope that the essays collectively will acquaint the reader with some features of an exciting and varied intellectual terrain. Indeed, we hope the essays will serve as an irresistible invitation to venture forth to new frontiers and help shape the future of the field.

John H. Flavell
Lee Ross

1 The "intuitive scientist" formulation and its developmental implications

Lee Ross

The concerns and research strategies of the developmental psychologist are bound to be influenced by the model of the human adult that is guiding the developmentalist's colleagues in cognitive, personality, and social psychology. In this chapter I shall discuss one such contemporary model (see also Nisbett & Ross, 1980; Ross, 1977, 1978), a model that portrays the adult human as an *intuitive social scientist* who, like the formal scientist, employs data and theories, and a variety of inferential tools, in attempting to understand, predict, and control the phenomena of everyday social experience.

The overall proficiency of the intuitive scientist hardly needs to be commented upon, for the general success of individual and collective human endeavor is eloquent testimony to this proficiency. But human folly and misunderstanding are also pervasive – too pervasive, and too consequential, to be dismissed. In fact, it has been the apparent shortcomings of the intuitive scientist that have received the lion's share of attention in contemporary research. In reviewing the intuitive scientist formulation, I shall try to highlight features that might be of particular interest to the developmental researcher. Afterwards, I hope to identify some developmental issues whose pursuit might add perspective to our portrait of the adult.[1] First, however, it may be helpful to consider the relationship between the intuitive scientist model, with its particular emphasis on human error, and the mainstream of social psychological thought in the 1970s.

I wish to acknowledge the helpful comments and suggestions by John Flavell and Mark Lepper, both of whom helped me to see (to a far greater extent than I have been able to convey in this chapter) that many of the developmental questions and implications raised in these pages are far from *terra incognita* for many of my colleagues in developmental psychology.

1

From attribution theory to intuitive psychology

To an unprecedented degree, social psychology in the late 1960s and 1970s abandoned such traditional concerns as group functioning and interpersonal influence and became preoccupied with the cognitive responses of the individual. Although the volume of research dealing with people's attempts to interpret information about their social environment has been tremendous, the increasing shift of emphasis has not been universally heralded. Many critics have expressed alarm at this "cognitive" preoccupation, taking their colleagues to task both for their neglect of affective and motivational processes and for their seeming reluctance to explore any real social *behavior.*

Much of the credit, or blame, for the contemporary state of social psychology rests with the attribution theorists, first Heider (1944, 1958), then Jones and Davis (1965), Kelley (1967, 1971, 1973), and their more recent associates (cf. Jones, Kanouse, Kelley, Nisbett, Valins, & Weiner, 1971; Weiner, 1974). These theorists focused on two closely related cognitive tasks confronting the social perceiver. The first task is that of *causal judgment,* whereby the perceiver seeks to assess the personal or situational causes to which some particular effect (i.e., action or outcome) may most reasonably be "attributed." The second task is that of *social inference,* whereby the perceiver deduces the "attributes" of the relevant entities, including the abilities, traits, or other dispositions of particular actors, and the demands and constraints of the situations to which those actors have responded.

Even though the label "attribution theory" and some of the jargon of its proponents were new, its broad concerns with naive epistemology and the processes of social inference already enjoyed a considerable and honorable history in social psychology. Asch (1952) and others within social psychology's Gestalt tradition long ago emphasized the subject's active role in "defining the situation," that is, in actively interpreting rather than passively registering the events that unfold in the laboratory and in everyday experience as well. Over thirty years ago, when the group dynamics movement was just dawning, Icheiser's (1949) analysis of stereotyping and prejudice focused on very general social perception biases and their origins (see also Allport, 1954). Soon after, George Kelly (1955, 1958) brought a social inference perspective to the study of psychopathology, even to the point of explicitly stating the layperson–scientist analogy. Similarly, Schachter and Singer (1962) and Bem (1965, 1967, 1972) independently anticipated and helped to stimulate attributional approaches in their respective analyses of emotional labeling and self-perception processes. And Cronbach (1955) and others (see review by Schneider, Hastorf, & Ellsworth, 1979, pp. 206–23) offered sophisticated analyses of the bases for accuracy and error in social perception. Nevertheless, it was the formalization of attribution theory by Jones, Kelley, and company that commanded social psychology's center stage during the 1970s, and it has been that perspective that increasingly has made its influence felt not only in developmental psychology (DiVitto & McArthur, 1978; Guttentag & Longfellow, 1977; Harris, 1977; Karniol & Ross, 1976, 1966, 1979; Kun, Parsons, & Ruble, 1974; Lepper, 1980; Lepper, Sagotsky, Dafoe, & Greene, 1980; Shultz & Butkowsky, 1977; Shultz, Butkowsky, Pearce, & Shanfield, 1975; Smith, M., 1975; Weiner & Kun, 1978; Weiner & Peter, 1973) but also in psychopathology (Abrahmson, Seligman, & Teasdale, 1978; Davison & Valins, 1969; Valins & Nisbett, 1972) and even in cognitive psychology (e.g., Bower, 1978).

I will not pause here to review mainstream attribution research and theory in any detail or to document its influence. Instead, I will outline a series of recent events that have shifted the focus of current attribution research and, I believe, have also broadened.the scope of contemporary "cognitive" social psychology in a manner that may offer some particularly exciting challenges for the developmentalist.

Logical attributional principles versus nonlogical biases

From its inception, attribution theory pursued the complementary, but in a sense competing, goals of accounting both for inferential accuracy and for inferential error (see Jones & Gerard, 1967; Kelley, 1967, 1973). Most early thinking and research however, was concerned more with people's successes than with their failures. To this end, theorists proposed a set of general principles that could reasonably be employed by people seeking to make correct causal judgments. These included, notably, the *covariation* principle (whereby effects are assigned to causes with which they covary) and the *discounting* principle (whereby the role of any causal candidate is "discounted" to the extent that the action or outcome to be explained is attended by other potentially sufficient candidates). Ensuing research provided ample evidence that subjects' causal attributions and inferences generally are at least directionally responsive to variables suggested by these normative principles (see McArthur, 1972, 1976; Orvis, Cunningham, & Kelley, 1975; Weiner, Heckhausen, Meyer, & Cook, 1972). What was less clear from such research was the layperson's capacity to give the relevant variables (i.e., "distinctiveness," "consistency," and especially "consensus") an appropriate or normatively optimal weighting, particularly when the data in question were not neatly "pre-packaged" in the laboratory but had to be derived from the flow of everyday experience (see Nisbett & Ross, 1980). In the last few years, however, interest in further demonstrating or clarifying the operation of rational attribution principles declined sharply. Investigators increasingly shifted their attention to sources of error in the attribution process – to various biases that might distort causal judgments and social inferences, thereby promoting seeming irrationalities and the risk of social dishar-mony (see reviews by Fischhoff, 1976; Ross, 1977, 1978; Schneider et al., 1979).

Much of the initial interest in attributional error was focused on the possibility of a consistent motivational or "ego-defensive" bias. This bias, as postulated, would lead people to take credit for their successes but to blame other people or the "situation" for their failures, would lead actors to give themselves more credit and less blame than they were given by observers, and would generally lead social participants to see themselves in more positive terms than would be warranted by totally dispassionate assessment. Evidence for such consistent self-serving biases, however, proved difficult to obtain. Actors sometimes did show asymmetries in their interpretations of success and failure, and sometimes did make attri-butions different from those made by disinterested observers, but these asymmetries were not found consistently and when they were found they were not consistently self-serving. Indeed, they sometimes seemed quite the opposite (e.g., Ross, Bierbrauer, & Polly, 1974)! More importantly, even when attributions objectively served to maintain or enhance actors' self-esteem, nonmotivational interpretations for these phenomena could easily be offered (see review by Bradley, 1978; Miller & M. Ross, 1975; Wortman, 1976).

Gradually, the concern with attributional biases and their origins shifted toward cognitive, perceptual, or informational factors (e.g., Arkin & Duvall, 1975; Fischhoff & Nisbett, 1972; Fischhoff, 1975; Langer, 1975, Newtson, 1973; M. Ross & Siccoly, 1979; Taylor & Fiske, 1978; Trope, 1978). One result of these shifts of emphasis, first from logical attributional principles to sources of attribution error and then from moti-vational to nonmotivation sources of bias, has been to encourage social psychologists to expose themselves to thinking and research in other areas of psychology where cognitive and perceptual deficiencies or biases have long been a central concern. And this exposure, inevitably, has led us to look beyond the specific tasks of social attribution to other, equally im-portant tasks involved in human inference and understanding.

Attribution and prediction

One inferential task in particular captured the attention of cognitively oriented social psychologists in the 1970s. This task was that of *prediction*, of inferring the future from the past or, more generally, of estimating the unknown from the known. In many circumstances, of course, the task of prediction is intimately related to the task of attribution. Assessing the causes of an action, and deducing the properties of the actor and his or her situation, obviously influences one's predictions both about the future behavior of that actor and about the behavior of other actors who might face the same situation. Any items of information that influence attributions are apt to influence related behavioral predictions. Conversely, any failures to make appropriate use of information in the attribution process are likely to be accompanied by parallel failures in intuitive prediction.

Research on the impact of "consensus" or "base-rate" information has been particularly provocative with respect to this parallel between attribution and prediction tasks. In the attribution camp, several investigators found that information about the relative commonness or uncommonness of particular responses in a given situation often has surprisingly little effect on people's causal assessments (McArthur, 1972, 1976) and even less effect on their willingness to make inferences about the relevant actors (Cooper, Jones & Tuller, 1972; Miller, Gillen, Schenker, & Radlove, 1973). This lack of impact of consensus information can be demonstrated even when the attributions concern assessments about the self (see Nisbett, Borgida, Crandall, & Reed, 1976). At roughly the same time as these contradictions to the normative principles of attribution theory were emerging, Daniel Kahneman and Amos Tversky, working from an entirely different perspective, were contributing a series of extraordinarily important papers on the role of judgmental heuristics in intuitive prediction and judgment (Kahneman & Tversky, 1972, 1973; Tversky & Kahneman, 1973, 1974, 1978). One of their most striking demonstrations involved the layperson's willingness to make predictions about category membership that reflected heavy use of specific information about the target case, even relatively nondiagnostic information, but little if any use of information about category frequencies or base rates. Thus, for example, in judging whether a particular individual described in a brief personality sketch was an engineer or a lawyer, subjects gave great weight to the similarity of the sketch to their prior conceptions of what a lawyer or engineer should look like, but virtually no weight to any information provided about the proportion of lawyers versus engineers in the population at hand.

The relevance of Kahneman and Tversky's work to the consensus findings and to other more general concerns of attribution theory was quick
to be noted (cf. Fischhoff, 1976). Perhaps most important were the efforts
of Nisbett and Borgida (1975). These investigators correctly anticipated
that base-rate data would be grossly underutilized by people in making
predictions about behavior. Specifically, subjects were asked to predict
the prior behavior of particular actors who had participated in psychology
experiments involving such responses as altruistic intervention and
willingness to receive electric shock. Not only did authentic base-rate
information fail to influence subjects' guesses about the behavior of particular participants, it also failed to influence their attributions about
causes of such behavior and, notably, their predictions about what their
own behavior might be in such situations. Borgida and Nisbett (1977)
followed up on these studies by contrasting the effects of base-rate data
with the effects of exposure to information about the responses of concrete individuals. In a series of experiments, students in introductory
courses received their peers' evaluations of several more advanced
courses and then were invited to state their own tentative preferences for
future enrollment in those courses. For some students, these peer evaluations came in the form of summarized ratings of a virtually exhaustive
sample of previous enrollees; for others, the evaluations were ratings
from only two or three individuals, presented on a face-to-face basis. As
anticipated, the students were more influenced in their selections, and
were more confident about those selections, when the small set of concrete face-to-face evaluations rather than the exhaustive and logically
more compelling base-rate data provided the basis for their judgments.

The related findings by Nisbett and Borgida and by Kahneman and
Tversky, and the seemingly gloomy portrait they painted of intuitive prediction in particular and human inference in general, almost immediately
prompted a flood of would-be rebuttal studies (Genosar & Trope, 1980;
Hansen & Donahue, 1977; Hansen & Stonner, 1978; Wells & Harvey,
1977, 1978). Inevitably, the issue of normativeness or rationality came to
the fore, and as it did the debate broadened to address more abstract
questions: How rational, *in general,* are the layperson's judgments, estimates, and inferences? What particular tasks, situations, instructions and
the like, promote rationality versus irrationality? And, of course, how
could or should we define the terms "rational" and "irrational"? That is,
by what criteria can we determine whether a particular judgment or judgmental strategy is optimal, or at least reasonable, in terms of the intellectual resources it demands and the outcomes it offers? Both the burgeon-
ing interest in attributional biases, and the more focused debates about

the psychology of prediction, forced social psychologists to ponder these issues and the phenomena that gave rise to them. Investigators increasingly began to expose themselves not only to the Kahneman and Tversky papers but also to the thinking and research of others (e.g., Dawes, 1964, 1976; Meehl, 1955; Simon, 1957; Slovic & Lichtenstein, 1971) whose concerns with human judgment and decision making had led them to ponder similar questions and problems. In my own case, it led to a collaboration with Richard Nisbett in which we tried, using the tasks and strategies of the formal scientist as our reference point, to examine systematically the tasks, tools, and outcomes of informal human inference (Nisbett & Ross, 1980).

Strategies for studying the intuitive scientist

Before discussing details of the intuitive scientist formulation, it is worth noting that two different research strategies can follow from such a formulation. One strategy involves specifying particular tasks, such as data coding or parameter estimation or theory testing, and then attempting to assess people's success in performing these tasks and to diagnose their methods and the source of any shortcomings in their performance. The other strategy is less direct. In a sense it demands "working backward," that is, starting with phenomena that seem to offer particularly dramatic evidence of people's success or failure in dealing with the inferential demands of everyday life and then attempting to discover the more specific scientific tasks and inferential strategies that produce such results.

The remainder of this chapter will explicate these strategies, trying always to pique the interest of the developmentalist. Some of the developmental questions raised will be immediately obvious, for they are essentially of the form: How would younger intuitive psychologists, who presumably have not yet learned all the tricks of the adult trade, fare in inferential or judgmental contexts similar to those that have been explored with adults? But I hope to show that other less obvious questions, and the additional issues they raise, are also worthy of the developmentalist's interest. Needless to say, I also hope that my developmental colleagues will be able to raise other questions, to spot further conceptual connections that go well beyond my own tentative steps.

Tasks of the intuitive scientist

It is hardly surprising that the layperson–scientist analogy occurs to those of us who wear the scientist's mantle in the laboratory but share the layperson's dilemmas and shortcomings when we must confront our fellows and the society outside our laboratory. Notably, both roles compel us to seek out and analyze data that may guide our behavior and increase our knowledge. The process, moreover, inevitably entails a kind of bootstrapping operation – using what we know or believe to aid in the collection and interpretation of data, while simultaneously using those data to update our knowledge and improve the accuracy of our beliefs. In fact, intuitive inference and judgment involve a number of steps, described below, which both the formal scientist and lay scientist must undertake.[2]

Characterizing the datum and the sample

Perhaps the most basic of all scientific undertakings is that of characterizing or "coding" the individual *datum*. To make inferences about the relationship between transgressions and the occurrence of punishment, or smiles and the dispersal of wrath, or social roles and social behaviors, one first must be able to identify the relevant actions or events and distinguish them from others that may be similar in some salient characteristics. No simple generalizations can be made about the layperson's overall performance at the task of "data coding," except for the obvious one that people make heavy use, often without any awareness that they are doing so, of prior theories, schemas, and other knowledge structures. As a consequence, the speed and generally the accuracy with which people code objects and events is greatly enhanced; but also as a consequence, they are exposed to the risk of miscoding experience – either because their theories and preconceptions are invalid or because they are willing to apply valid theories and schemas beyond their realm of applicability. (See review by Taylor & Crocker, 1980.)

A second very basic task of the intuitive scientist involves characterizing not an individual datum but a *sample* of data. Again generalizations are risky, but everyday experience and laboratory research (see Peterson & Beach, 1967) attest to the fact that people are often quite proficient at estimating frequencies, proportions, or averages when the objects or events in question are immediately at hand or readily retrievable from memory. But when the retrieval process becomes more difficult, the possibilities for bias and error increase dramatically. The initial salience of objects or events, and a host of factors that similarly are imperfectly related to actual frequency or likelihood but that nevertheless influence retrievability from memory, all may distort the data samples available for more complex inferential processes (see Kahneman & Tversky, 1973; Rothbart, Fulero, Jensen, Howard, & Birrell, 1978; Taylor & Fiske, 1978; Trope, 1978).

Generalizing from the sample

Many important social judgments and the actions they foster essentially require the individual to make an inductive generalization – to infer population parameters from sample information or to infer the overall nature of the entity from a sample of its attributes. Whether such inferences are made by the scientist or the layperson, their accuracy generally depends on two considerations: the *size* of the sample and its *freedom from bias*. Evidence seems to be mounting that people have little general appreciation of the importance of either consideration. They seem to underestimate the relative stability shown by the characteristics of any large sample of observations and, conversely, the instability and unreliability shown by the characteristics of very small samples. (See Borgida & Nisbett, 1977; Nisbett & Borgida, 1977; Tversky & Kahneman, 1971.) More damaging still, people often seem to be oblivious, or at best extremely unresponsive, to the perils of generalizing from samples known or strongly suspected to be biased. (See Hamill, Wilson, & Nisbett, 1980; Slovic, Fischhoff, & Lichtenstein, 1976.)

In fairness, it should be noted that, in their behavior as well as in their explicit statements, people frequently do manifest insights about the importance of sample size and sample bias. Even at very early ages, they understand the distinction between random and nonrandom events (Piaget & Inhelder, 1975). But such insights seem particularistic and restricted to relatively familiar contexts. Thus well-learned maxims, or "scripts," warn us about generalizing from the potentially biased data provided by such self-serving and sometimes mendacious informants as used-car salesmen or politicians. But defenses against other, equally serious, sources of bias introduced by accidents of perspective or selective experience are lacking. What the lay scientist suffers from most, perhaps, is the absence of a general appreciation of the normative dictates involved in sampling theory, an appreciation that could guide the making of generalization even in new and unfamiliar contexts (see Nisbett and Ross, 1980, pp. 77–89, 256–63).

Covariation assessment

The layperson's success as an intuitive scientist obviously depends heavily upon an ability to detect relationships or *covariations* among events – between early symptoms of problems and later manifestations, between behavioral or cognitive strategies employed and outcomes obtained, and between relatively overt characteristics of people or situations and relatively covert ones. Indeed, learning the lessons and adapting to the demands of everyday social experience require that we not only detect covariations but that we also assess their relative magnitudes and make appropriate use of such assessments in judgments, inferences, and actions. (See Shultz & Mendelson, 1975; Siegler & Liebert, 1974.)

Notwithstanding the central role that covariation assessment could play in human adaptation, most research dealing explicitly with this ability has been rather unflattering to the layperson (e.g., Smedslund, 1963; Ward & Jenkins, 1965; Wason & Johnson-Laird, 1972). There is mounting evidence that under many circumstances people may be extremely poor at detecting and assessing empirical covariations. In particular, it appears that a priori theories or expectations may be more important than actual data configurations in determining people's impressions of relatedness between variables. If the individual has a plausible theory that predicts covariation between classes of events, then a substantial degree of covariation will be perceived – or at least its existence will continue to be assumed and reported – even if no such covariation is actually present in the data at hand. Conversely, even relatively powerful empirical relationships are apt to go undetected, or be assessed as trivial in their magnitude, if they could not be predicted from the intuitive scientist's prior theories and preconceptions (see Jennings, Amabile, & Ross, 1980; and Nisbett & Ross, 1980; also, earlier work including Chapman & Chapman, 1967, 1969).

Causal assessment and prediction

Given the layperson's limitation as a covariation assessor, the implications for prediction and causal-assessment tasks are all too clear. Preconceptions, arising from a host of invalid sources as well as valid ones, exert a profound influence on intuitive assessments of causality and predictions. At the same time, important lessons contained in the objective data of experience are apt to go unlearned.

The layperson's shortcomings in making causal assessments do not arise only because of deficiencies in covariation assessment. Social observers may go astray simply because they are too ready to see causal connections where none exist (see Langer, 1975; Langer & Roth, 1975; Wortman, 1976). They may also be misled because they inappropriately treat the perceptual salience of causal candidates as indicative of their impact (see Taylor & Fiske, 1978), because they wrongly assume that causes and effects should somehow resemble each other on various qualitative dimensions (see Nisbett & Ross, 1980, pp. 115–8), or because they apply misguided hydraulic assumptions and notions of "parsimony" (see Kanouse, 1972; Simon, 1967). The parsimony problem, which refers to the fact that once individuals have discerned one satisfactory explanation or "sufficient cause" for a phenomena they essentially stop looking and/or fail to recognize other equally sufficient causes, may be particularly pertinent to a finding on self-perception that is familiar to many developmentalists. Several investigators have shown that the introduction of a salient extrinsic factor, such as the possibility of a reward or the presence of surveillance, may undermine the actor's "intrinsic interest" in, and willingness to perform, a task that he or she otherwise would have performed willingly in the *absence* of the extrinsic factor (see Deci, 1971, 1972a, 1972b; Karniol & Ross, 1977; Kruglanski, Friedman, & Zeevi, 1971; Lepper, 1980; Lepper & Greene, 1978; Lepper, Greene, & Nisbett, 1973; Lepper, Sagotsky, Dafoe, & Greene, 1980).

The layperson's shortcomings at intuitive prediction similarly can be traced to some deficiencies other than those involved in covariation analysis. Most critically, people appear to have little intuitive appreciation of the regression phenomenon. That is, even when they recognize the relationship between two variables to be quite weak, they often make nonregressive predictions of the sort that would be justified only by virtually perfect relationships (see Kahneman & Tversky, 1973). As in the case of generalizing from small or biased samples, lay insights about regression phenomena are not nonexistent; but they tend to be situation-specific and insufficiently general to be readily applied to new outcomes or events.

Testing and revising theories

There can be no doubt that intuitive psychologists, of all ages, assimilate the data of everyday experience to their theories, schemas, and other preconceptions about the world around them. Indeed, there can be little *general* normative objection to the practice (see Ross & Lepper, 1980); for the application of old knowledge and experience to new settings is essential to social adaptation and efficient information processing. But the *assimilation* of data to preexisting impressions and schemas is normatively appropriate, and fully adaptive, only if it is accompanied by the continual *accommodation* of such "theories" to subsequent experience.

Over three and a half centuries ago, when formal scientific inquiry was in its infancy, Francis Bacon decried the human tendency to maintain preconceptions in the face of seemingly overwhelming logical or empirical challenges to their validity. Few complaints about human frailty are as consistently confirmed, both by everyday experience and by empirical research. Opinions (Abelson, 1959; Hovland, Janis, & Kelley, 1953), personality impressions (Asch, 1957; Jones & Goethals, 1972), and a variety of racial, religious, ethnic, and sex-role stereotypes (Allport, 1954; Katz, 1960; Taynor & Deaux, 1973) all have been shown to be highly resistant to the effects of new evidence and argumentation. Even the formal scientist has been indicted on this charge (e.g., Barber, 1952; Kuhn, 1962; Mahoney, 1976, 1977; McGuigan, 1963).

Much of my own recent work, with Mark Lepper, has involved an attempt to demonstrate and explicate such perseverance phenomena. Two paradigms have been employed. The first and more obvious one exposes people to information that is potentially ambiguous or "mixed" with respect to their existing beliefs. We found, as hypothesized, that subjects tend to accept information at face value and shift their attitudes in the indicated direction only if that information ostensibly supports or strengthens their existing beliefs. When the information ostensibly opposes their beliefs, they evaluate it more critically. They seek to formulate alternative, less damaging, interpretations and they tend to shift their beliefs only slightly. As a result (cf. Lord, Ross, & Lepper, 1979), a mixed set of evidence does not lead the contending factions in debates about controversial issues of social policy to become more tolerant of their adversaries' views and less confident of their own. Rather, it leads to increased polarization, as both factions become more confident and extreme in their positions on the basis of the same set of objectively inconclusive information.

The second and less obvious research paradigm that Lepper and I have used to demonstrate belief perseverance deals not with the addition of new evidence, but with the discrediting of old evidence. We have found that, once formed, beliefs about the self or others (see Ross, Lepper, & Hubbard, 1975; Jennings, Lepper, & Ross, 1980; Lepper, Ross, & Lau, 1980), and theories about functional relationships in the world (cf. Anderson, Lepper, & Ross, 1980), can survive even the most logically compelling of challenges to the evidence that initially gave rise to such beliefs. For example, subjects initially induced by false feedback to believe that they had performed superbly at a particular discrimination task continued to believe that they were blessed with unusual ability at the task, *even after being totally debriefed* about the random and noncontingent nature of the feedback they had received. Similarly, those subjects initially induced to believe they had performed badly continued, after debriefing, to believe themselves lacking in the relevant ability (Ross et al., 1975).

No less important than the phenomenon of belief perseverance are the cognitive mechanisms that underlie it. One mechanism we have already noted – the operation of *biased assimilation*, whereby newly obtained or recalled evidence is either accepted at face value or subjected to critical scrutiny as a function of its consistency with one's existing beliefs. The other mechanism is a bit subtler. It involves the capacity of people to readily invent causal explanations or scenarios in which they then place inappropriate confidence (see Anderson et al., 1980; Ross, Lepper, Strack, & Steinmetz, 1977). As a result of these two mechanisms, intuitive scientists gain the illusion that their theories are more logical and empirically buttressed than is really the case. They are even apt to believe that their theories enjoy "independent support" and to rely on such support in maintaining those theories when their original evidential basis is challenged and discounted.

Tools of the intuitive scientist

Discovering, describing, and critically evaluating the tools of human inference has, of course, been a major preoccupation of philosophers and psychologists for over two millenia. Much of this self-examination has been prompted by the desire to resolve a very old and central paradox – the seeming contradiction between the great triumphs and the dramatic failures of the human mind. Increasingly, we have come to recognize that human inferential strengths and weaknesses may be intimately linked, that the occasional failings may directly or indirectly reflect the operation of the same tools that more typically produce our species' success in mastering the various tasks of everyday inference.

Two broad classes of inferential tools have been receiving particular attention from contemporary researchers. These are *knowledge structures* or *schemas*, which embody the individual's generic knowledge about the world and aid him in recognizing and anticipating events in the flow of experience, and *judgmental heuristics*, which reduce many complex inferential undertakings to relatively simple judgmental operations.

Knowledge structures

Few if any social stimuli are approached for the first time by the adult. Instead they are processed through preexisting systems of schematized and abstracted knowledge, that is, beliefs, theories, propositions, and schemas. These structures are critical to the active or constructive nature of perception to which Bruner (1957), among others, has constantly alerted us. They allow us to categorize objects quickly and, for the most part, accurately. They further allow us to "go beyond the information given," to infer and expect properties that we cannot see, and often to suggest appropriate responses. Inevitably, however, this mental economy exacts a price. Knowledge structures, despite their value, are far from infallible guides to the nature of reality. Some beliefs, theories, and schemas are relatively poor and inaccurate representations of the external world – they sometimes "package" together attributes or events that are only modestly, if at all, correlated in the world. Furthermore, schemas that are invaluable in their place may be applied inappropriately, because objects or events are prematurely and incorrectly labeled on the basis of an insufficient or biased sample of evidence.

The term "schema" is far from new, of course, and the role of knowledge structures in general has long been appreciated by psychologists working within several traditions (see Bartlett, 1932; Piaget, 1936). Recent years, however, have brought an unparalleled explosion of interest in this topic. The lexicon of terms has expanded to include "frames" (Minsky, 1975), "scripts" (Abelson, 1976; Schank & Abelson, 1977), "prototypes" (Cantor & Mischel, 1977, 1979; Rosch, 1978), and "scenes" (Tomkins, 1979); and the old standby "schemas" has gained some vigorous new champions (e.g., Rumelhart, 1976). Nevertheless, at the time of this writing, real progress in understanding the role of schemas in fostering inferential accuracy and error remains disappointingly slow (although perhaps not nonexistent; e.g., Cantor & Mischel, 1977; Markus, 1977). What we seem to lack most acutely is an adequate theory of schema *recruitment*. We remain ignorant about what it is that makes a perceiver or actor likely to *apply* a given schema in a given setting. Freud, of course, made a valiant attempt in this direction by proposing theories of mental structure and process and suggesting a method for studying them. But neither his theories nor his analytic case studies seem to have provided a solid foundation for contemporary cognitive scientists to build on. In short, we still await, with eagerness if not optimism, both an adequate theory of psychic association and an adequate account of the links between cognition and action.

Judgmental heuristics

Beyond theories and schemas that encompass knowledge about specific classes of objects and events, certain very simple and general cognitive strategies seem to play a major role in the layperson's inferential performances. Kahneman and Tversky have used the term "heuristics" to characterize these strategies; and they have tried to illustrate the operation of these heuristics in a continuing series of provocative demonstration experiments (see Kahneman & Tversky, 1972, 1973; Tversky & Kahneman, 1971, 1973, 1974, 1978).

Heuristics, we should note, are not irrational or even nonrational devices. Although they are primitive, they probably produce vastly more correct or partially correct inferences than erroneous ones and, like specific knowledge schemas, they do so with great speed and little effort. However, the application, or more properly the misapplication, of these heuristics may lead people astray in some important inferential tasks. Two heuristics in particular have been emphasized by Kahneman and Tversky, and the operation of each has already been noted in introducing the tasks of the informal scientist.

The *representativeness heuristic* allows the individual to reduce many logically complex inferential tasks to what are essentially similarity or "goodness of fit" judgments. An object or event is assigned to one conceptual category rather than to another by assessing the extent to which its defining or most salient features match those of the categories in question, in much the same way that a botanist assigns plants to one species or another. This procedure serves one well when the available features are reliable and unique guides to classification; but it serves one rather poorly when such features are not unique or defining, or when various statistical considerations, such as category frequencies, are logically entitled to some weight in one's judgments. The reader may recall how Kahneman and Tversky's subjects predicted the occupations of people described in thumbnail personality sketches by relying exclusively upon representativeness criteria with virtually no regard for the "base rates" associated with those professions. Many other inferential tasks in which representativeness criteria seem to be applied could similarly be cited (see Nisbett & Ross, 1980, pp. 17–28 for a review). For example, lay assessments of causality and predictions may both be heavily influenced by judgments about the conceptual similarity between antecedents and consequences. Thus, personal motives are the preferred explanation for actions or outcomes that have motivational consequences, personal actions are attributed to personal dispositions, and outcomes are expected to share the features of the processes that generated them.

The *availability heuristic* similarly both facilitates a variety of inferential performances and leads the intuitive scientist to a variety of inferential errors. Through its application, objects or events are judged probable or causally efficacious to the extent that they are cognitively and/or perceptually "available," that is, readily accessible to the individual through the senses, recall from memory, or construction from imagination. Once again, this heuristic can be a useful tool. In general, the objects and events that are most readily noted perceptually or most readily recalled from memory are apt to be those that are relatively numerous and likely to occur. It is even reasonable to assume that, on the average, those actors and environmental features that are most prominent and likely to capture our attention are also the ones that, on the average, will prove most consistently to be powerful causal agents. But the indiscriminate use of the availability heuristic exposes the user to obvious risks, because both our experiences and the processes for attending to, storing, and retrieving those experiences are subject to many biases. For example, the relative likelihood of events that are prominently reported in the news media is apt to be overestimated while that of rarely reported events is underestimated (e.g., Slovic, Fischhoff, & Lichtenstein, 1979). Ratings of the causal impact of actors who are distinctive or nondistinctive because of their seating position or their racial or sexual status within a group (see Taylor & Fiske, 1978) are similarly apt to be distorted.

To review the rapidly expanding literature on the uses and abuses of the availability and representativeness heuristics would increase the length of this chapter beyond reasonable limits. (Obviously, any psychologist intent on understanding and applying new developments in cognitive and cognitive-social psychology would be well advised to consult some of the sources previously cited.) Instead, I would like to venture a guess about future developments. I anticipate a concerted effort to apply the notions of availability and representativeness criteria to the problem of schema recruitment and application, that is, an attempt to specify both the criteria for schema "availability" and the principles for judging the "representativeness" of such generic knowledge to particular objects or events. I further anticipate that a concept something like schema availability will play a major role in attempts to characterize individual differences in belief systems, cognitive styles, and behavior.

An overview of developmental implications

If the central problem of developmental psychology is a systematic understanding of the individual's journey from ignorant and helpless infant to wise and competent adult, then a special challenge is offered by the intuitive scientist formulation summarized in this chapter. For human adults, despite their impressive success in dealing with most everyday events, and despite their rich store of knowledge about the actors and situations that comprise their social experience, have proven to be far from paragons in their inferential methods and performances. An adequate developmental account, accordingly, must help us to reconcile the growth of inferential capacities with the existence, persistence, and perhaps even the growth of inferential shortcomings. The broad outlines of some of the questions and issues that will have to be addressed in this account are already apparent.

The origins of adult shortcomings

The first and most basic questions are those of origin. To what extent, and for which tasks or for which domains, do adult shortcomings reflect deficiences that are also apparent, perhaps even more apparent, in the child – deficiencies that, in a sense, have never been totally "overcome" by the adult? Alternately, to what extent, and for which tasks or domains, are adult shortcomings a consequence of development itself, that is, a by-product of the adult's ever-developing inferential strategies and ever-expanding knowledge structures?

To address these questions we first need to collect (or abstract from previous research) evidence about the performances of intuitive scientists far younger than those typically scrutinized by investigators concerned with failings of human inference. Are children any less "theory-driven" than adults in the way they code individual events or assess covariations? Are they any more willing to accommodate heretofore useful theories and schemas to new evidence or to the discrediting of old evidence? Are children simply blessed, or cursed, with fewer and less encompassing preconceptions about what "hangs together" in the world (but equally or more willing to apply and preserve the theories and schemas that they do possess)?

Kahneman and Tversky have sometimes characterized the availability and representativeness heuristics as "primitive" tools of inference. Are they, perhaps, primitive in the sense that they are acquired very early or are even somehow linked to basic and inevitable cognitive and perceptual processes? Are children genetically predisposed, in some Chomskian fashion, to develop and use these heuristics? Certainly, there is ample anecdotal and experimental evidence that very young children readily perform the exercises involved in applying the representativeness heuristic. That is, they seem spontaneously to note similarities and dissimilarities in the salient features of the entities and events they experience: A cloud may be likened to a dragon or a ship, the contours of a piece of wood may allow it to be used by the child as a truck, a rocketship, or a submachine gun. Indeed, the literal-minded adult may be less likely than the child to spontaneously respond to such similarities. Freudian accounts of so-called primary process thinking in the child, or the childlike adult, are similarly replete with seeming instances of representativeness-based association.

The operation of the availability heuristic also seems to be well documented in developmental observation and experimental research, although different terms have been employed by the investigators. Discussions of egocentrism in role taking (see Selman, 1971, 1976) seem especially relevant here. Children may fail at "perspective taking" primarily because the data of their own past and immediate experiences are too salient or too "available" to be ignored in favor of less salient data (cf. Flavell, 1977, pp. 124–5). What adults have learned to do, albeit imperfectly, is to recognize that in certain contexts their own experiences, feelings, or thoughts, despite their immediate availability, may not be the best data for predicting the responses of others.

Many of the adult's advantages over the child in inferential performance may reflect the operation of domain-specific insights and acquired knowledge that *protect* the adult from the excesses of indiscriminate application of availability and representativeness criteria. For instance, as adults we have acquired a rich set of person schemas or prototypes that inhibit egocentrism by leading us to focus on the unique nature of the actor rather than on our own response to the situation facing that actor ("I am a male, a psychologist, a Canadian, and a liberal, while she is female, a musician, an Italian, and an anarchist – so she may see things differently and act differently than I do"). Similarly, the adult is armed with cultural maxims ("you can't tell a book by its cover") and reinforced by experiences that inhibit unbridled exercise of the representativeness heuristic. Such schema-based insights, of course, are only as good as the accuracy of their content and the appropriateness of their application. Accordingly, as we shall see in this chapter, they can sometimes promote error instead of accuracy.

The acquisition of knowledge content

A second basic set of developmental issues that arise from the intuitive scientist formulation focuses on the distinction between cognitive *processes* and cognitive *content*. Formal scientists' methods of inference and hypothesis testing are apt to change far less over their careers than is the content of either their specific theories or of the data bases upon which such theories rest. Nevertheless, from time to time newer and more sophisticated tools – methods of analysis, new data-collection techniques, even new constraints and standards for making inferences – are apt to be added to the scientist's repertoire. Generally this occurs not because of some independent personal insight but because someone has educated the scientist about the advantages of the new tools or the deficiencies of the old ones. Without prejudging what is ultimately an empirical question, it seems a reasonable working hypothesis that the career of the intuitive scientist follows a similar course of development.

The intuitive scientist acquires an ever-richer and more encompassing set of theories and beliefs to which, in turn, an ever-broader data base of experience is assimilated. To the extent that such "theories" are increasingly more accurate, and to the extent that the data samples relevant to those theories are increasingly large and increasingly free of (or at least *not* increasingly subject to) sampling biases, the quality of inferential performance should increase throughout the life span. And where new inferential insights or tools are acquired – such as an appreciation of how some *formal* normative principles operate within a given domain, or the knowledge of how to resolve an empirical question by performing an "experiment" – the rate of increase in quality of inferential performance should be accelerated (see Inhelder & Piaget, ·1958). But this optimistic developmental portrait is by no means the only, or even the most accurate one that could be painted. For everyday social experience can lead us to acquire *erroneous* theories – because our culture, family, or social class indoctrinates us with them, or because our experiences lead us to them by presenting biased data, or simply because our inductive and deductive capacities are imperfect. And, through the perseverance mechanisms described in this chapter, social experience can promote illusions about the broadening domain to which our existing theories and schemas seem to apply, and can promote marked "overconfidence" about the validity of imperfect judgments and beliefs (see Einhorn & Hogarth, 1978).

At present, researchers possess little data concerning differences between the theories held by older and younger intuitive scientists or their relative merits. (Mischel's contribution to this volume offers a start in this direction.) We similarly know little about the differing biases that influence the data to which people are exposed at different periods in their lives. Thus, we run the constant risk of misattributing adult superiority in inferential performance to supposed superiority in the quality of their inferential processes or strategies. We also run the risk of being unduly surprised when, as I shall document, the younger intuitive scientist "paradoxically" proves to be wiser than his elders. But both phenomena may verify the refrain that has now been sounded several times in this chapter. Becoming an ever more theory-rich and theory-biased processor of information may dramatically improve the economy of our inferential performances, and it may (less dramatically, perhaps) improve the average quality of such performances. But in domains where erroneous theories are apt to abound, an increasing reliance on theoretical preconceptions and preexisting knowledge schemas may cost us dearly. One such domain, I suggest, is that of interpersonal perception. For erroneous theories about human nature in general, and especially erroneous theories about the characteristics of particular classes of people, are all too readily offered by our culture. And the behavior that we observe is sufficiently ambiguous, constrained by situational factors, and even biased by our own preconceptions and behavior (see Snyder & Swann, 1978; Snyder, Tanke, & Berscheid, 1977), for erroneous theories to survive and flourish.

Metacognitive psychology – the study of the human's developing ability to reflect on human cognitive processes and capacities – is, as the emphasis of several chapters in this volume attests, a flourishing endeavor (see especially Chapters 9, 10, and 11). I would suggest that some shift or expansion of emphasis is needed, so that the study of the child's developing awareness of cognitive *content* – of his theories, beliefs, and knowledge schemas, of the data samples that are salient to him, and of the role that each plays in his everyday judgments and inferences – begins to receive greater attention.

The analysis of specific inferential biases

To add perspective to our portrait of the intuitive psychologist, and to illustrate some of the developmental concerns brought into focus by that portrait, we shall now consider more specific phenomena. In each case I shall describe a familiar bias in everyday judgment and then attempt to "work backwards," from the phenomenon to an analysis of underlying inferential strategies and shortcomings, and thence to some specific developmental possibilities and issues. Each case, as we shall see, underscores the classic problem of situational versus dispositional attribution; and it is this problem – or more specifically the performances of intuitive scientists of varying ages who wrestled with this problem – that will be the subject of the one piece of developmental research that I shall report in any detail.

The divergent attributions of actors and observers

One of the most provocative phenomena illustrating bias in the process of social inference was captured in Jones and Nisbett's (1971) generalization regarding the "divergent" perceptions of actors and observers. These investigators cited a mixture of laboratory and anecdotal evidence that suggested that in many situations in which actors attribute their own behavior to situational forces and constraints, observers are likely to attribute the same choices to the actors' stable abilities, attitudes, traits, or other personal dispositions. Indeed, there appears to be a consistent tendency for people to believe that, in general, "other people" can be characterized in terms of stable personal dispositions that manifest themselves across many situations, whereas we, ourselves, lack such broad and cross-situationally consistent dispositions.

In a sense, Jones and Nisbett's generalization was a qualification of an attributional bias that was first identified by Heider (1958) and Lewin (1935) and has been the one perhaps most frequently cited ever since. This bias, which I have elsewhere referred to as the "fundamental" attribution error (see Anderson & Ross, 1980; Nisbett & Ross, 1980; Ross, 1977) is the tendency for people to underestimate the impact of situational factors relative to personal dispositions in controlling behavior, to thereby expect consistency in the behavior of any individual across widely disparate situations and contexts, and to jump to hasty dispositional inferences upon witnessing behavior in any particular situation. Jones and Nisbett's contention, therefore, was essentially that actors – in accounting for their own behavior and making inferences about themselves – are *less* susceptible than observers to this "fundamental" dispositionalist bias.

Why should actors and observers differ in this manner? More specifically, what basic inferential tasks and strategies are implicated in these phenomena? Jones and Nisbett proposed that differences exist both in the relevant data sample that actors and observers draw upon and in the salience or availiability of contending causal candidates. First, in the actor's case, any general bias that favors dispositional accounts of behavior is apt to be countered by an available data sample that shows considerable variability in actual behavior (evidence of "generosity" or "aggressiveness" or "optimism," for instance, in situations that seemed to demand such responses, but not in situations where situational forces and constraints dictated otherwise). By contrast, Nisbett and Jones reasoned, the observer typically deals with a much more restricted data sample, often a single relevant episode. No variance in the data sample, accordingly, inhibits the observer's dispositionalist bias. The second source of the divergence between actor and observer attributions arises from the simple fact that the actors cannot see themselves when they act. It is the immediate situation, and any shifts in the properties of that situation that command the actor's attention – in no small part because it is the opportunities and constraints of the situation that are motivating and guiding the actor's behavior. The observer's perspective is quite different; for the observer, the actor is "figural" and the situational context merely "ground." In short, the observer's predisposition to cite the actor as the cause of his or her action is reinforced by the simple fact that it is the actor who is seen doing the acting.

One clear and quickly appreciated implication of Jones and Nisbett's analysis concerned the factors that might *shift* either actors' or observers' attributions. If differences in the perceptual availability of particular causal candidates are responsible for the differences in attribution, then it should be possible to make actors' perceptions more "observerlike" and observers' perceptions more "actorlike" simply by *manipulating* their particular perspectives via videotape replays (Storms, 1973) or other procedures. A further, more general, implication was also quick to be recognized: Any actor or object that one can be made to focus one's attention on can thereby be made to seem a more potent causal agent. This finding has now been obtained in a wide variety of contexts through manipulation of many different types of factors, including the presence of mirrors to make actors more "self conscious" or "self-aware," seating arrangements to control what observers look at, the relative amount of movement shown by actors and by their environments, and actors' racial, sexual, or physical distinctiveness (cf. Arkin & Duval, 1975; McArthur & Post, 1977; McArthur & Solomon, 1978; Regan & Totten, 1975; Taylor & Fiske, 1975). Even subtle linguistic manipulations of availability have proven capable of influencing causal explanations (cf. Pryor & Kriss, 1977; Salancik, 1974, 1976; Salancik & Conway, 1975).

The class of attributional biases cited, and the analyses of perceptual and cognitive mechanisms that underlie them, seem to offer rich possibilities for developmental inquiry. Susceptibility to the relevant sampling and availability biases in observer attributions, age-related differences in the development of domain-specific insights that might sometimes protect observers from such dispositionalist biases, and children's developing ability to *resist* making the fundamental attribution error regarding their own outcomes and actions furnish some of the more obvious targets for such inquiry.

The false consensus or "egocentric" attribution bias

The second inferential bias I shall discuss again relates to the issue of situational versus dispositional attributions. It concerns people's tendencies to perceive a "false consensus" for their own responses, that is, to see their own behavioral choices and judgments as relatively common, and relatively appropriate to existing circumstances, while seeing alternative responses as relatively uncommon, inappropriate, and reflective of the actors' specific disposition.[3]

Passing references to "egocentric attribution" (Heider, 1958), to "attributional projection" (Holmes, 1968), and to several specific findings related to false consensus biases (e.g., Katz & Allport, 1931; Kelley & Stahelski, 1970) have appeared sporadically in the social perception literature. More recently, my colleagues and I have focused on these phenomena in a series of studies (Ross, Greene, & House, 1977) that presented subjects with various real or hypothetical behavior dilemmas and asked them to predict the responses of their peers. In perhaps the most compelling of these demonstrations, subjects were asked if they would be willing to walk around campus for thirty minutes wearing a large sandwich-board sign bearing a simple message (e.g., "Eat at Joe's"). After making their own decision they were then asked to estimate the proportion of other subjects who would agree or refuse to do likewise, and to make trait inferences about particular peers who ostensibly had opted for the compliant or noncompliant choice.

The results of this study provided clear evidence for the hypothesized false-consensus effect. Overall, subjects who agreed to wear the sandwich-board sign estimated that almost two-thirds of their peers would make the same choice. By contrast, subjects who refused to wear the sign estimated that less than one-third of their peers would agree to wear it. Furthermore, as predicted, compliant subjects made more confident and more extreme inferences about the personal characteristics of a noncompliant peer, while noncompliant subjects made stronger inferences about a compliant peer.

Some of the broader implications of the false-consensus effect for our conception of the intuitive scientist and his development should be clear. Intuitive estimates of relative deviance, and the host of social inferences and interpersonal responses dictated by such estimates, are systematically and egocentrically biased. Other people, who necessarily behave differently than we do in at least some contexts, are bound to be seen as creatures whose behavior (unlike our own) reveals distinguishing dispositions and perversities. In part, then, the Jones and Nisbett generalization about self-perceptions versus social perceptions can be *derived* from the false consensus effect: Observers are bound to be more susceptible than actors to the fundamental error – at least in many particular contexts where the observers are accounting for responses that are different from those that they have shown, or believe they would show, in similar circumstances.

What accounts for the intuitive scientist's susceptibility to the false consensus or egocentric attribution bias? One obvious factor involves the biased data samples upon which consensus estimates generally are based. Usually, we know and associate with people who share our background, experiences, interests, values, and outlook. Our associates *do,* in disproportionate numbers, respond as we would in a wide variety of circumstances. Such shared characteristics may, in fact, provide the basis for association; indeed, we may be inclined to deliberately avoid those whom we believe unlikely to share our judgments and responses. Related, but more subtle and more cognitive in character, are the various factors that increase our ability to recall, visualize, or imagine paradigmatic instances of behavior. In a given situation the specific behaviors that we have chosen, or would choose, are likely to be more readily retrievable from memory and more easily imagined than opposite behaviors. In Kahneman and Tversky's (1973) terms, the behavioral choices we favor may be more cognitively "available"; and we are apt to be misled by this ease or difficulty of access in estimating the likelihood of relevant behavioral options.

A second major source of the false consensus effect arises from the intuitive psychologist's response to ambiguity – both about the nature and magnitude of situational forces and about the meaning and implications of the various response alternatives. Attempts to resolve such ambiguity involve interpretation, estimation, and guesswork, all of which can exert a parallel effect on the attributor's own behavior choices and upon his predictions and inferences about the choices of others. Thus, subjects who anticipated and feared the ridicule of peers for wearing the "Eat at Joe's" sign, and who regarded the experimenter's wishes and expectations as trivial, were likely to refuse to wear the sign, to assume similar refusals by their peers, and to draw strong inferences about the traits of any subjects who chose to wear the sign in the face of such "unequal" situation forces. Opposite expectations, perceptions, and priorities, of course, would have produced opposite personal choices and opposite social estimates and inferences.

How might adults and children compare in their susceptibility to the false-consensus mechanisms? Certainly, the view that children are egocentric relative to adults – that they are less able to anticipate discrepancies between their own view of the world and that of other people – might lead one to expect false-consensus effects to be more pronounced among the young. However, in some respects, children may also be uniquely shielded from the false-consensus effect. Generally, they have less capacity than their parents to surround themselves with people who share their values, priorities, impressions, and interests. The child's neighborhood play group, classmates at school, and even the children of parental friends, are apt to vary quite widely in their outlooks and actions; in a sense, they constitute a more random sample of their species than the adult's co-workers and friends. The question is an empirical one, of course, but it is reasonable to expect that no simple adult versus child difference will emerge. The nature of the behavioral domain in question, and the bases upon which consensus predictions are made within that domain, may determine whether it is the child or the parent who is more "egocentric" (and more or less accurate) in assessing the probable responses of other people.

Evaluating role-biased actions and outcomes

The course of a social encounter is often shaped and constrained by the formal and informal roles that the various actors must play. Accurate social inferences about these actors, accordingly, will depend upon the evaluator's ability to separate the actor from the role, that is, to recognize and make allowance for the "biased" nature of the data presented by role-constrained interactions. Prompted by these concerns, Ross, Amabile, & Steinmetz (1977) suggested that social perceivers characteristically may *fail* to make the necessary allowances and, consequently, may draw inaccurate social inferences about role-advantaged and role-disadvantaged actors. In one sense this suggestion simply proposed a special case of the fundamental attribution error described in this chapter. Whereas the fundamental error is a tendency to underestimate the impact of situational determinants and overestimate the degree to which actions and outcomes reflect the actor's dispositions, the special case proposed by Ross et al. involves the intuitive scientist's insensitivity to the impact of social roles.

The particular roles dealt with in the Ross et al. study were those of "questioner" and "contestant" in a general knowledge quiz game. After random assignment to these roles (by a flip of the coin in their presence) both subjects heard a description of their own role and that of their coparticipant. The questioner's duties consisted of preparing ten "challenging but not impossible" questions from his or her own store of general knowledge, and then posing them to the contestant whose only duty was to try to answer those questions. As the session proceeded, the substantial advantage of the questioner's role in self-presentation asserted itself. Again and again, the questioner displayed esoteric knowledge in the questions asked and the answers supplied when the contestant failed to respond correctly. Finally, at the conclusion of the session, the two participants, and in a subsequent reenactment observers as well, were required to rate the questioner's and the contestant's general knowledge.

It should be emphasized that the source of the bias in the respective "samples" of general knowledge displayed by questioners and contestants could hardly have been more blatant. The questioners' role guaranteed that they would reveal no area of ignorance, whereas the contestants' role gave no opportunity for such selective, self-serving displays. Instead, it made displays of ignorance by the contestant virtually inevitable.

What were the effects of these biased displays of knowledge? Notwithstanding the obviousness of the questioners's "advantage" and the explicitness of the random role assignments that conferred such advantage, contestants judged themselves to be well below average and their questioners to be well above average in general knowledge. Observers agreed with those relative assessments but offered a somewhat different verdict about the participants' probable standing within the student population as a whole. They concluded that the contestants, overall, were no worse than average but that the questioners were truly exceptional. Interestingly, the questioners themselves did not seem to share any such illusions; their mean rating for both their own knowledge and that of the contestant was simply "average."

To clarify these findings, and direct attention to more general issues of inferential performance, it is helpful to focus on the inferential task facing each participant in the Ross et al. study. Note specifically that each participant essentially had been invited to use two data *samples* (i.e., the knowledge overtly displayed by the contestant and questioner) to make inferences about the broader stores of knowledge from which those samples were derived. From this perspective, it is clear that both the contestant and observer were forced to rely upon a highly *biased* sample of the questioner's knowledge – specifically a sample of facts that the questioner happened to know but thought sufficiently obscure and esoteric to be unknown to other people. On the other hand, they both had a reasonably *unbiased* sample of the contestant's own knowledge, that is, a more or less random sample of the contestant's knowledge of obscure information. Observers, however, enjoyed one additional clue to help them decide whether the questioner was unusually knowledgeable or the contestant unusually ignorant, for observers knew that they *shared* the contestant's inability to match the questioner's knowledge. Accordingly, observers rated the questioners even more positively than the contestants had rated them, and they rated the contestant less negatively than the contestants had rated themselves.

The ratings offered by the questioners, specifically their failure to be misled by their role-conferred advantage in self-presentation, can similarly be understood from this perspective. Given their essentially random sample of the contestant's knowledge, and given their awareness of the many, many gaps in their own knowledge that were not apparent in the biased sample presented by their questions, it is not surprising that, on the average, they rated both themselves and their contestants as "merely average."

Both the adult's apparent insensitivity to the impact of social roles, and the adult's more basic difficulties in recognizing the limited inferential value of biased data (see also Hamill et al., 1980; Nisbett & Ross, 1980) may be of potential interest to the developmentalist. Children's particular susceptibility to media advertising has been a topic of considerable interest during the past decade (e.g., Robertson & Rossiter, 1974, 1977). There is already considerable evidence, both anecdotal and experimental, suggesting that young children have difficulty in recognizing that teachers, police officers, doctors, and other actors they encounter may have personal dispositions that are unpredictable from, and even incongruent with, their professional performances. For that reason, perhaps they are apt to be surprised, and even a bit disturbed, to see such actors temporarily freed of the pressures and constraints of their roles, such as when they see their teacher on the beach in a bathing suit, or their doctor cheering on his or her own children at a Little League baseball game. Even older intuitive scientists may share this tendency. My colleagues Sandra and Daryl Bem recount how their undergraduates do a "double take" when encountering them in a pizza parlor, or in a park with their children, or when engaged in any other such "unprofessional" pursuits.

There are many factors that may contribute to these inferential deficiencies beyond the very basic difficulties (e.g., Saltz & Medow, 1971) that young children may have in recognizing that one person or object can belong to two different categories. First, children simply have less opportunity than their parents to see different roles produce different behavior samples. They rarely get to see particular actors (with the possible exception of their parents) performing different roles in different settings. They are too young to have seen actors change their roles, and thus the dominant impression they present to others, over the life span. Furthermore, they themselves do not play as many different and divergent roles as their parents do. Perhaps most importantly, children may be at a disadvantage because they lack specific personally acquired or culturally transmitted knowledge that, in at least some common situations, serves to warn the adult about the pitfalls of generalizing from biased data. Thus, adults who have little general or abstract appreciation of the inferential advantages of random data samples, and who in a great many contexts may be misled by samples that are not random, may nevertheless be far from defenseless in particular situations where biased data are apt to be presented. Adults have schematic knowledge (which children acquire only gradually) that alerts them to the data-presentation tactics of deceptive politicians and salespeople, to the fact that certain crises cause people to behave uncharacteristically, and even to the existence of particular individuals who are rogues in their personal lives but pillars of respectability in their professional lives (or vice-versa).

Research is needed to disentangle some of these factors. How do children at different ages and stages of development fare in recognizing the pitfalls of generalizing from biased data when their familiarity with the specific domain is held constant? How much and in what domains do they differ in the specific knowledge they have learned or acquired from their culture about such pitfalls? And how much do they differ in their capacity to understand, apply, and generalize from the domain-specific knowledge with which they are presented?

Studying the intuitive scientist developmentally: age-related susceptibility to the fundamental attribution error

Each of the specific phenomena highlighted thus far has revealed the intuitive scientist's difficulties in distinguishing situationally caused actions and outcomes from dispositionally caused ones. Each, in fact, has addressed some aspect of the so-called fundamental attribution error. It is this error, or more specifically the susceptibility of intuitive scientists of various ages to it, that we shall now examine in some detail.

Conceptual analysis and hypotheses

Before discussing specific procedures or results, it may be helpful to remind the reader of a general contention offered in this chapter about age-related changes in inferential accuracy. This contention was that although the acquisition of theories, schemas, and other types of generic knowledge generally promotes increased inferential accuracy, it occasionally can promote error. Specifically, where the acquired theories and schemas are only slightly valid, or where they are apt to be misapplied, we may expect to see what appear to be age-related *decrements* in inferential performance.

It was this expectation that prompted my colleagues and I (Ross, Turiel, Josephson, & Lepper, 1978; Josephson, 1977) to assess the magnitude of the fundamental attribution error in children and young adults from five to twenty years of age. Our working hypothesis was that trait theorists are made and not born, that the knowledge structures and schemas that prompt adults to anticipate and "see" cross-situational consistency in the behavior of their peers are culturally transmitted, or at least are the product of continuing experience in a cultural context.

Certainly, there can be little doubt that our own culture, that is, American, or more generally Western culture, transmits such a dispositionalist bias. For our ideology, our popular literature, even our language with its incredibly rich supply of personal descriptors and its relatively impoverished vocabulary for characterizing situations (see Bem & Funder, 1978; Bem & Lord, 1979), all seem to offer the same basic set of interrelated messages: that people are responsible for their own actions and outcomes, that personal qualities ultimately matter more than luck or advantages of station, and more generally that people are blessed, or cursed, with distinguishing personal characteristics that are consistently manifested in their everyday behavior. If the sources of the dispositionalist bias we have termed the fundamental attribution error are primarily cultural and experiential, a straightforward prediction follows: Younger children should prove to be less like "trait theorists" than their older peers. More specifically, we postulated that younger children would manifest a behaviorist or "situationalist" outlook, leading them to believe that actors' behavior could best be predicted from the nature of the particular situation at hand, rather than from any evidence about the actor's distinguishing personal "dispositions."

Our second prediction was grounded in the conviction that as intuitive scientists begin to reach early adulthood in our society – particularly in our colleges and universities – they are apt to be exposed to a new and rather different set of theories about human nature and human behavior. This view is more egalitarian, relativistic, and situationalist. It stresses the essential uniformity of the human family – uniformity in needs, in capacities for good and evil, and in susceptibility to the influence of one's environment. We therefore predicted (with more than a little trepidation) that our oldest subjects, the twenty-year-olds, might "revert" or "regress" toward the type of situationalist inferences and predictions that we expected from our youngest subjects, the five-year-olds.

In short, our overall prediction was the occurrence of a quadratic relationship between subjects' ages and their preference for dispositionally based behavioral predictions over situationally based ones.

Procedures

Subjects at five age levels (five, eight, eleven, fifteen, and twenty years) were presented with four versions of three basic stories in a "within-subject" design. Each version of each story described one of two actors, offered one of two descriptions of the particular situation facing that actor, and then asked the subject to predict the relevant actor's response. In one story, for instance, in which a little boy confronts a large dog, the subjects' task was to predict whether the child in question would run away from the animal. The descriptions of each boy presented information about his behavior in loosely related situations that would either make his running away from the dog more likely or less likely from the viewpoint of a "dispositionalist," but would be irrelevant from the viewpoint of a pure situationalist. Similarly, the description of each situation presented information about the dog that would make running away either more likely or less likely from the viewpoint of a situationalist but would be irrelevant to a pure dispositionalist. Thus, in the "Boy Meets Dog" story the little boy whose past behavior suggested a "personality" that might *promote* the target response of "running away" was described as follows:

This is a picture of Johnny. [E shows S a photograph of a child.] When Johnny goes to the park with his mother, he doesn't go on the high slippery slide, because he's scared. When he's at school, he doesn't play with kids who are bigger than he is, because sometimes they push him around. Johnny is also scared of the dark.

By contrast, the little boy whose past behavior suggested a personality that might *inhibit* running away was described quite differently:

This is a picture of Billy. [E shows S a photograph of a child.] When Billy goes to the park, he swings really high on the big swings, and he isn't scared. He plays football with the big kids at school, and he doesn't care if he gets hurt a little. Billy doesn't mind being in dark places.

After the relevant actor was introduced, information about the dog or "situation" that might *promote* a timid response was offered.

Now here's a picture of a dog. [E shows S a photograph of a large German Shepherd.] Suppose Johnny was playing by himself in front of his house one day, and this dog in the picture came running up to him and barked and growled pretty loudly.

And the description of the situation that might *inhibit* that target response was again quite different:

Now here's a picture of a dog. [E shows S a photograph of a fluffy white Samoyed.] Suppose Billy was playing by himself in front of his house one day, and this dog in the picture came running up and wanted to play with him.

Following the presentation of each of the four actor–situation pairings (e.g., "timid" Johnny meets "fierce" dog) subjects were asked to predict how the actor in question would respond, then to indicate how sure they were about their answer. Three such stories were presented, each featuring a different pair of actors and a different pair of stimulus situations.

Results and interpretation

The specific techniques used to score answers and the details of data analysis were fairly complicated, and need not concern us here (see Josephson, 1977). But the main findings, both for the "Boy Meets Dog" story and for the three stories combined, were straightforward and can be summarized briefly.

First, it was evident that all five age groups knew how to make inferential use of both the "person" information and the "situation" information. Almost without exception, individual subjects' ratings showed a "main effect" of both types of information. Holding constant the description of the dog, for instance, they consistently expressed greater confidence that the child would run away if his past behavior suggested timidity than if it suggested boldness; and holding constant the description of the child, they consistently expressed more confidence that the actor would run away if it was the "fierce" dog that was described than if it was the friendly one.

Second, as predicted, although all actors gave some weight to both the person information and the situation, it was the youngest children, the five-year-olds, whose ratings gave the greatest weight to the situation and the least weight to the person.

Third, also as predicted, it was the oldest subjects, the twenty-year-old college students, whose responses were most like those of the five-year-olds. The eight-, eleven-, and fifteen-year-olds were more inclined than *either* the five-year olds or the twenty-year-olds to give heavy weight to past behavioral information suggesting stable personality traits on the part of the actor and relatively light weight to the specific nature of the situation to which the actor responded. The predicted quadratic relationship between age and dispositionalism was thus confirmed.

Finally, by looking at our young subjects' answers when they asked how they personally would respond to the various situations described, it is possible to comment on the probable *accuracy* of the various age groups. Almost without exception, the youngsters' assertions about their *own* probable responses were a simple reflection of the stimulus situation described. For instance, virtually all youngsters confidently predicted (probably correctly) that they personally would run away from the fierce dog but not from the friendly one. In other words, the youngest and oldest subjects

seemed less inclined than their "middle-aged" peers to commit the fundamental attribution error.

It seems reasonable to conclude that when our maturing intuitive scientists began to make use of person schemas, and to resist the "egocentric" tendency to assume that others would share their feelings and reactions, they thereby went astray. And only when a newer, subtler, and
more accurate set of knowledge structures came into play could they
begin to match the inferential accuracy of our five-year-olds. This facile
summary, of course, leaves a number of important questions unanswered:
Were the twenty-year-olds' insights a passing phase, one that would be
abandoned along with other vestiges of liberal and relativistic ideology
when these twenty-year-olds reached their thirties and forties? Did their
insights really reflect any abstract or general appreciation of the wisdom
of situationalism or the folly of unbridled dispositionalism; or were they
merely the product of more sophisticated knowledge about how little
boys respond to such stimulus situations as fierce versus friendly dogs?
Last but not least, were our provocative results totally or partially a
consequence of the struggle of subjects of different ages to master the
subtleties of outguessing experimenters?

Rarely has the cliché "more research is needed" been so appropriate.
But I have little doubt that in carefully controlled research, as in everyday
encounters with the social world, the young intuitive psychologist may be
immune to at least some of the failings of the old one. For, as another
cliché aptly states, "A little learning" (or better still, a little theory) "can
be a dangerous thing."

Summary

The model of the adult human as an intuitive scientist, one whose high
level of overall proficiency is marred by specific inferential shortcomings,
may be a particularly fruitful one for students of cognitive social development. This model, which has its origins in the study of attributional
strategies and biases, leads to a specification of particular judgmental or
inferential tasks that must be mastered by younger and older social perceivers alike. Principal among these tasks are data coding, generalizing
from data samples, assessing covariations among events, making causal
inferences and predictions, and testing and updating one's theories or
beliefs about the world. The intuitive scientist model further leads to
consideration of very general inferential tools that are employed in the
performance of many different "scientific" tasks. One set of tools, long
familiar to developmentalists but of particular interest to contemporary

cognitive scientists, includes schemas or knowledge structures. Another, less familiar, pair of tools consists of judgmental "heuristics" – specifically the availability heuristic and the representativeness heuristic – which serve to reduce many complex inferential undertakings to relatively crude judgmental operations.

Research on these tasks and tools highlights the close relationship between human inferential strengths and weaknesses; it also challenges us to reconcile the obvious growth of inferential capacities with the existence, persistence, and seeming development of inferential shortcomings. Developmental research is needed on the one hand to clarify the respects in which adult shortcomings reflect deficiencies that are apparent in the child and in a sense are never totally "overcome" by the adult, and on the other hand to reveal tasks or domains where adult shortcomings may be an inevitable by-product of the adult's ever-developing inferential strategies and ever-increasing store of generic knowledge. In this context the distinction between the quality of the perceiver's information and theories and the quality of that perceiver's inferential performance becomes critical. Specifically, the generally superior inferential performances of the adult over the child (and the perplexing cases where adults or older children seem less proficient than relatively young children) may reflect less about differences in inferential methods than about differences in the theories and data samples that are brought to bear by perceivers of different ages.

The analysis of specific attributional biases, including asymmetries between actors' and observers' perceptions of the causes of behavior, "egocentrism" in estimates of behavioral consensus, and inadequate allowance for the impact of social roles on social actions, may prove to be similarly provocative for the developmentalist. These biases, each of which involves social perceivers' difficulties in weighing the relative impact of situational versus dispositional influences, once again can be traced to various deficiencies in the types of data, theories, and inferential strategies available to the relevant perceivers. And for each case, the developmental progression from child to adult introduces differences in data and theories, if not in strategies, that promise to exert complex effects on age-related susceptibilities to the biases in question. Indeed, for one particular inferential error – the so-called fundamental attribution error, whereby actions are incorrectly seen as evidence of the actor's traits rather than as results of situational forces and constraints – it is possible to show a nonlinear developmental trend that reveals that the youngest and oldest of children are most alike in their judgments and inferences, and that both differ from their "middle-aged" peers.

Notes

1 No attempt, however, will be made here to review the considerable, and ever-expanding literature on cognitive social development – much of which has implicitly or explicitly made use of the analogy between the endeavors of the scientist and those of the young human who is exploring and gaining increasing understanding of the physical and social world. Beyond the various chapters of the present volume that review and expand this literature, the reader will recognize some clear continuities between present concerns and those discussed earlier by Piaget (1936, 1972; Inhelder & Piaget, 1958; see Flavell, 1963) and more recently by Flavell (1977) Siegler (1976) and especially Schantz (1977). A new and very pertinent paper by Shaklee (1980) further testifies to convergences between contemporary cognitive social psychology and some longstanding interests of developmentalists.

2 My discussion will emphasize the parallels between the layperson's tasks and those of the formal scientist conducting research. For a discussion of dissimilarities and their implications – many of which can be anticipated by noting that the layperson's immediate needs and priorities often make his role more closely akin to that of the applied scientist or practitioner than to that of the pure researcher – see Nisbett and Ross, 1980, especially pp. 274–6.

3 The relative terms of the false-consensus effect merit some emphasis, and perhaps some further explication. Obviously people who endorse the legalization of cocaine use, launch revolutions, or adopt clerical celibacy recognize that their choices would not be shared by the majority of their peers. The relative terms of the false-consensus hypothesis suggest only that such people would see their persona choices as less deviant, and more in tune with environmental forces and constraints, than would those of us who oppose the legalization of cocaine, advocate less traumatic methods of political change, or never dream of becoming celibate clerics.

References

Abelson, R. P. Modes of resolution of belief dilemmas. *Conflict Resolution,* 1959, *3,* 343–52.

Script processing in attitude formation and decision-making. In J. S. Carroll and J. W. Payne (Eds.), *Cognition and social behavior.* Hillsdale, N.J.: Lawrence Erlbaum Associates, 1976.

Abrahamson, L. Y., Seligman, M. E. P., & Teasdale, J. D. Learned helplessness in humans. Critique and reformulation. *Journal of Abnormal Psychology,* 1978, *87,* 49–74.

Allport, G. W. *The nature of prejudice.* Reading, Massachusets: Addison-Wesley, 1954.

Anderson, C. A., Lepper, M. R., & Ross, L. The perseverance of social theories: The role of explanation in the persistence of discredited information. *Journal of Personality and Social Psychology,* in press.

Arkin, R., & Duval, S. Focus of attention and causal attributions of actors and observers. *Journal of Experimental Social Psychology,* 1975, *11,* 427–38.

Asch, S. *Social psychology.* Englewood Cliffs, N.J.: Prentice-Hall, 1952.

Barber, B. *Science and the social order.* New York: Collier, 1952.

Bartlett, F. C. *Remembering.* New York: Cambridge University Press, 1932.

Bem, D. J. An experimental analysis of self-persuasion. *Journal of Experimental Social Psychology,* 1965, *1,* 199–218.

Self-perception: An alternative interpretation of cognitive dissonance phenomena. *Psychological Review,* 1967, *74,* 183–200.

Self-perception: The dependent variable of human performance. *Organizational Behavior and Human Performance*, 1967, *22*, 105–21.

Self-perception theory. In L. Berkowitz (Ed.), *Advances in experimental social psychology* (Vol. 6). New York: Academic Press, 1972.

Bem, D. J., & Funder, D. C. Predicting more of the people more of the time: Assessing the personality of situations. *Psychological Review*, 1978, *85*, 485–501.

Bem, D. J., & Lord, C. G. Template matching: A proposal for probing the ecological validity of experimental settings in social psychology. *Journal of Personality and Social Psychology*, 1979, *37*, 833–46.

Borgida, E., & Nisbett, R. E. The differential impact of abstract vs. concrete information on decisions. *Journal of Applied Social Psychology*, 1977, *7*, 258–71.

Bower, G. Experiments on story comprehension and recall. *Discourse Processes*, 1978, *1*, 211–31.

Bradley, G. W. Self-serving biases in the attribution process: A reexaminatin of the fact or fiction question. *Journal of Personality and Social Psychology*, 1978, *36*, 56–71.

Bruner, J. S. Going beyond the information given. In H. Gruber, K. R. Hammond, & R. Jesser (Eds.), *Contemporary approaches to cognition*. Cambridge, Mass.: Harvard University Press, 1957.

Cantor, N. & Mischel, W. Traits as prototypes: Effects on recognition memory. *Journal of Personality and Social Psychology*, 1977, *35*, 38–49.

Prototypicality and personality: Effects on free recall and personality impressions. *Journal of Research in Personality*, 1979, *13*, 187–205.

Chapman, L. J., & Chapman, J. P. The genesis of popular but erroneous psychodiagnostic observations. *Journal of Abnormal Psychology*, 1967, *72*, 193–204.

Illusory correlation as an obstacle to the use of valid psychodiagnostic signs. *Journal of Abnormal Psychology*, 1969, *74*, 271–80.

Cooper, J., Jones, E. E., & Tuller, S. M. Attribution, dissonance and the illusion of uniqueness. *Journal of Experimental Social Psychology*, 1972, *8*, 45–7.

Cronbach, L. J. Processes affecting scores on "understanding of others" and "assumed similarity." *Psychological Bulletin*, 1955, *52*, 177–93.

Davison, G. C., & Valins, S. Maintenance of self attributed and drug attributed behavior change. *Journal of Personality and Social Psychology*, 1969, *11*, 25–33.

Dawes, R. M. Social selection based on multidimensional criteria. *Journal of Abnormal and Social Psychology*, 1964, *68*, 104–9.

Shallow psychology. In J. Carroll & J. Payne (Eds.), *Cognition and social behavior*. Potomac, Maryland: Lawrence Erlbaum Associates, 1976.

Deci, E. L. Effects of externally mediated rewards on intrinsic motivation. *Journal of Personality and Social Psychology*, 1971, *18*, 105–55.

Intrinsic motivation, extrinsic reinforcement, and inequity. *Journal of Personality and Social Psychology*, 1972, *22*, 113–20. (a)

The effects of contingent and non-contingent rewards and controls on intrinsic motivation. *Organizational Behavior and Human Performance*, 1972, *8*, 217–29. (b)

DiVitto, B., & McArthur, L. Z. Developmental differences in the use of distinctiveness, consensus, and consistency information for making causal attributions. *Developmental Psychology*, 1978, *14*, 474–82.

Einhorn, H. J., & Hogarth, R. M. Confidence in judgment: Persistence of the illusion of validity. *Psychological Review*, 1978, *85*, 395–416.

Fischhoff, B. Hindsight ≠ foresight: The effect of outcome knowledge on judgment under uncertainty. *Journal of Experimental Psychology: Human Perception and Performance*, 1975, *1*, 288–99.

Attribution theory and judgment under uncertainty. In J. H. Harvey, W. J. Ickes, & R.

F. Kidd (Eds.), *New directions in attribution research* (Vol. 1). Hillsdale, N.J.: Lawrence Erlbaum Associates, 1976.

Flavell, J. H. *The developmental psychology of Jean Piaget.* New York: Van Nostrand Co., 1963.

Cognitive development. Englewood Cliffs, N.J.: Prentice-Hall, 1977.

Genosar, L., & Trope, Y. The effects of base rates and individuating information on judgments about another person. *Journal of Experimental Social Psychology,* 1980, *16,* 228–42.

Guttentag, M., & Longfellow, C. Children's social attributions: Development and change. In H. E. Howe & C. B. Keasey (Eds.), *Nebraska symposium on motivation,* 1977, *25,* 305–41.

Hamill, R., Wilson, T. D., & Nisbett, R. E. Insensitivity to sample bias: Generalizing from atypical cases. *Journal of Personality and Social Psychology,* in press.

Hansen, R. D., & Donoghue, J. M. The power of consensus: Information derived from one's own and other's behavior. *Journal of Personality and Social Psychology,* 1977, *35,* 294–302.

Hansen, R. D., & Stonner, D. M. Attributes and attributions: Inferring stimulus properties, actors' dispositions, and causes. *Journal of Personality and Social Psychology,* 1978, *36,* 657–67.

Harris, B. Developmental differences in the attribution of responsibility. *Developmental Psychology,* 1977, *13,* 257–65.

Heider, F. Social perception and phenomenal causality. *Psychological Review,* 1944, *51,* 358–74.

The psychology of interpersonal relations. New York: Wiley, 1958.

Holmes, D. S. *Dimensions of projection. The psychology of interpersonal relations.* New York: Wiley, 1958.

Hovland, C. I., Janis, I. L., & Kelley, H. H. *Communication and persuasion.* New Haven, Conn.: Yale University Press, 1953.

Icheiser, G. Misunderstanding in human relations: A study in false social perception. *American Journal of Sociology,* 1949, *55,* 1–70.

Inhelder, B., & Piaget, J. *The growth of logical thinking from childhood to adolescence.* New York: Basic Books, 1958.

Jennings, D., Amabile, T. M., & Ross, L. Informal covariation assessment: Data-based vs. theory-based judgments. In D. Kahneman, P. Slovic, & A. Tversky (Eds.), *Judgment under uncertainty: Heuristics and biases.* New York: Cambridge University Press, 1980.

Jennings, Dennis L., Lepper, Mark R., & Ross, Lee. Persistence of impressions of personal persuasiveness: Perseverance of erroneous self-assessments outside the debriefing paradigm. *Personality and Social Psychology Bulletin,* in press.

Jones, E. E., & Davis, K. E. From acts to dispositions. In L. Berkowitz (Ed.), *Advances in experimental social psychology* (Vol. 2). New York: Academic Press, 1965.

Jones, E. E., & Gerard, H. B. *Foundations of social psychology.* New York: Wiley, 1967.

Jones, E. E., & Goethals, G. R. Order effects in impression formation: Attribution context and the nature of the entity. In E. E. Jones, D. E. Kanouse, H. H. Kelley, R. E. Nisbett, S. Valins, & B. Weiner (Eds.), *Attribution : Perceiving the causes of behavior.* Morristown, N.J.: General Learning Press, 1971.

Jones, E. E., Kanouse, D. E., Kelley, H. H., Nisbett, R. E., Valins, S., & Weiner, B. (Eds.). *Attribution: Perceiving the causes of behavior.* Morristown, N.J.: General Learning Press, 1971.

Jones, E. E., & Nisbett, R. E. The action and the observer: Divergent perceptions of the causes of behavior. In E. E. Jones, et al. (Eds.), *Attribution: Perceiving the causes of behavior.* Morristown, N.J.: General Learning Press, 1971.

Josephson, J. *The child's use of situational and personal information in predicting the behavior of another.* Unpublished doctoral dissertation, Stanford University, 1977.

Kahneman, D., & Tversky, A. Subjective probability: A judgment of representativeness. *Cognitive Psychology*, 1972, *3*, 430–54.

Kahneman, D., & Tversky, A. On the psychology of prediction. *Psychological Review*, 1973, *80*, 237–51.

Kanouse, D. E. Language, labeling, and attribution. In E. E. Jones et al. (Eds.), *Attribution: Perceiving the causes of behavior.* Morristown, N.J.: General Learning Press, 1971.

Karniol, R., & Ross, M. The development of causal attributions in social perception. *Journal of Personality and Social Psychology*, 1976, *34*, 455–64.

The effect of performance-relevant and performance-irrelevant rewards on children's intrinsic motivation. *Child Development*, 1977, *48*, 482–7.

Children's use of a causal attribution schema and the inference of manipulative intentions. *Child Development*, 1979, *50*, 463–8.

Katz, D. The functional approach to the study of attitudes. *Public Opinion Quarterly*, 1960, *24*, 163–204.

Katz, D., & Allport, F. *Students' attitudes.* Syracuse: Craftsman Press, 1931.

Kelley, H. H. Attribution theory in social psychology. In D. Levine (Ed.), *Nebraska symposium on motivation* (Vol. 15). Lincoln, Nebraska: University of Nebraska Press, 1967.

Attribution in social interaction. In E. E. Jones et al. (Eds.), *Attribution: Perceiving the causes of behavior.* Morristown, N.J.: General Learning Press, 1971.

The processes of causal attribution. *American Psychologist*, 1973, *28*, 107–28.

Kelley, H. H. & Stahelski, A. J. Social interaction basis of cooperators' and competitors' beliefs about others. *Journal of Personality and Social Psychology*, 1970, *16*, 66–91.

Kelly, G. *The psychology of personal constructs* (2 vols.). New York: Norton, 1955.

Man's construction of his alternatives. In G. Lindzey (Ed.), *Assessment of human motives.* New York: Holt, Rinehart & Winston, 1958.

Kruglanski, A. W., Friedman, I., & Zeevi, G. The effects of extrinsic incentives on some qualitative aspects of task performance. *Journal of Personality*, 1971, *39*, 606–17.

Kuhn, T. S. *The structure of scientific revolutions.* Chicago: University of Chicago Press, 1962.

Kun, A., Parsons, J., & Ruble, D. Development of integration processses using ability and effort information to predict outcome. *Developmental Psychology*, 1974, *10*, 721–32.

Langer, E. J. The illusion of control. *Journal of Personality and Social Psychology*, 1975, *32*, 311–28.

Langer, E. J., & Roth, S. Heads I win, tails it's chance: The illusion of control as a function of the sequence of outcomes in a purely chance task. *Journal of Personality and Social Psychology*, 1975, *32*, 951–5.

Lepper, M. R. Intrinsic and extrinsic motivation in children: Detrimental effects of superfluous social controls. In W. A. Collins (Ed.), *Minnesota symposium on child psychology* (Vol. 14). Hillsdale, N.J.: Lawrence Erlbaum Associates, 1980.

Social control processes, attributions of motivation, and the internalization of social values. In T. E. Higgins, D. N. Ruble, & W. W. Hartup (Eds.), *Social cognition and social behavior: A developmental perspective.* New York: Cambridge University Press, in press.

Lepper, M. R., & Greene, D. (Eds.). *The hidden costs of reward.* Hillsdale, N.J.: Lawrence Erlbaum Associates, 1978. (a)

Overjustification research and beyond: Toward a means-ends analysis of intrinsic and extrinsic motivation. In M. R. Lepper & D. Greene (Eds.), *The hidden costs of reward.* Hillsdale, N.J.: Lawrence Erlbaum Associates, 1978. (b)

Divergent approaches to the study of rewards. In M. R. Lepper & D. Greene (Eds.), *The hidden costs of reward.* Hillsdale, N.J.: Lawrence Erlbaum Associates, 1978. (c)

Lepper, M. R., Greene, D., & Nisbett, R. E. Undermining children's intrinsic interest with extrinsic rewards: A test of the "overjustification" hypothesis. *Journal of Personality and Social Psychology,* 1973, *28,* 129–37.

Lepper, M. R., Ross, L., & Lau, R. R. *Persistence of inaccurate and discredited personal impressions: Field demonstrations of attributional perseverance in educational contexts.* Unpublished manuscript, Stanford University, 1980.

Lepper, M. R., Sagotsky, G., Dafoe, J., & Greene, D. *Effects of a nominal contingency on children's subsequent intrinsic interest: A means-ends analysis.* Unpublished manuscript, Stanford University, 1980.

Lewin, K. *A dynamic theory of personality.* New York: McGraw-Hill, 1935.

Lord, C., Ross, L., & Lepper, M. R. Biased assimilation and attitude polarization: The effects of prior theories on subsequently considered evidence. *Journal of Personality and Social Psychology,* 1979, *37,* 2098–109.

Mahoney, M. J. *Scientist as subject: The psychological imperative.* Cambridge, Mass.: Ballinger Publishing Co., 1976.

Publication prejudices: An experimental study of confirmatory bias in the peer review system. *Cognitive Therapy and Research,* 1977, *1,* 161–75.

Markus, H. Self-schemata and processing information about the self. *Journal of Personality and Social Psychology,* 1977, *35,* 63–78.

McArthur, L. Z. The how and what of why: Some determinants and consequences of causal attribution. *Journal of Personality and Social Psychology,* 1972, *22,* 171–93.

The lesser influence of consensus than distinctiveness information on causal attributions: A test of the person-thing hypothesis. *Journal of Personality and Social Psychology,* 1976, *33,* 733–42.

McArthur, L. Z., & Post, D. Figural emphasis and person perception. *Journal of Experimental Social Psychology,* 1977, *13,* 520–35.

McArthur, L. Z., & Solomon, L. K. Perceptions of an aggressive encounter as a function of the victim's salience and the perceiver's arousal. *Journal of Personality and Social Psychology,* 1978, *36,* 1278–90.

McGuigan, F. J. The experimenter: A neglected stimulus object. *Psychological Bulletin,* 1963, *60,* 421–8.

Meehl, P. *Clinical vs. statistical prediction.* Minneapolis: University of Minnesota Press, 1955.

Miller, A. G., Gillen, B., Schenker, C., & Radlove, S. Perception of obedience to authority. *Proceedings of the 81st Annual Convention of the American Psychological Association,* 1973, *8,* 127–8.

Miller, D. T., & Ross, M. Self-serving biases in the attribution of causality: Fact or fiction? *Psychological Bulletin,* 1975, *82,* 213–25.

Minsky, M. A framework for representing knowledge. In P. H. Winston (Ed.), *The psychology of computer vision.* New York: McGraw-Hill, 1975.

Newtson, D. Attribution and the unit of perception of ongoing behavior. *Journal of Personality and Social Psychology,* 1973, *28,* 28–38.

Nisbett, R. E., & Borgida, E. Attribution and the psychology of prediction. *Journal of Personality and Social Psychology,* 1975, *32,* 932–43.

Nisbett, R. E., Borgida, E., Crandall, R., & Reed, H. Popular induction: Information is not always informative. In J. Carroll & J. Payne (Eds.), *Cognitive and social behavior.* Potomac, Md.: Lawrence Erlbaum Associates, 1976.

Nisbett, R. E. & Ross, L. *Human inference: Strategies and shortcomings of social judgment.* Englewood Cliffs, N.J.: Prentice-Hall, 1980.

Orvis, B. R., Cunningham, J. D., & Kelley, H. H. A closer examination of causal inference: The roles of consensus, distinctiveness, and consistency information *Journal of Personality and Social Psychology, 1975, 32,* 605–16.

Peterson, C. R., & Beach, L. R. Man as an intuitive statistician. *Psychological Bulletin,* 1967, *68,* 29–46.

Piaget, J. *La naissance de l'intelligence chez l'enfant.* Neuchatel et Paris: Delachau et Niestle, 1936.

Intellectual evolution from adolescence to adulthood. *Human Development,* 1972, *15,* 1–12.

Piaget, J., & Inhelder, B. *The origin of the idea of chance in children.* New York: Norton, 1975.

Pryor, J. B., & Kriss, M. The cognitive dynamics of salience in the attribution process. *Journal of Personality and Social Psychology,* 1977, *35,* 49–55.

Regan, D. T., & Totten, J. Empathy and attribution: Turning observers into actors. *Journal of Personality and Social Psychology, 1975, 32,* 850–6.

Robertson, T. S., & Rossiter, J. R. Children and commercial persuasion: An attribution theory analysis. *Journal of Consumer Research,* 1974, *1,* 13–20.

Short-run advertising effects on children: A field study. *Journal of Marketing Research,* 1976, *13,* 68–70.

Rosch, E. Principles of categorization. In E. Rosch & B. Lloyd (Eds.), *Cognition and categorization.* Hillsdale, N.J.: Lawrence Erlbaum, 1978.

Ross, L. The intuitive psychologist and his shortcomings: Distortions in the attribution process. In L. Berkowitz (Ed.), *Advances in experimental social psychology* (Vol. 10). New York: Academic Press, 1977.

Afterthoughts on the intuitive psychologist. In L. Berkowitz (Ed.), *Cognitive theories in social psychology.* New York: Academic Press, 1978.

Ross, L., Amabile, T. M., & Steinmetz, J. L. Social roles, social control, and biases in the social perception process. *Journal of Personality and Social Psychology,* 1977, *35,* 485–94.

Ross, L., Bierbrauer, G., & Polly, S. Attribution of educational outcomes by professional and nonprofessional instructors. *Journal of Personality and Social Psychology,* 1974, *29,* 609–18.

Ross, L., Greene, D., & House, P. The false consensus phenomenon: An attributional bias in self-perception and social perception processes. *Journal of Experimental Social Psychology,* 1977, *13,* 279–301.

Ross, L., & Lepper, M. R. The perseverance of beliefs: Empirical and normative considerations. In R. A. Shweder (Ed.), *New directions for methodology of social and behavioral science: Fallible judgment in behavioral research.* San Francisco: Jossey-Bass, 1980.

Ross, L., Lepper, M. R., & Hubbard, M. Perseverance in self-perception and social perception: Biased attributional processes in the debriefing paradigm. *Journal of Personality and Social Psychology,* 1975, *32,* 880–92.

Ross, L., Lepper, M. R., Strack, F., & Steinmetz, J. Social explanation and social expectation: The effects of real and hypothetical explanations upon subjective likelihood. *Journal of Personality and Social Psychology,* 1977, *35,* 817–29.

Ross, L., Turiel, E., Josephson, J., & Lepper, M. R. *Developmental perspectives on the fundamental attribution error.* Unpublished manuscript, Stanford University, 1978.

Ross, M., & Sicoly, F. Egocentric biases in availability and attribution. *Journal of Personality and Social Psychology,* 1979, *37,* 322–36.

Rothbart, M., Fulero, S., Jensen, C., Howard, J., & Birrell, B. From individual to group impressions: Availability heuristics in stereotype formation. *Journal of Experimental Social Psychology,* 1978, *14,* 237–55.

Rumelhart, D. E. Understanding and summarizing brief stories. In D. LaBerge & S. J. Samuels (Eds.), *Basic process in reading: Perception and comprehension.* Hillsdale, N.J.: Lawrence Erlbaum, 1976.

Salancik, G. R. Inference of one's attitude from behavior recalled under linguistically manipulated cognitive sets. *Journal of Experimental Social Psychology,* 1974, *10,* 415– 27.

Extrinsic attribution and the use of behavioral information to infer attitudes. *Journal of Personality and Social Psychology,* 1976, *34,* 1302– 12.

Salancik, G. R., & Conway, M. Attitude inferences from salient and relevant cognitive content about behavior. *Journal of Personality and Social Psychology,* 1975, *32,* 829– 40.

Saltz, E., & Medow, M. L. Concept conservation in children: The dependence of belief systems on semantic representation. *Child Development,* 1971, *6,* 1533–42.

Schachter, S., & Singer, J. E. Cognitive, social and physiological determinants of emotional state. *Psychological Review,* 1962, *69,* 379–99.

Schank, R., & Abelson, R. P. *Scripts, plans, goals, and understanding.* Hillsdale, N.J.: Lawrence Erlbaum Associates, 1977.

Schneider, D. J., Hastorf, A. H., & Ellsworth, P. C. *Person Perception.* Reading, Mass.: Addison-Wesley, 1979.

Selman, R. The relation of role-taking to the development of moral judgment in children. *Child Development,* 1971, *42,* 79–92.

Social-cognitive understanding: A guide to educational and clinical practice. In T. Lickona (Ed.), *Moral development and behavior.* New York: Holt, Rinehart & Winston, 1976.

Shaklee, H. Bounded rationality and cognitive development: Upper limits on growth? *Cognitive Psychology,* 1979, *11,* 327–45.

Shantz, C. The development of social cognition. In E. M. Heatherington (Ed.), *Review of child development and research* (Vol. 5). Chicago: University of Chicago Press, 1975.

Shultz, T. R., & Butkowsky, I. Young children's use of the scheme for multiple sufficient causes in the attribution of real and hypothetical behavior. *Child Development,* 1977, *48,* 464–9.

Shultz, T. R., Butkowsky, I., Pearce, J. W., & Shanfield, H. Development of schemes for the attribution of multiple psychological causes. *Developmental Psychology,* 1975, *11,* 502–10.

Shultz, T. R., & Mendelson, R. The use of covariation as a principle of causal analysis. *Child Development,* 1975, *46,* 394–8.

Siegler, R. Three aspects of cognitive development. *Cognitive Psychology,* 1976, *4,* 481– 520.

Siegler, R. S., & Liebert, R. M. Effects of contiguity, regularity, and age on children's causal inferences. *Developmental Psychology,* 1974, *10,* 574–9.

Simon, H. *Models of man.* New York: Wiley, 1957.

Simon, H. A. Motivational and emotional controls of cognition. *Psychological Review,* 1967, *74,* 29–39.

Slovic, P., Fischhoff, B., & Lichtenstein, S. Rating the risks. *Environment,* 1979, *21,* 14– 39.

Cognitive processes and societal risk taking. In J. S. Carroll and J. W. Payne (Eds.), *Cognition and social behavior.* Hillsdale, N.J.: Lawrence Erlbaum, 1976.

Slovic, P., & Lichtenstein, S. Comparison of Bayesian and regression approaches to the study of information processing in judgment. *Organizational Behavior and Human Performance,* 1971, *6,* 649–744.

Smedslund, J. The concept of correlation in adults. *Scandinavian Journal of Psychology,* 1963, *4,* 165–73.

Smith, M. C. Children's use of the multiple sufficient cause schema in social perception. *Journal of Personality and Social Psychology,* 1975, *32,* 737–47.

Snyder, M., & Swann, W. B., Jr. Behavioral confirmation in social interaction: From social perception to social reality. *Journal of Experimental Social Psychology,* 1978, *14,* 148–62.

Snyder, M., Tanke, E. D., & Berscheid, E. Social perception and interpersonal behavior: On the self-fulfilling nature of social stereotypes. *Journal of Personality and Social Psychology,* 1977, *35,* 656–66.

Storms, M. D. Videotape and the attribution process: Reversing actors' and observers' points of view. *Journal of Personality and Social Psychology,* 1973, *22,* 165–75.

Taylor, S. E., & Crocker, J. C. Schematic bases of social information processing. In E. T. Higgins, P. Herman, & M. P. Zanna (Eds.), *The Ontario symposium on personality and social psychology* (Vol. 1). Hillsdale, N.J.: Lawrence Erlbaum, 1980.

Taylor, S. E., & Fiske, S. T. Point of view and perceptions of causality. *Journal of Personality and Social Psychology,* 1975, *32,* 439–45.

Salience, attention and attribution: Top of the head phenomena. In L. Berkowitz (Ed.), *Advances in experimental social psychology* (Vol. 11). New York: Academic Press, 1978.

Taynor, J., & Deaux, K. When women are more deserving than men: Equity, attribution, and perceived sex differences. *Journal of Personality and Social Psychology,* 1973, *28,* 360–7.

Tomkins, A. Script theory: Differential magnification of affects. In H. E. Howes & R. A Dienstbier (Eds.), *Nebraska symposium on motivation* (Vol. 26). Lincoln, Neb.: University of Nebraska Press, 1979.

Tversky, A., & Kahneman, D. Belief in the law of small numbers. *Psychological Bulletin,* 1971, *76,* 105–10.

Availability: A heuristic for judging frequency and probability. *Cognitive Psychology,* 1973, *5,* 207–32.

Judgment under uncertainty: Heuristics and biases. *Science,* 1974, *185,* 1124–31.

Causal schemata in judgments under uncertainty. In M. Fishbein (Ed.), *Progress in social psychology.* Hillsdale, N.J.: Lawrence Erlbaum 1978.

Valins, S., & Nisbett, R. E. Attribution processes in the development and treatment of emotional disorders. In E. E. Jones et al. (Eds.), *Attribution: Perceiving the causes of behavior.* Morristown, N.J.: General Learning Press, 1972.

Ward, W. D., & Jenkins, H. M. The display of information and the judgment of contingency. *Canadian Journal of Psychology,* 1965, *19,* 231–41.

Wason, P., & Johnson-Laird, P. *Psychology of reasoning.* Cambridge, Mass.: Harvard University Press, 1972.

Weiner, B. (Ed.). *Achievement motivation and attribution theory.* Morristown, N.J.: General Learning Press, 1974.

Weiner, B. Achievement motivation as conceptualized by an attribution theorist. In B. Weiner (Ed.), *Achievement motivation and attribution theory.* Morristown, N.J.: General Learning Press, 1974.

Weiner, B. (Ed.), *Cognitive views of human motivation.* New York: Academic Press, 1974.

Weiner, B., Heckhausen, H., Meyer, W. U., & Cook, R. E. Causal ascriptions and achievement behavior: The conceptual analysis of effort and reanalysis of locus of control. *Journal of Personality and Social Psychology,* 1972, *21,* 239–48.

Weiner, B., & Kun, A. The development of causal attributions and the growth of achievement and social motivation. In S. Feldman & D. Bush (Eds.), *Cognitive development and social development: Relationships and implications*. Hillsdale, N.J.: Lawrence Erlbaum Associates, in press.

Weiner, B., & Peter, N. A cognitive-developmental analysis of achievement and moral judgments. *Developmental Psychology*, 1973, *9*, 290–309.

Wells, G. L., & Harvey, J. H. Do people use consensus information in making causal attributions? *Journal of Personality and Social Psychology*, 1977, *35*, 279–93.

Naive attributors' attributions and predictions: What is informative and when is an effect an effect? *Journal of Personality and Social Psychology*, 1978, *36*, 483–90.

Wortman, C. B. Causal attributions and personal control. In J. H. Harvey, W. J. Ickes, and R. F. Kidd (Eds.), *New directions in attribution research* (Vol. 1). Hillsdale, N.J.: Lawrence Erlbaum, 1976.

2   The development of thoughts about animate and inanimate objects: implications for research on social cognition

Rochel Gelman and Elizabeth Spelke

The soul is characterized by two faculties, (a) the faculty of discrimination which is the work of thought and sense, and (b) the faculty of originating local movement.

> From Aristotle's *De Anima*, Book III, Chapter 8, as presented in McKeon, 1941.

This chapter was motivated by a very general question: How is the development of social cognition related to the development of cognition of the nonsocial world? It directly addresses a different but, we believe, prior question: How does a child understand the distinction between animate and inanimate objects? Adults distinguish between the animate and inanimate domains, while recognizing that all objects share certain fundamental properties. They know that some thoughts and actions can be directed to objects of any kind, but that certain other thoughts and acts should be reserved for the class of animates or inanimates alone. In this chapter we consider the development of knowledge of the animate–inanimate distinction, especially the distinction between people and manipulable objects. We hope to show that this interesting, rarely studied question can be easily investigated and that it can shed light on the larger question of the relation between social and nonsocial cognition. For a fundamental difference between social and nonsocial events is that the former involve animate objects – especially people – whereas the latter do not.

We begin with a preliminary analysis of animate and inanimate objects

We thank all the Penn graduate students who participated in our Spring 1979 seminar on the development of social cognition. They gave us the opportunity to discuss many of the ideas presented here. We are especially grateful to Jon Baron, Merry Bullock, Diane Evans, John Flavell, Randy Gallistel, Molly Logan, Betty Meck, Al Pepitone, Lee Ross, John Sabini, Prentice Starkey, and Judy Stewart, who read critically one or more of the previous drafts of this paper. Preparation of this manuscript was partially supported by Grant NSF BNS-03327 and NICH HD-10965 to Rochel Gelman and Grant NICH HD-13428 to Elizabeth Spelke. Authors are listed in alphabetical order.

as they appear to be known to adults. Based on this analysis, and on a variety of experimental investigations, we then consider the child's developing understanding of the animate–inanimate distinction, and the child's ability to think appropriately about objects in each domain. We next illustrate how an analysis of the child's concept of animate and inanimate may shed light on the relationship between social and nonsocial cognition. Our discussion focuses on the development of object permanence and the development of causal reasoning. We conjecture that at least part of what develops over infancy and childhood is not a concept of permanence or causation per se but an ability to apply these concepts to a world of animate and inanimate objects that behave in very different ways. We speculate that the child's understanding of objects and of causal principles advances when he or she comes to understand the distinctive properties of animate and inanimate objects. The chapter concludes with some hypotheses about the development of social cognition.

A theme will recur throughout this chapter. Children's understanding of a given domain depends not only on the logical structure of the tasks used to assess competence and the level of development of some general set of cognitive structures. Their competence depends as well on the nature of the objects about which they must reason. Different structures and processes may be used on different objects, depending on the child's conception of those objects. Therefore, we consider the distinctive properties of animate objects and the child's understanding of those properties.

A beginning analysis of the animate–inanimate distinction

We focus on clear examples of animate and inanimate objects. The reader should understand *animate* to refer primarily to people and *inanimate* to refer to such three-dimensional, nonliving things as rocks, machines, books, furniture, clothing, and toys. It is not our goal to attempt to specify the necessary and sufficient conditions for animacy and the proper classification of ambiguous cases. However difficult and philosophically interesting ambiguous cases such as viruses and chess-playing computers may be, we take it for granted that the distinction is central to a good deal of everyday reasoning in adults. By considering how people react to clear instances of animate and inanimate objects we hope to formulate more precise research questions. To this end, we discuss the adult's analysis of animate and inanimate objects as: (1) collections of properties; (2) objects of perception; (3) recipients of action; and (4) domains of systematic knowledge.

Animate and inanimate objects as different natural kinds

Animate and inanimate objects share many properties: They both have physical dimensions, specifiable in terms of size, shape, color, and so forth. They are subject to similar transformations such as displacement in space and occlusion. Despite their similarities, there is a fundamental difference between them that is expressed in several ways. We consider four of its expressions. First, animate objects can act: The source of the transformations in which they engage can be internal as well as external. The same is not true of inanimate objects: They move only when something or someone initiates the transformation.

Second, animate and inanimate objects may both change over time, but they change in different ways. Animate objects grow and reproduce, acting to sustain themselves and their offspring. Inanimate objects may change in size or number if they undergo certain transformations (e.g., ice melts in warm temperatures, and glass may shatter if it is dropped), but they cannot bring these changes on themselves. Nor can they regulate through actions or internal processes the changes that occur in them.

Third, animate objects are entities that know, perceive, emote, learn, and think. In these respects, inanimate objects have no counterpart. A machine may undergo complex transformations of states that are internal and unseen. But it lacks the capacity for any mental representations or processes.[1]

Finally, although most animate and some inanimate objects have internal structures that relate their parts, the structures of animate and inanimate objects differ in certain respects. Animate objects are made up of structures that function to maintain life, foster growth, and allow reproduction. The parts that are common to animate objects are directly related to the kinds of things they can do: Limbs permit movement, digestive and respiratory systems support eating and breathing, reproductive systems create offspring, and brains and nervous systems support sensation, perception, learning, emotion, motivation, and the acquisition of knowledge. Inanimate objects do not eat, grow, reproduce, or think. They lack the life-sustaining, reproductive, and nervous structures that make these functions possible. Nevertheless, they may be comprised of parts that are structurally related. The clearest examples are machines, whose parts serve specific functions and whose organization obeys certain structural constraints. Only in science fiction, however, do machines have structures that permit reproduction, emotion, and intention.

Animate and inanimate objects as objects of perception

Both animate and inanimate objects can be perceived. Objects in both categories have a definite size, shape, substance, and other properties that may be specified to the eye, ear, and hand. Nevertheless, perceivers usually abstract different sorts of information from animate and inanimate objects. When we perceive an inanimate object, we focus on its physical properties. Perception is usually quite determinate (an object usually does or does not look round) and accurate (an object usually is round if it looks so). When we perceive an animate object, we note its physical properties, but are more likely to focus on the object's actions and intentions, motives, and feelings. The appreciation of intentions and feelings is often indeterminate (a person may not look clearly happy or unhappy), even deceptive (a person may look happy without being so).

The process of acquiring information about animate and inanimate objects also differs, because animate objects have the potential to deliver communications. Perceivers evaluate these communications along with all the other information they receive about the object. Perceivers may also communicate with an animate object, requesting information and eliciting certain reactions from the object. Inanimate objects neither communicate with perceivers nor respond to communications from them.

Animate and inanimate objects as recipients of action

Animate and inanimate objects may be acted on in many of the same ways: Both can be pushed, tapped, kissed, and so forth. Actions on animate and on inanimate objects nevertheless differ in certain respects. First, the consequences of such actions are different. Animate objects usually respond to an action by acting in turn, and their reactions are not fully predictable. Inanimate objects cannot respond with independent action. What they do can usually be predicted by a consideration of their physical characteristics and the characteristics of the action on them.

Second, an actor can use a second animate object as an agent; he or she may use an inanimate object as an instrument but never as an agent. One uses an instrument by acting directly on it. It is necessary to coordinate instrument action with goal action. One uses an agent, however, by communicating one's intent to the agent. It often suffices to look at someone in a certain way to get that individual to do something. One could stare at a rock forever, and nothing would happen.

Third, the action of one person can be similar in kind to that of another person. This has several implications. Animate objects have the potential for acting reciprocally and for reversing roles. Reversals occur in communication (A speaks to B after B speaks to A), in action (A may push B after being pushed by B), and in socially organized situations (A may alternately lead and be led by B). Role reversals and reciprocal interactions do not occur between animates and inanimates, although one may mimic such reversals in play.

In addition, an actor and a second animate object can pursue common or conflicting goals. They can cooperate and they can compete. In either case, each actor must take account of the intentions of the other. An inanimate object may at times be a prop or an obstacle for an actor, but it has no goals of its own.

Systems of knowledge about animate and inanimate objects

Thinking about objects, both animate and inanimate, appears to be systematic and principled. We draw on our systematic knowledge to organize our understanding of properties of objects and the dynamics of events. Different systems of knowledge appear to be used, depending on whether the objects and events that we know are animate or inanimate. Knowledge of inanimate objects is organized according to a set of physical laws. To understand what an object is, what states it can enter, and what transformations it can undergo, we must develop some formal or informal understanding of the laws of physics. Knowledge of animate objects is organized as well according to psychological principles and social conventions. To understand the states and predict the actions of a person, we usually appeal to the person's feelings and intentions, to theories about others, and to the conventions of society, as well as to the physical forces that act on him or her.

These different systems of knowledge provide information about what we can and cannot do. They serve to regulate our actions. For example, our knowledge of physical laws keeps us from attempting to move a mountain, part the seas, or lift a building. Our knowledge of social conventions keeps us from undressing in public or driving on the wrong side of the road. Our grasp of moral principles is presumably involved when we help those in distress.

The development of the distinction between people and inanimate objects

When does a child first appreciate that animate and inanimate objects differ in some properties, that they are perceived and acted on in different ways, and that some knowledge about them is organized differently?

Evidence for the development of this distinction comes from a variety of sources. We will review some of the evidence, following the format set forth in our analysis of the adult's distinction between animate and inanimate objects.

The child's understanding of the properties of animate and inanimate objects

To understand the differences between the properties of animate and inanimate objects, children must come to realize that only animate objects act independently, grow, reproduce, possess certain structures, and think. Piaget (1930) suggested that children attribute the capacity for independent action to some inanimate objects – clouds, rivers, the moon – throughout the preschool years. When presented with well-known objects, however, even very young children seem to know that only animate objects act on their own. Golinkoff and Harding (1980) noted that infants of twenty-four months were surprised when a real chair seemed to move on its own; they showed no surprise when the chair was moved by a person. Infants of sixteen months failed to be surprised by any of these events. Thus the understanding that people – but not chairs – are capable of independent movement may develop in the first two years of life.

We know of little work that addresses the question of when children first understand that only animate objects can grow, reproduce, and die. Even seven-month-old infants appear to be responsive to the age of another person: They are more interested in and less fearful of people who are young (Brooks & Lewis, 1976). Likewise, children of four years are sensitive to age differences; they communicate differently with two-year-olds than with peers or adults (Shatz & Gelman, 1973). Work by Piaget (1969) suggests that an understanding of growth develops. By four or five years, children appreciate that they were once as little as an infant; by five or six years, they acknowledge that an adult was once as young as they. These findings raise a critical question: Do young children appreciate that unlike people, rocks and chairs do *not* grow? That a small stone is no younger or less competent than a large one? That a large stone was not once small? In play, young children sometimes appear to treat inanimate objects like animate objects; for example, the smallest-sized block may be called "the baby." We do not know whether this game reflects a metaphorical extension or a genuine failure to appreciate that growth and reproduction are capacities reserved for animate objects.

Children as young as four years appear to appreciate that only animate objects have certain kinds of parts. Carey (1978) taught preschool-aged children that a given animal (for example, a cow or a human) had an omentum. An omentum is a membrane that holds the intestines in place, but surely none of the children were aware of this. Children were then asked whether each of a series of objects – for example, aardvark, fish, or bug – had an omentum. Children's willingness to grant this organ to other animals depended somewhat on the similarity of that animal to a cow or human. In general, however, all children were much more willing to attribute this organ to any animal than to any inanimate object. Children of four years implicitly may understand that animate and inanimate objects are made up of different kinds of parts or substances.

Johnson and Wellman (1979) studied young children's beliefs about the brain. Even the youngest subjects reported that they and the experimenter had brains. Most of the four- and five-year-olds and many of the youngest children further believed that the brain was not visible and was located inside the head. In contrast, most four- and five-year-olds declared that a doll does not have a brain. Here the three-year-olds disagreed. Those who attributed a brain to the experimenter were likely to grant one to the doll as well. The understanding that only animate objects have brains may develop after the third year.

Perhaps the most interesting aspect of the animate–inanimate distinction is the fact that only animate objects have minds. When does a child appreciate that animate objects, and only animate objects, can perceive, think, know, feel, and act in response to motives and/or intents?

Studies of perspective-taking abilities suggest that young children distinguish between animate and inanimate objects as objects that can perceive. Lempers, Flavell, and Flavell (1977) have shown that very young children know that humans have perceptions. There are hints in this research that young children also know that inanimate objects do not have perceptions. Lempers et al. report that one child tried to get an adult to see an object by bringing the object close to the eyes, and that the child did not do this with a doll. Similarly, Flavell, Shipstead, and Croft (1979) reported that some young children say they cannot see a person if his or her eyes are closed; the children did not say this about a doll with closed eyes. These scattered findings are worth pursuing.

When do children know that humans think and dream whereas rocks do not? Johnson and Wellman (1979) provide indirect evidence that such knowledge exists at five years of age. Kindergarten children report that thinking and dreaming are functions of mind, and that they themselves have minds and brains. Because they deny brains to dolls they may further believe that dolls and other inanimate objects lack minds and related mental functions. Other investigations with more demanding tasks suggest that preschool children have no consistent understanding of thinking and dreaming (Broughton, 1978; Piaget, 1929).

Quite early in life children may appreciate that only animate objects have knowledge. Gelman and Shatz (1977) show that four-year-olds attribute different capacities and/or knowledge states to other humans as a function of age. Recent work by Flavell et al. (1979) further suggests that they do not attribute such knowledge to inanimate objects. Children reported that a person can know his or her name, but that a doll cannot. These findings contrast with early work by Piaget (1929) in which young children asserted, for example, that the sun "knows when it sets." These discrepancies invite further studies on the child's treatment of animate and inanimate objects as knowing creatures.

Young children seem to learn quickly that only animate objects have feelings. In an extensive study of semantic and conceptual development, Keil (1979) asked children whether certain statements about objects made sense. Children as young as three years consistently distinguished between animate and inanimate objects when those statements involved feelings. For example, they judged that sentences like "the lady is sorry" are sensible whereas sentences like "the door is sorry" are not.

Finally, by about three years of age, children will grant people intentions and motives (see Keasey, 1978, for a review). Whether they restrict such attributions to people is in dispute. Piaget's subjects sometimes explained the movements of clouds by referring to intentions. Bullock (1979) finds no comparable explanations when three- and four-year-olds reason about the movements of simple, familiar inanimate objects.

There is a clear rift in research on the child's theory of mind. Some investigators find evidence of a coherent, developing theory early in the preschool years, whereas others, notably Piaget, find no consistent and coherent theory before the period of concrete operations. Furthermore, the former group of investigators finds that the child restricts "minds" to animate objects early in life, whereas the latter group finds no such restriction. Piaget (1929) reported that young children grant knowledge, feelings, and intentions to at least some inanimate objects, like the moon. He also reported that preschool children do not grant perception to people and other animate objects exclusively. These discrepancies may reflect in part the nature of the inanimate objects that Piaget asked young children about. The moon and the clouds are not objects that children know well. As Piaget notes, these objects also appear to share one characteristic of animate objects – independent movement – because the wind, the earth's rotations, and interplanetary gravitational forces are not perceptible to humans. Children may distinguish people from familiar inanimate objects like toys and furniture before they can think appropriately about less well-known and less clear cases of inanimate objects like the moon and machines that mimic human actions.

A second difference between the Piagetian work and the work of Flavell, Wellman, and others concerns the nature of the tasks given to children. In his work on animism, Piaget asked children some questions that an adult would have trouble answering. For example, he asked whether "the sun knows where it is moving." The answer seems to be neither "yes" nor "no." The sun is neither knowledgeable nor ignorant; indeed, as Keil points out, these are anomalous questions. Accordingly, children may have been understandably confused by Piaget's questions.

In summary, the case can be made that, at least by age four, children appear to begin to develop a systematic set of beliefs about the thoughts, feelings, intentions, motives, knowledge, and capacities of other people. In other words, following Premack and Woodruff (1978), they develop a theory of mind. Young children do not seem inclined to attribute mind or its functions to inanimate objects – as long as they are asked to use their theory to guide some action or simple judgment, and not to reflect on it or state it explicitly. The differentiation of many key properties of animate and inanimate objects may begin early in life.

The child's understanding of animate and inanimate objects as objects of perception

As noted, the adult's perception of animate objects differs from his perception of inanimate objects in at least two ways: (1) the focus of perception of a person is in part on the intentions and feelings of the person, and (2) the adult gets information from a person in part by communicating with him or her. Observational studies of young infants give every indication that they, too, perceive animate and inanimate objects in different ways.

Young infants have been reported to be sensitive to the manifestations of emotion in another person. They react in kind to expressions of positive and negative emotion at five months (Kreutzer & Charlesworth, 1973). Infants of two months may also distinguish a person who intends to communicate with them from one who speaks to someone else (Trevarthen, 1977). Finally, infants of eight months are sensitive to the direction of gaze of another person and appear to attempt to look in the same direction (Scaife & Bruner, 1975). Thus we may speculate that infants as well as adults attempt to discover what others are doing or feeling. We do not know whether they investigate inanimate objects in the same ways.

It has been claimed that very young infants attempt to communicate with animate objects and not with inanimate objects. Faced with a graspable ball, a prereaching child may engage in intense activity of the fingers, hands, and arms (Bower, 1972; Bruner & Koslowski, 1972; Dodwell, Muir, & DiFranco, 1976; Trevarthen, 1977). Faced with a responsive person, an infant may be more apt to gesture with its face and make "prespeech" sounds, while its hands are inactive (Trevarthen, 1977). This contrast suggests that infants differentiate between objects in the two classes. Of course, these studies do not demonstrate that infants respond to the animate–inanimate distinction rather than to other distinctions between people and toys, such as differences in size.

More striking evidence that infants expect people to act in a communicative setting comes from studies of responses to the impassive face of a parent or other person. Very young infants are upset if someone faces them without moving or speaking (Trevarthen, 1977; Tronick, Adamson, Wise, Als, & Brazelton, 1975; Bloom, 1977). Although systematic comparisons have not been made, it seems unlikely that a static inanimate object could evoke a comparable response. The infant's distress may reflect in part his expectation that a person will engage in reciprocal acts of communication with him.

Regardless of the weight of these early observations, it seems clear that once children can talk, they talk to people in order to exchange information, and they do not do this with inanimate objects. Young children sometimes speak when they are alone at play with toys, and they may even "converse" with a doll or other toy. It seems very unlikely, however, that they expect the toy to answer and engage in reciprocal conversation. A child who addresses an adult and is not answered will persist with greater and greater insistence. A child who also talks to a doll appears to accept the doll's nonresponse as a matter of course. These observations suggest a clear differentiation between animate and inanimate objects for purposes of communication. Nevertheless, this differentiation needs to be documented experimentally.

The child's understanding of animate and inanimate objects as recipients of action

Animate objects behave differently from inanimate objects in three major ways: (1) only animate objects respond to an action with an act of their own; (2) only animate objects can serve as agents; and (3) only animate objects can act reciprocally, reverse roles, cooperate, and compete.

Even young infants are sensitive to contingencies between their actions and movements of an inanimate object (Papoušek, 1969; Watson, 1972), or an animate object (e.g., Trevarthen, 1977; Weisberg, 1963). We know of no research, however, on the infant's ability to distinguish between contingent responses of animate and inanimate objects. We also do not know if infants expect the contingent responses of animate objects to be more variable and less predictable than those of inanimate objects. Other than the work on infancy, there is no research on these questions.

When do children appreciate that a person can be used either as an agent or an instrument whereas an inanimate object can be used only as an instrument? Piaget observes that infants of eight months or more will use one inanimate object in order to move or attain another. For example, they may use a blanket to pull nearer a toy that lies on it. Bates (1976) finds that infants of the same age treat people differently. People are appealed to; they are used implicitly as agents in the attainment of the child's goals. Young infants soon become adept at communicating their needs to a person who then satisfies them; no one has suggested that they systematically communicate their needs to inanimate objects. None of these findings are based on systematic comparisons of actions on animate and inanimate objects: Such comparisons are needed.

Once the child can talk, he or she can use knowledge of agent–instrument object relationships in various ways. For example, preschoolers can be shown the initial and final states of a transformed object and select the instrument that brought about the transformation (Gelman, Bullock, & Meck, 1980). We do not know whether they can do such a task with transformations that are brought about by a human agent and (most interestingly) whether they reason about agents and instruments in different ways. When do children first know, for example, that use of an instrument to achieve a goal implies some agent, but that the use of an agent need imply no separate instrument? When do they first understand that two separate agents can cooperate or compete, but that two instruments (or an agent and an instrument) can do neither? Once again, a study that pitted animate against inanimate objects in tasks such as this would greatly enhance our understanding of the developing agent–instrument distinction.

Concerning the reciprocal nature of actions on animate objects, Piaget (1952) grants that a rudimentary understanding of reciprocity is achieved by the end of infancy. Recent studies lead to the suggestion that this understanding develops even earlier. Very young infants have been reported to imitate some of the facial and manual gestures of an adult (Church, 1970; Meltzoff & Moore, 1977). If these findings are substantiated – two attempted replications have failed (Hamm, Russell, &

Koepke, 1979; Hayes & Watson, 1979) – they will suggest that a baby implicitly "knows" that he and another person can act in kind. They do not reveal whether babies also know that inanimate objects cannot do what they do. Infants have been observed to "imitate" with tongue protrusion the movements of a pencil as well as those of the mouth (Jacobson & Kagan, 1978). One of us has observed four-month-old infants to "imitate" with hand movements the movements of toy animals and blocks. The tendency to imitate may thus reflect no consistent differentiation of animate and inanimate events.

Finally, observations of children's play suggest a developing understanding of turn taking, role reversals, cooperation, and competition (Garvey, 1977). As children grow, their social network becomes increasingly complex. However, even young children appear to distinguish in their play between animate and inanimate objects. A young child who wishes to play may approach another person, perhaps with toys and social overtures; children are rarely seen to approach inanimate objects in these ways.

When we consider all the evidence on the understanding of the different principles of action that apply to the animate and inanimate domains, we are impressed with how early in life this distinction may be worked out.

The child's developing systems of knowledge

When do children first distinguish physical laws from psychological laws and social conventions? Lockhart, Abrahams, and Osherson (1977) questioned children about the possibility of changing physical laws, social conventions, and moral principles. Apparently children do not distinguish among these domains until eight or nine years of age (cf. Piaget, 1932). Preschoolers claimed that the laws of all domains were immutable. Surprisingly, older children were willing to indicate that physical laws as well as social conventions could be changed. Thus, if everybody in the state of California were to agree, we could not only decide to drive on the left and eat with our hands but could also decide that rocks can float in water! By contrast, work by Turiel (this volume) suggests that children begin very early to distinguish at least between social conventions and moral principles. In Turiel's study, children of all ages state that it is "all right" for a school or society to change its rules to permit public nudity (a presumed violation of conventions of the children's own society), but that it would never be all right for a school or society to permit hitting (a presumed violation of a moral principle).

Turiel's studies suggest an earlier distinction among systems of knowledge than do the studies by Piaget and Lockhart et al. One difference between the studies is in the questions that children were asked. Lockhart asked whether it is *possible* for society to decide that we can drive on the left and hit each other, whereas Turiel asked whether it is *right* for society to make such decisions. Turiel's questions are thus moral questions, and they test the child's understanding of the various sets of principles that constrain his actions. A comparison of Turiel's and Lockhart's work suggests that children may develop an ability to think about what is right before they can think about what is possible. To our knowledge, however, there have been no studies that focus on the distinction between the possible, the permissible, and the ethical. The following anecdote suggests that children may think in terms of the permissibility or the morality of actions at an early age. This conversation with a young child illustrates the way one can contrast animate and inanimate objects in questions that are ambiguous as regards the possible and permissible:

R.G.: Can you kick a table?
Adam: (3 years, 7 months) Shakes head yes.
R.G.: Can you hit a table?
Adam: Yes.
R.G.: Can a table cry?
Adam: No, hasn't got a mouth.
R.G.: Can you kick me?
Adam: No. Can't kick people.
R.G. Can you kick a kitten?
Adam: No!
R.G.: A wall?
Adam: Yes.

We draw attention to the fact that Adam is a three-year-old; at least a rudimentary understanding of what are permissible acts on people appears to develop early in life. Do very young children distinguish between actions on animate versus inanimate objects with regard to judgments of permissibility?

We have asked friends and colleagues whether they believe infants show anything resembling moral restraint in their actions on animate objects. Will an infant who, at some stage, attempts to play with all his toys by hitting them with a stick also hit a person with a stick? The intuitions of our informants widely differed. Some took the view of Hobbes, maintaining that infants will hit, scratch, and pinch people indiscriminately, in blissful freedom from moral inhibitions. Others were more Rousseauian and strongly felt that infants are much gentler with other people, perhaps especially other infants. Those in the former group pointed to the "terrible two's" as incontrovertible support for the hypothesis of an amoral infant. Those of the latter group saw the two's as an age when infants begin to feel out implicit rules that have always constrained their actions – such as the ban on hitting animate objects – by systematically violating these principles and observing the consequences. In view of these sharply divergent and heated opinions there would seem to be a special need for research on this question.

Summary

This review of research supports three conclusions about the child's developing understanding of the animate–inanimate distinction. First, the beginnings of this distinction seem to appear very early in life: Even one-month-old infants appear to treat animate and inanimate objects as different in some respects and for some purposes. Second, an understanding of the differences between animate and inanimate objects appears not to develop in a unitary fashion. A child of three may understand some aspects of this distinction – for example, that only animate objects can communicate – and yet fail to comprehend other aspects of the distinction – for example, that only animate objects have brains. Third, it seems possible that children come to understand that only animate objects can act in certain ways before they understand that only animate objects have certain static properties and organs. Children may also understand that different systems of knowledge constrain their own actions on objects before they understand that different systems of knowledge are used to predict the behavior of another object. In general, children may draw distinctions between animate and inanimate objects for purposes of action and communication before they draw these distinctions for other ends.

These conclusions are offered tentatively, because the development of the animate–inanimate distinction has received little systematic study. The most productive experimental approach, we believe, is one in which animate and inanimate objects are pitted against each other in a single experimental paradigm. A child may be asked the same questions about a person and a doll (e.g., "What made it move?" "Does it breathe?"). A child may also be asked to perform the same action or bring about the same result with a person and a chair (e.g., "bring it to me."). An infant may be systematically observed with a person and a toy under comparable conditions (e.g., conditions in which neither – or both – responds contingently to any action by the infant). In any of these cases, we may observe whether the child treats the animate and the inanimate object differently. By varying the tasks that a child is given, experiments may reveal the child's understanding of the ramifications of the animate–inanimate distinction. By varying the objects to which each task is applied, experiments may elucidate the child's categories of animate and inanimate, their definition and their organization.

The development of social and nonsocial cognition

As we reviewed evidence concerning the child's differentiation of the animate from the inanimate, one investigator towered over all others in his contribution. Piaget has addressed this question time and again in his studies of animism, causality, moral judgment, perspective taking, and communication. Many of Piaget's analyses in these domains turn on the distinction between animate and inanimate objects. Yet Piaget believed that animate and inanimate objects alike come to be known through the development of a unitary set of abstract cognitive structures and processes.

We believe that this assumption needs to be scrutinized. There is reason to think that the child's developing cognitive structures are far less general, and more task specific, than Piaget holds. For example, the child's concept of number may be mediated by structures that differ from those that underlie perspective taking (Gelman, 1978). Such observations point to the possibility that social and nonsocial cognitions also derive, at least in part, from separate cognitive systems (cf. Glick, 1978). We explore this possibility by looking at the development of concepts of object permanence and causality.

The development of object permanence and attachment

During the first years of life, striking changes are observed in infants' responses to hidden objects. If a toy is moved out of view, five-month-old infants act as if it is no longer there (cf. Harris, 1975; Piaget, 1954), unless perhaps one observes them under special and restricted conditions (Bower, 1967). Their attention is likely to turn immediately to something else and they make no effort to remove the toy's cover – an action that need not be beyond their motor capacities. A few months later, however, infants continue to orient to the hidden object and search for it under or behind the cover. Their ability to search consistently and effectively for variously displaced objects continues to grow throughout infancy and, indeed, childhood (Wellman, Somerville, & Haake, 1979). The development of search in infancy is thought to reflect the achievement of an ability to represent objects as independent entities in an objective spatial layout: the development of the "object concept" (Piaget, 1954).

During the first year, dramatic changes also occur in the child's emotional response to others. Young infants generally respond positively to all people, and they react with equanimity to separations from any of them. Infants in the second six months come to respond most positively to a small number of people, to monitor their movements with care, and sometimes to protest their departures. This developmental change appears to reflect the development of specific attachments (cf., Bowlby, 1969, 1973; Ainsworth, 1973). That development in turn has been thought to depend in part on the child's growing ability to appreciate the persisting existence of an absent person: the development of "person permanence" (Bell, 1970).

What is the relationship between the development of attachment behavior and the development of systematic search for inanimate objects? Many have felt that the two developments are closely linked. People, like toys, can move from the child's view. Surely children will not attempt to prevent a person's departure or hasten his or her return until they can represent that person as an independent, enduring object. Attachment behavior and object search therefore might both depend on the same underlying capacity. This view has received little experimental support (cf. Flavell, 1977). Does it make sense in principle, in light of the similarities and differences between animate and inanimate objects? To address this question, we compare the two classes of objects as things that can disappear and be recovered.

Animate and inanimate objects occupy definite locations in space. Both exist in the world, not just in the experience of some perceiver, and they continue to exist when they are out of perceptual contact. Neither is basically dependent for its existence on any action by the child. These are the properties that Piaget emphasized in discussing the development of the object concept. He did not discuss three differences between animate and inanimate objects.

First, an animate object that is out of visual contact appears to be "gone" in ways that an inanimate object is not, even if the animate and inanimate objects are equally near or far. As ethologists and social psychologists remind us, perceptual acts directed at an animate object can have enormous social consequences. A given action may mean different things if it is acompanied by eye contact than if it is not (Ekman, Friesen, & Ellsworth, 1972; Smith, 1977). A person to whom the child is not looking, and who is not looking to the child, is not as "talkable-to" or as "playable-with" as one who faces the child with full attention. In his discussion of the object concept, Piaget proposed that the child must learn that out-of-sight transformations do not affect the status of an object as a recipient for action: Objects are unaffected by the child's acts of perception. It is clear that this general rule does not hold if the object is animate and the perceptual action functions as a communication.

Second, different kinds of transformations alter the position of out-of-sight animate and inanimate objects. An inanimate object, because it does not move from within, will remain in a hiding place unless it is displaced by some external force. An infant can keep track of it by representing and interpreting the effect of external actions on it. An animate object can move at will. Once the mother has disappeared behind the front door, she is not likely to remain there. An ability to take account of unseen, external actions on an object will rarely help an infant to keep track of a person who leaves his view. The unseen displacements of animate objects will usually be better predicted by taking account of the object's habits and customs (e.g., mother usually returns after an hour when she leaves at nap time) than by attempting to keep track of every unseen displacement.

A third difference concerns the actions by which an out-of-sight object is recovered. To recover any object that moves from view, one must act in some way to reverse the transformation that takes it from sight. If the object is inanimate, the transformation that made it disappear was external to the object: A person placed a barrier in front of the object, or knocked the object over so that it fell behind a pillow. Thus, the child must detour to avoid the obstruction, or act on the obstructor, or act on the person that manipulated it, in order to recover the object. He cannot act on the object directly until he has done something else. Recovering inanimate objects thus requires a coordination of means with ends, an ability that Piaget believes is attained rather late in infancy, at Piaget's fourth stage of sensorimotor development. If the object is animate, however, the transformation that took it from view probably came from within that object: The person walked out of the child's room. The best way – and often the only way – to reverse such a transformation is to act on the motivational system of the person. The child can do this by calling, cajoling, or crying. These are immediate emotional responses to the disappearance of the desired object. Thus, a child may become accomplished at activities that bring back the mother without representing her as an independent object at all. In terms of Piaget's stage theory of development in infancy, protest on separation bears a closer semblance to stage two functioning (attained at about 1 month of age) than to stage four (attained at about 8 months). Indeed, Piaget cites just this activity as an example of stage-two behavior (1954, p. 12).

Let us return to the question of how searching for objects and attachment to people develop. Do both developments depend on the achievement of a general understanding of the objectivity of all things? Although Piaget's theory remains tenable, we offer an alternative hypothesis. Infants may come to search adaptively for animate and inanimate objects as they learn to sort out their commonalities and differences. The development of object search and attachment may reflect not a general decline of egocentrism but (in part) the acquisition of knowledge of objects – and of the crucial distinctions among them.

Early in life, the disappearances of a person might very well be of greater consequence to a child than the disappearances of an inanimate object. Infants may begin to first develop abilities to perceive the disappearance of people, to anticipate their reappearance and to recover them by calling and crying. When faced with similar disappearances of inanimate objects, infants may do nothing – if they have not yet developed any comparable understanding of inanimate objects – or they may generalize what they have learned about animate to inanimate objects. Some such generalizations will be appropriate; for example, if the child learns to attend to the point of departure of a parent, such a strategy will apply well to the point of departure of a toy. Other generalizations may be inappropriate. For example, a child who learns that a parent out of visible contact cannot be played with easily may fail to play with unseen toys as well. And a child who learns that a parent can move independently from one near place to another may come to expect falsely that a toy will do this as well, and hence he may not attempt to deduce where such a toy is. Many of Piaget's examples of bizarre searching for inanimate objects, such as persistent tracking and searching in habitual hiding places, could derive from inappropriate generalizations from the animate to the inanimate. Such generalizations might be expected if the child fails to appreciate some of the properties of inanimate objects and some of the ramifications of the animate–inanimate distinction. The child who generalizes inappropriately across these domains may appear to be guided by false and bizarre beliefs about the world, and thus may be branded "egocentric." In fact, the child may simply be reasoning about objects whose properties are insufficiently understood.

We are speculating, in brief, that young infants do not fail an object permanence task because of a generalized "egocentrism" or because they lack any understanding of the objectivity of things in the world. They fail in part because they do not understand that different kinds of objects are transformed and returned to view in different ways. These are only speculations and have not been thoroughly evaluated. They may be addressed, however, by investigations of the infant's understanding of the animate–inanimate distinction.

The development of causal reasoning: physical mechanisms and social attributions

Beginning in infancy and continuing into the school years, children appear to develop an increasingly elaborated and adaptive understanding of causal relationships. This development may be observed in two domains. First, children come to interpret physical events by appeal to increasingly sophisticated causal principles and mechanisms. They invoke such mechanisms in their explanations of why a particular event came about and in their efforts to bring about an event themselves. Second, children come to analyze social events – in particular, the actions of other people – by appealing to social and psychological principles and mechanisms. These causal principles are involved when children explain why people do what they do and when they anticipate what people will do next. Are the child's developing understandings of physical and social causality related? Again, we approach this question by comparing the causal properties of animate and inanimate objects.

There appear to be two overriding similarities between the causal properties of the animate and the inanimate, as they are conceived by human adults. First, both animate and inanimate events are believed to have causes of some kind. Second, for both types of events, the cause is believed to precede the effect or occur simultaneously with it; cause cannot follow effect. The causes of animate events otherwise differ greatly from the causes of inanimate events. The largest difference, we believe, concerns the nature of a causal mechanism.

Inanimate events are usually brought about by mechanisms that can be taken apart and analyzed. The puppet's movements are really controlled by strings that can be pulled, cut, or replaced to discover how they work. Animate events are brought about by mechanisms of a different kind. A person's actions are caused by intentions, habits, or dispositions. These cannot be seen or taken apart. In the case of animate events, we make attributions regarding intent and motive. In the case of inanimate we perceive or infer physical mechanisms. Because different mechanisms underlie animate and inanimate events, different information will be used in judging the causes of these events. For example, the cue of spatial contiguity is probably only used in the inanimate domain. This follows from the fact that psychological states have no spatial properties. Thus, children must develop some causal principles that apply both to the animate and to the inanimate, and some that are restricted to one of these domains.

Early research by Piaget (1930) suggests that the preschool child's concept of physical causality is sketchy at best. The child begins with a diffuse sense that events are caused, but he may attribute all causes to things inside himself; he may endow inanimate objects with intentions, and he may think "magically" about the sources of events. In contrast, more recent reports show that children as young as four years have a concept of causality for inanimate events that goes considerably beyond what Piaget described. Bullock (1979; Bullock & Gelman, 1977) found that four-year-olds appear to understand that inanimate events have causes, that causes precede their effects, and that causes are spatially and temporally contiguous with their effects. They also infer unseen, intervening mechanisms when none are visible. Moreover, children expect certain kinds of events to have causes of certain types: The impact of a ball is considered a reasonable cause for the popping of a jack-in-the-box, while an intention to jump is not. Four-year-olds will also analyze systematically a simple causal mechanism that has broken down. If one object, attached to another by a partly hidden string, initially moves when the second object is pulled, and then fails to do so, four-year-olds will look for a break in the string (Bullock, 1979).

Four-year-olds seem, then, to reason appropriately about the causes of inanimate events and do not appear to grant inanimate objects animate-like causal mechanisms. Although we know of no direct studies, we suspect that young children know that people can move without being pulled, pushed, or propelled by another, although toys cannot. It is known that children as young as three ascribe intents and motives to explain acts of people (Keasey, 1978). It appears likely that the four-year-old reasons differently about the causes of animate and inanimate events.

Bullock has also studied three-year-olds, and their reasoning appears somewhat different. Although they appear to understand that events have causes and that causes precede their effects, they do little apparent analysis of causal mechanisms. A three-year-old who confronts the display with two objects and a string will not infer that the string is broken once the two objects no longer move in tandem. Asked "what happened?" the three-year-old might say "won't work," and no probing can bring a further illumination.

What are we to make of these findings? Are three-year-olds the "precausal" creatures that Piaget described all preschoolers to be? We doubt it, because they do not appeal to intentions or other psychological attributes when asked to explain why a mechanical device no longer works. We offer an alternative possibility. Three-year-olds may well appreciate the causal principles that apply to all objects: principles such as "events have causes" and "causes precede their effects." Indeed Kun (1978), working within the framework of attribution theory, has demonstrated that children this young honor the principle of temporal ordering when deciding about social events. Young children may also understand that animate and inanimate events have causes of different kinds. They may even know that people have intents and motives (cf. Keasey, 1978; Guttentag & Longfellow, 1978). But they may be ignorant of the principles that are restricted to an inanimate event: principles like spatial contiguity and analyzability of a mechanism. They may treat a causal mechanism as an underlying property of the whole object itself – as the mechanism may be if the object is animate. In brief, what may develop over childhood is a clear understanding of the distinction between the psychological and physical mechanisms that govern animate and inanimate events respectively.

Conclusions

In developmental psychology, the study of social cognition, like the study of cognition in general, has been dominated by the view that all cognitive development derives from the growth of a unitary system of cognitive structures. These structures are thought to apply to all objects and all tasks. Students of social cognition have asked how the structures and processes that underlie cognition of the physical world are applied to the social world. Our considerations of the nature of thoughts about the animate and inanimate worlds lead us to conclude that this a priori view may be unwarranted. The relation of thinking about animate objects to thinking about inanimate objects is likely not to be simple, and no simple assumptions about it seem justified. Rather than making such assumptions, psychologists should make the relationship between thinking about animate objects and thinking about inanimate objects itself a primary area of investigation.

We have suggested one focus for research: studies of children's ability to distinguish between animate and inanimate objects, and studies of their understanding of the implications of this distinction for perception, action, and thought. Experimental tasks need to be designed that pit reactions to the animate and the inanimate domains against each other. Similarities and differences in the child's thinking about the two kinds of objects can be noted. Then students of social cognition may begin to map the child's understanding of the animate–inanimate distinction onto his conceptions of the social world.

Our review of the development of the animate–inanimate distinction provides more questions than answers. However, it appears that humans of all ages – even newborns – make this distinction to some degree and for certain purposes. But the distinction is by no means fully formed at an early age; the child's understanding of animate and inanimate objects appears to grow and deepen with development. There appears to be much that a young child has to learn about the animate–inanimate distinction.

We now need to understand this developmental progression. As psychologists come to learn more about the child's developing understanding of the animate–inanimate distinction, we should be able to make better sense of the development of social cognition, the development of cognition of the physical world, and of the relation of social cognition to the larger enterprise of cognitive psychology.

We end with a speculation about what such a study of social cognition may find. We suggest that for many purposes, an understanding of animate objects and their properties will develop before any comparable understanding of inanimate objects is achieved. Suggestions that cognitions about animate objects develop first have come from many quarters. Children have been seen to be sometimes remarkably sophisticated in their approach to problems that are clearly social. The young infant who searches ineptly, even bizarrely, for a hidden toy may be much more adept at bringing back a departing parent. The communication and perspective-taking abilities of children improve immensely when they are tested in a truly interpersonal situation. Even the perceptual capacities of infants may be best revealed when they must perceive animate events.

If these speculations have any truth, then an investigation of cognition about animate and inanimate objects should be of interest to all students of cognitive development. The animate world will provide a rich domain in which to study not only the child's developing social understanding, but also some of the most advanced aspects of his innate and early developing cognitive capacities.

Note

1 Here, as elsewhere in the text, the reader will surely ponder the status of a computer. For purposes of exposition, we disregard or set aside modern man-made machines that mimic in one or more ways the characteristics of man.

References

Ainsworth, M. D. S. The development of infant–mother attachment. In B. M. Caldwell & H. N. Ricciuti (Eds.), *Review of child development research* (Vol. III). Chicago: University of Chicago Press, 1973.

Bates, E. *Language and context: The acquisition of pragmatics.* New York: Academic Press, 1976.

Bell, S. M. The development of the concept of object as related to infant–mother attachment. *Child Development*, 1970, *41*, 291–311.

Bloom, K. Operant baseline procedures suppress infant social behavior. *Journal of Experimental Child Psychology*, 1977, *23*, 128–32.

Bower, T. G. R. The development of object permanence: Some studies of existence constancy. *Perception and Psychophysics*, 1967, *2*, 411–18.

  Object perception in infants. *Perception*, 1972, *1*, 15–30.

Bowlby, J. *Attachment*. New York: Basic Books, 1969.

  Separation. New York: Basic Books, 1973.

Brooks, J., & Lewis, M. Infants' responses to strangers: Midget, adult, and child. *Child Development*, 1976, *47*, 323–32.

Broughton, J. Development of concepts of self, mind, reality, and knowledge. In W. Danon (Ed.), *New directions for child development* (Vol. I). San Francisco: Jossey-Bass, 1978.

Bruner, H. S., & Koslowski, B. Visually preadapted constituents of manipulatory action. *Perception*, 1972, *1*, 3–14.

Bullock, M. *Aspects of the young child's theory of causation*. Unpublished doctoral thesis, University of Pennsylvania, 1979.

Bullock, M., & Gelman, R. Preschool children's assumptions about cause and effect: Temporal ordering. *Child Development*, 1979, *50*, 89–96.

Carey, S. *The child's concept of animal*. Paper presented at the annual meeting of the Psychonomic Society, San Antonio, Texas, 1978.

Church, J. Techniques for the differential study of cognition in early childhood. In J. Hellmuth (Ed.), *Cognitive Studies I*. New York: Brunner-Mazel, Inc., 1970.

Dodwell, P. C., Muir, D., & DiFranco, D. Responses of infants to visually presented objects. *Science*, 1976, *194*, 209–11.

Ekman, P., Friesen, W. V., & Ellsworth, P. *Emotion in the human face*. Elmsford, N.Y.: Pergamon Press, 1972.

Flavell, J. H. *Cognitive development*. Englewood Cliffs, N.J.: Prentice-Hall, 1977.

Flavell, J. H., Shipstead, S. G., & Croft, K. *What young children think you see when their eyes are closed*. Unpublished manuscript, Stanford University, 1979.

Garvey, C. *Play*. Cambridge, Mass.: Harvard University Press, 1977.

Gelman, R. Cognitive development. *Annual Review of Psychology*, 1978, *29*, 297–332.

Gelman, R., Bullock, M., & Meck, E. Preschoolers' understanding of simple object transformations. *Child Development*, 1980, *51*, 691–9.

Gelman, R., & Shatz, M. Appropriate speech adjustments: The operation of conversational constraints on talk to two-year-olds. In M. Lewis & L. Rosenblum (Eds.), *Interaction, conversation, and the development of language*. New York: Wiley, 1977.

Glick, J. Cognition and social cognition: An introduction. In J. Glick and K. A. Clarke-Stewart, *The development of social understanding*. New York: Gardner Press, Inc., 1978.

Golinkoff, R. M., & Harding, C. G. *The development of causality: The distinction between animates and inanimates*. Paper presented at the International Conference on Infant Studies, New Haven, April 1980.

Guttentag, M., & Longfellow, C. Children's social attributions: Development and change. In C. B. Keasey (Ed.), *Nebraska symposium on motivation* (Vol. 25). Lincoln, Neb.: University of Nebraska Press, 1978.

Hamm, M., Russell, M., & Koepke, J. *Neonatal imitation?* Paper presented at the Society for Research in Child Development, San Francisco, March 1979.

Harris, P. L. Development of search and object permanence during infancy. *Psychological Bulletin*, 1975, *82*, 332–44.

Hayes, L. A., & Watson, J. S. *Neonatal imitation: Fact or artifact?* Paper presented at the Society for Research in Child Development, San Francisco, March 1979.

Jacobson, S. W., & Kagan, J. *Released responses in early infancy: Evidence contradicting selective imitation.* Paper presented at the International Conference on Infant Studies, Providence, March 1978.

Johnson, C. N., & Wellman, H. M. *Children's conception of the brain: A developmental study of knowledge about cognitive processes.* Unpublished manuscript, 1979.

Keasey, C. B. Children's developing awareness and usage of intentionality and motives. In C. B. Keasey (Ed.), *Nebraska symposium on motivation* (Vol. 25). Lincoln, Neb.: University of Nebraska Press, 1978.

Keil, F. *Semantic and conceptual development.* Cambridge, Mass.: Harvard University Press, 1979.

Kreutzer, M. A., & Charlesworth, W. R. *Infants' reactions to different expressions of emotion.* Paper presented at the Society for Research in Child Development, Philadelphia, March 1973.

Kun, A. Evidence for preschooler's understanding of causal direction in extended causal sequences. *Child Development,* 1978, *49,* 218–22.

Lempers, J. D., Flavell, E. R., & Flavell, J. H. The development in very young children of tacit knowledge concerning visual perception. *Genetic Psychology Monographs,* 1977, *95,* 3–53.

Lockart, K. L., Abrahams, B., & Osherson, D. N. Children's understanding of uniformity in the environment. *Child Development,* 1977, *48,* 1521–31.

McKeon, R. (Ed.), *The basic works of Aristotle.* New York: Random House, 1941.

Meltzoff, A. N., & Moore, M. K. Imitation of facial and manual gestures by human neonates. *Science,* 1977, *198,* 75–8.

Papoušek, H. Individual variability in learned responses in human infants. In R. J. Robinson (Ed.), *Brain and early behavior.* New York: Academic Press, 1969.

Piaget, J. *The child's conception of the world.* London: Routledge & Kegan Paul, 1929.
The child's conception of physical causality. London: Routledge & Kegan Paul, 1930.
The moral judgment of the child. London: Routledge & Kegan Paul, 1932.
The origins of intelligence in children. New York: International Universities Press, 1952.
The construction of reality in the child. New York: Basic Books, 1954.
Epistémologie et psychologie de l'identité. Volume XXIV des études d'épistemologie génétique. Paris: Presses Universitaires de France, 1969.

Premack, D. & Woodruff, G. Does the chimpanzee have a theory of mind? *The Behavioral and Brain Sciences,* 1978, *4,* 515–26.

Scaife, M., & Bruner, J. S. The capacity for joint visual attention in the infant. *Nature,* 1975, *253,* 265–6.

Shatz, M., & Gelman, R. The development of communication skills: Modifications in the speech of young children as a function of listener. *Monographs of the Society for Research in Child Development,* 1973, *38* (2, Serial No. 152), 1–37.

Smith, W. J. *Behavior of communicating.* Cambridge, Mass.: Harvard University Press, 1977.

Trevarthen, C. Descriptive analyses of infant communicative behavior. In H. R. Schaffer (Ed.), *Studies in mother-infant interaction.* London: Academic Press, 1977.

Tronick, E., Adamson, L., Wise, S., Als, H., & Brazelton, T. B. *The infant's response to entrapment between contradictory messages in face-to-face interaction.* Paper presented at the Society for Research in Child Development, Denver, April 1975.

Watson, J. S. Smiling, coding, and "the game." *Merrill-Palmer Quarterly,* 1972, *18,* 323–39.

Weisberg, P. Social and nonsocial conditioning of infant vocalizations. *Child Development,* 1963, *34,* 377–88.

Wellman, H. M., Somerville, S. C., & Haake, R. C. Development of search procedures in real-life spatial environments. *Developmental Psychology,* 1979, *15,* 530–42.

3 Perspectives on the difference between understanding people and understanding things: the role of affect

It has traditionally been assumed that cognition is unitary, and that the cognitive processes used in dealing with the physical world are the same as those employed in the social domain. According to Piaget, for example, social cognition parallels physical cognition. ("The reaction of intelligence . . . to the social environment is exactly parallel to its reaction to the physical environment" [Piaget, 1963, p. 60].) Recent writers question this. Glick (1978) views the two domains as substantially different. Thus whereas the movement of things is predictable from a knowledge of the physical forces acting upon them, people can move themselves. People are also sensitive to subtle variations in context, and their behavior is only loosely predictable from the social forces acting upon them. Consequently, social cognition must operate under different rules. It is based less on logic and more on probability, shared cultural belief systems, cultural stereotypes, and scripts. These bases of social cognition, moreover, are often nonveridical because they tend to override immediately available data. For example, when we use stereotypes we often overlook the idiosyncratic properties of a particular person.

Gelman and Spelke (this volume) point to a number of distinctions that adults make between people and things. In addition to the differences mentioned by Glick, they note, for example, that although people and things both change over time, only people reproduce, and act to sustain themselves and their offspring. Things may change (e.g., ice melts,) but they cannot do this by themselves. Only people can know, perceive, emote, learn, think, and mentally represent. Gelman and Spelke also note that apart from differences in their properties, people and things are perceived differently. Although both may have a definite size and shape, for example, it is only when perceiving a thing that one focuses exclusively on physical properties. When perceiving a person one may note his physical properties but one's focus is often on his inner states, which are more indeterminate and deceptive. And although both people and things may be acted on in similar ways (e.g. pushed), the response of people is far less predictable.

There are several other factors that contribute to the complexity, hence the difficulties involved in social cognition. These factors derive from the interactional context within which social cognition usually operates. First, people are not only acted upon but, unlike most physical objects, they act back. Furthermore, how they react is not a simple function of how one acted toward them. Rather, how they react is mediated by their inner states, which are unpredictable and unobservable, such as how they interpreted one's act and what they hope to accomplish by their response. Second, the people one encounters behave differently, and the meaning of their action differs depending on the nature of one's relationship to them. There are any number of relationships that are possible (e.g., relationships based on kinship, friendship, power, contract, chance encounters). Furthermore, one's relationship with a particular person may change dramatically over time. Finally, not only do the relationships with people vary, but there are a variety of emotions associated with these different relationships. The emotions aroused in interacting with physical objects are far less varied, revolving, for example, around such matters as whether one succeeded or failed on tasks involving the objects. The emotions aroused in social interactions are also apt to be more intense; the intensity may operate against effective cognitive processing. There is evidence, for example, that intense arousal directs one's attention to the physical features of verbal communications, to the relative neglect of semantic content (Mueller, 1979) and, more generally, that it interferes with one's effort to derive meaning from verbal and other cues (Kahneman, 1973).

Development of social and nonsocial cognition

For all these reasons, people are more complex to deal with than physical objects, and their responses would appear to be less predictable than those made by physical objects. We might reasonably conclude that social cognition is less effective, and that its development must lag behind the development of physical cognition. Yet the evidence, weak as it is, seems to point in the opposite direction.

Permanence

Person permanence, for example, appears to precede object permanence. That is, the research indicates that children are capable of carrying an internal representation of a person, in the person's absence, long before they can do the same with physical objects (e.g., Bell 1970). It is true in this research that the two tasks are not comparable; for example, in the study by Bell, the person was larger than the physical object, more familiar to the child, and moved herself from one position to the next; the object of course was moved by the experimenter. If size, animation, and familiarity were controlled, the difference might disappear. A study by Jackson, Campos, & Fisher (1978) suggests this would happen. Bell's design, however, appears to be ecologically valid, because persons *are* animated in the real world and most persons with whom the child interacts are apt to be larger and more familiar than the objects with which he deals. The Jackson et al. findings may thus be viewed as giving us some of the reasons why person permanence precedes object permanence.

Person permanence may also precede object permanence because infants normally have a far greater emotional investment in the persons in their lives than in the objects they encounter. Permanence is a combination of constructing a representation of an object, divorcing the representation from the immediate stimulus, and remembering the representation. When the infant first becomes capable of these cognitive operations, they may be mobilized in relation to an object because of the infant's motivation and emotional investment in that object. That is, the first objects that lead the infant to mobilize these newly acquired capabilities may be objects in which he has a strong emotional investment. (The adaptive function of early person permanence may be that it enables the infant to tolerate increasing periods of separation from the caretaker, thus freeing the infant to engage in exploratory behaviors that contribute to cognitive development – including perhaps object permanence.)

There is no evidence yet that an emotional investment in an object can enhance the processes of constructing a representation of it or of divorcing the representation from the immediate stimulus, but there is evidence that positive emotion may aid memory (Isen, Shalker, Clark & Karp, 1978). This suggests that the infant's involvement with persons may contribute to his ability to keep them in mind even in their absence. It would be interesting to see if the permanence of "transitional objects," objects that are invested with emotion and help tide the child over in the parent's absence (e.g. Winnicott, 1960), precedes the permanence of other objects.

Causality

In a study by Fein (1972) subjects of five age groups were asked to judge the causality or noncausality of physical and social picture sequences. Young children tended to perceive all sequences as causal, this tendency decreasing with age. Accurate discrimination between social causal and social noncausal sequences was established by age seven. For the physical sequences, this skill was not fully established until age eleven. There is no reason to assume that the social task is easier than the physical. Indeed, the reverse appears true, because the difference between the causal and noncausal physical sequence is defined by the presence or absence of direct visible contact between the agent and the consequent action (e.g., "ball moves to bottle, contact made, bottle shown broken on floor" versus "ball on floor, moves slightly, picture on wall falls to floor"). There is no such obvious contact in the social sequence, but rather a norm-interpretive element ("boy breaks window, is sent into house" versus "boy pulls girl's hair, is given bicycle"). Why then should the young child comprehend social or moral causality before physical causality? Piaget (1970) suggests that all laws are moral rather than physical until about eight or nine years of age; judgments of physical causes are thus often incorrect because of the child's precausal moral thinking. However, precausal thinking was virtually absent in Fein's study (only three cases were found).

Fein's explanation of why children understand social before physical causality is that although social rules are learned early, the child is exposed to violations of them and can therefore discriminate between instances of social causation and violations of social causation. This is not true for physical situations, where the young child does not observe violations of causal laws. His ability to discriminate between occurring and nonoccurring situations (laws and violations) may thus be hampered, and he may tend to attribute causality relatively indiscriminately. I would add that the child has not only observed but also experienced instances of social causality, that is, he has acted in certain ways and been rewarded, and acted in other ways and been punished. In other words, the child's direct experience of how people respond to his own actions may help him to understand how people respond to the actions of others. And, because his observations of how people respond to his own actions has an affective as well as a cognitive dimension, emotion may contribute further to the ability to distinguish between causal and noncausal sequences in the moral sphere.

There are two other possibly pertinent findings that I will mention briefly. First, there is evidence that children have the ability to recognize two independent causes as simultaneously determining a person's behavior, somewhat earlier in life than they can recognize a physical object's action as being codetermined by two independent causes. (Compare the findings obtained by Kuhn and Ho, 1977, with those obtained by Erwin and Kuhn, 1979). Second, Van der Lee and Oppenheimer (1979) found that children seven to nine years of age were adept at backward temporal ordering of social events (each event depicted in a series of five pictures) before they were able to conserve length or quantity. This finding, which was contrary to expectation, indicates that reversibility in the conservation of the attributes of things is not, as previously thought, a prerequisite for reversibility in the social domain.

Assessing inner states

Thus far I have been talking about cognitive competencies in the social domain that have a more or less exact parallel in the physical domain. There are also social cognitive competencies that do not have such a parallel. One of these pertains to the processes involved in assessing other people's inner states and thought processes. As already noted, humans are more apt to attend to the inner states of people than to the inner states of things. There is also a more fundamental difference: Whereas knowledge or ignorance of the inner workings of a class of things predicts to knowledge or ignorance of any item in that class (if you know how steam engines work, you know what is happening inside any steam engine you encounter), this is not true of people. Until recently it was generally assumed that children had to be capable of concrete operations before they could assess another person's inner states. This view fit well with Piaget's early research showing that children below seven or eight years of age typically made the egocentric error of attributing their own viewpoint to a doll situated in various locations around a papier-mâché landscape. Recent research shows that by modifying the design, children as young as three years make few such errors. Two-year-olds will turn a picture toward another person who asks to see it, and even one-year-olds rarely orient a picture so that only they can see it (Lempers, Flavell, & Flavell, 1977).

Concerning more complex assessments of other people's inner states, I have elsewhere presented anecdotal evidence indicating that children below two years of age are capable of deceiving or manipulating others (Hoffman, 1975). The prime example cited was the following: Marcy, aged twenty months, was in the playroom of her home and wanted a toy that her sister was playing with. She asked for it but her sister refused vehemently. Marcy paused for a moment, as if reflecting on what to do, and then ran straight to her sister's favorite rocking horse – which her sister never allowed anyone to touch – climbed on it and began yelling "Nice horsey! Nice horsey!" keeping her eye on her sister all

the time. Her sister put down the toy and came running angrily, where-
upon Marcy immediately climbed down, ran directly to the toy, and
grabbed it.

It may be useful to speculate about what went on in Marcy's head.
One possibility is that she engaged in a logical role-taking sequence in
which she first realized that to get the toy she had to induce her sister to
leave it, then figured out that this could be accomplished by arousing
her sister's concern about something more important to her than the
toy, and finally thought of climbing on the horse. Another, more egocentric possibility is that Marcy thought about what she would do if she
were in her sister's place, realized that she would give up the toy only if
suitably distracted, assumed her sister would do the same, remembered
how strongly her sister felt about the horse, and utilized this knowledge
to lure her sister away from the toy. More likely, in view of her age,
Marcy's thought process was less formal-operational – based more on
imagery and association, perhaps, than either of these. For example, she
may have first noticed the horse, which triggered an image (or script)
derived from past experiences in which she climbed on the horse and
her sister came running and pushed her off, and then realized that
getting on the horse was a way of getting her sister away from the toy.
Whatever the precise cognitive operations involved, it seems safe to
assume at the very least that Marcy realized that her sister would not
give up the toy voluntarily, that to get the toy she had to lure her sister
away from it, and that a way to lure her was to climb on her horse. In
other words, this child showed awareness of another's inner states that
differed from her own even though she probably was too young to
understand the instructions in the simplest of role-taking experiments. If
we may generalize tentatively from this instance, it would appear that
some kind of rapid processing of information about other people's feelings, at least in familiar, highly motivating natural settings is possible in
children who are still in the sensory-motor period as regards the physical
domain.

Facilitators of social cognition

I mention these comparisons not because my argument requires that social cognition precedes physical cognition. It does not. The comparisons
are not definitive in any case because in none of them were the tasks
strictly comparable. The comparisons do point out, however, that there is
no evidence yet that development of social cognition seriously lags behind

the development of cognition in the physical domain. The question may be raised, how is this possible in view of the high degree of complexity and unpredictability of people relative to things, discussed earlier?

Interactional context

I have already suggested certain qualities about people that may facilitate social cognition (e.g., they are animated and they are objects of emotional investment). Are there any more general characteristics about people that serve to facilitate social cognition? One possible answer is the interactional context in which social cognition often takes place. Although the interactional context may contribute to the complexity of social cognition, the interactional context may also compensate for the complexity because it presents the child with occasional discrepancies from the behavior he expects of others. These discrepancies provide the child with continuous corrective feedback about the interpretations he makes of the other's behavior and inner states, and they motivate him to attempt a reassessment. An example from real life illustrates how this process may work.

Michael, aged fifteen months, and his friend Paul were fighting over a toy and Paul started to cry. Michael looked worried and let go, but Paul still cried. Michael paused, then brought his teddy bear to Paul, but Paul continued to cry. Michael paused again, and then finally succeeded in stopping Paul's crying by fetching Paul's security blanket from an adjoining room. Let us examine this incident from Michael's perspective. First, it is clear that Michael first assumed that his own teddy bear, which often comforts him, would also comfort Paul. Second, Paul's continued crying served as corrective feedback that led Michael to consider alternatives and come up with an appropriate response. Third, Michael's final successful act has several possible explanations. One is that he simply imitated what he had observed in the past. This is unlikely, because his parents were certain he had never seen Paul being comforted with a blanket. A second explanation is that Michael remembered seeing another child soothed by a blanket, which reminded him of Paul's blanket. This is more complex than it first appears, because Paul's blanket was out of Michael's perceptual field at the time. A third explanation is that Michael was somehow able to reason by analogy that Paul would be comforted by something he loved in the same way that Michael loved his own teddy bear. Whatever interpretation is correct, this incident, as well as a strikingly similar one reported by Borke (1972), suggests that a child less than one and a half years of age can, with the most general kind of feedback, correct his initial, erroneous hunch about another person's needs and then act in a way that alters the other's behavior in the desired manner.

Similarities among people

Social cognition has another advantage. As I have noted (Hoffman, 1975), the observer and the model are both humans – with the same nervous system and a shared background of similar experiences especially during the long period of socialization. Given this similarity in organizational structure, the observer and the model are apt to respond to stimuli in very similar ways. Thus, if the observer does nothing more than rely on social scripts and shared belief systems, and attributes his own interpretation of events to the model, he will generally be correct. Furthermore, when he does this he can act more quickly than if he considers all the currently available data about the person with whom he is interacting. And, acting quickly may generally be as adaptive as acting more slowly on the basis of all the data, at least in the social world, in which one ordinarily has little time for cognitive appraisal and reflection.

Although the role-taking research has stressed the ability to assess another's view when it *differs* from one's own, in real life egocentric and normatively based attributions are more apt to be right than wrong. In other words, the process may not be entirely veridical, based on reality testing, but it may usually be effective. It will not be effective, of course, when others behave contrary to the norm, when they deviate from the script, or when they attempt to deceive the observer by acting in ways that differ from their intentions. In these cases, being flexible and able to use all the currently available data, such as information about the model's personality and past behavior, would be more adaptive. But these types of unexpected behavior by others are apt to be less frequent than behavior that is in keeping with the norm. In the course of most people's lives, therefore, behavior based on hurriedly made "egocentric" attributions, shared belief systems, and scripts may generally lead to accurate predictions and in most instances be adaptive.

Empathy

Concerning the observer's understanding of the model's feelings, I have suggested (Hoffman, 1977, in press) that affect is often aroused vicariously, or empathically, in humans through involuntary, minimally cognitive mechanisms that may be described briefly as follows:

1. According to Lipps (1906), empathy is an innate, isomorphic response to another person's expression of emotion. There are two steps: The observer automatically imitates the other with slight movements in facial expression and posture ("motor mimicry"). This then creates kinesthetic cues in the observer that contribute (through afferent feedback) to his feeling the same emotion. Although this mechanism has been neglected in the literature, there is recent research that suggests its plausibility (see review by Hoffman, 1977).

2. The second mechanism is the direct classical conditioning of empathy that results when one observes another person who is experiencing an emotion, at the same time that one is having a direct experience of the same emotion. The result is that cues reflecting the other's emotion become conditioned stimuli that evoke the same emotion in the self. The necessary co-occurence of emotion in the self and cues of the same emotion in someone else has been produced in the laboratory (Aronfreed & Paskal, 1966). It also occurs in real life, such as when the mother's affective state is transferred to the infant through physical handling. If the mother feels anxious or tense, for example, her body may stiffen and the child consequently experiences distress. Subsequently, the mother's facial and verbal expressions that accompanied her distress can serve as conditioned stimuli that evoke distress in the child even in the absence of physical contact. Furthermore, through stimulus generalization, similar expressions by other persons may evoke distress feelings in the child.

3. The third mechanism was described by Humphrey (1922). When we observe someone experiencing an emotion, his facial expression, his voice, posture, or any other cue in the situation that reminds us of past situations in which we experienced that emotion, may evoke a similar emotion in us. The usual example cited is the boy who sees another child cut himself and cry. The sight of the blood, the sound of the cry, or any cue from the victim or the situation that reminds the boy of his own past experiences of pain may evoke an empathic distress response. This mechanism does not require the co-occurrence of direct affect in self and cues of the same affect in another. The only requirement is that the observer have *past* experiences of the affect. The affect can then be evoked in the observer by cues of the other's affect in the immediate situation that have elements in common with the observer's past experiences. It is thus a far more general mechanism than the second and it provides the basis for a variety of affective experiences with which children and adults may empathize.

4. The fourth mechanism is like the third except that the cues of affect in the immediate situation evoke an empathic response not because of their physical or expressive properties but because they symbolically indi-

cate the other's feelings. For example, one can respond empathically to someone by listening to a verbal description of what is happening to him. This is obviously a relatively advanced mechanism because it requires language. It is still largely involuntary, however, because the language serves mainly as a mediator between the model's affective state and the observer's empathic response.

Regardless of which mechanism operates, the vicariously aroused affect provides nonverbal, kinesthetic cues from the viscera and the somatic musculature. These cues are linked to the actor's own past experience and thus give him information about the affect experienced by the model. The actor's visceral arousal may not provide *distinctive* cues about the model's feelings (it has long been known that visceral arousal is general, i.e., it does not reflect discrete emotions), but the visceral cues do serve to inform the observer at least that the model is emotionally aroused.

Furthermore, there is recent research suggesting that distinctive cues about the other's affect may be provided by feedback from the actor's somatic musculature. For example, the different emotions appear to be accompanied by different degrees of tone in the skeletal muscles (e.g., the loss in muscle tone that accompanies sadness is associated with characteristic postures that are diametrically opposed to those seen in a happy mood) and by different patterns of facial muscle activity (Gelhorn, 1964, Izard, 1971). And there is evidence that cues from one's facial musculature, at least, may contribute to the actual experience of an emotion. In a series of experiments by Laird (1974), subjects were instructed to arrange their facial muscles, one at a time, into positions that corresponded to "smiles" or "frowns," without knowing that their faces were set in smile or frown positions. This was done by asking the subject to contract various muscles (e.g., the experimenter touched the subject lightly between the eyebrows with an electrode and said, "Pull your brows down and together . . . good, now hold it like that"). The subjects reported feeling more angry when their faces were set in the frown position and more happy when their faces were set in the smile position, even though they were unaware of frowning or smiling. They also reported that cartoons viewed when "smiling" were more humorous than cartoons viewed when "frowning."

We may tentatively conclude that the observer's visceral and somatic responses together provide cues about the fact that another person is affectively aroused and they also provide some rough cues about the particular affect the other is experiencing. This may put a new light on Michael's act, in the example cited earlier, of bringing his own teddy bear to comfort his friend. Although Michael acted in a seemingly egocentric manner, he also showed by this same act that he had received the basically correct emotional message that his friend was sad and needed comforting. Although he was probably not capable of making a cognitive assessment of the other child's state, he was able, probably through empathic arousal and feedback mechanisms, to know something important about the other child's feelings. It may be true of people in general that they become aware of the harmful or beneficial effects of their actions partly through nonverbal cues from others that both reflect the other's internal state and produce empathic responses in the actor.[1]

Empathy may thus alert one to the fact that someone is having an affective response in a situation and it may provide initial information about what that affect is. In this way empathy provides cues about one of the major sources of people's unpredictability, namely, their feelings. A person's empathic response may also at times give him cues about the other's feelings that contradict his words, because people's feelings are often "leaked" through changes in their facial response, posture, or tone of voice. (Changes in facial response may be less revealing in older children and adults than in younger children, because people are often socialized to mask their true feelings and this is best accomplished through controlling one's facial responses [Ekman & Friesen, 1974; Littlepage & Pineault, 1979].) Although these cues are not likely to be precise they may be an accurate enough reflection of the other's true feelings to make the observer uncomfortable and thus alert him to possibilities of deception that might otherwise be overlooked. Social cognition may thus gain valuable assistance from empathy, and this may compensate for the complexity and relative unpredictability of its subject matter that I discussed earlier.

There are developmental implications of this argument. In my theoretical model of empathy (Hoffman, 1975), I stressed the idea that the subjective experience of one's vicarious affective response to others is expanded as one develops a cognitive sense of others and becomes capable of understanding the causes of the other's condition. In light of the present discussion, it would appear that, because of simple empathic arousal mechanisms, the ability to be aroused vicariously may not only precede the development of the cognitive sense of others, it may actually contribute to that development by alerting the child to affective arousal in others, providing him with initial cues about what affects they are experiencing, and mobilizing his efforts to assess cognitively just what their condition is. The usual role of social cognition, then, may be to help the observer know that the affect he is experiencing is a response to someone else's situation, to give the observer a more precise idea of just what affect the other is experiencing, and to provide information about causes that may further shape the observer's response. In short, social cognition serves to fine tune the observer's assessment of what the other person is feeling. (Social cognition is also, of course, necessary for understanding complex emotions in others, such as disappointment).

Social cognition may at times serve more than a fine-tuning role, that is, it may actually initiate the empathic process. A person may, for example, believe it is important to comprehend someone's feelings (perhaps because one is a parent or a therapist). One may then try to imagine that what is happening to the other person is happening to the self. This process, whether intended or not, may produce a vicarious affective response because of the associative connections between the resulting image of oneself in the other's situation, and one's actual experiences in similar situations in the past (Hoffman, 1977). The vicarious affective response then contributes cues that give additional meaning to one's initial cognitive assessment of the other's feeling. In general, then, the empathic, hence also the nonverbal communication process under discussion may originate either through (1) simple mechanisms like conditioning, association, and mimicry that arouse affect, followed by cognitive elaboration or (2) through a more deliberate cognitive process that in turn triggers a vicarious affective reaction. Either way, the cues of the model's affective state or situation serve as stimuli for arousing a similar affective state in the observer, which in turn provides the observer with information about the model's affective state.

To summarize, social cognition, to a far greater degree than cognition in the physical domain, operates not alone but in the context of a complex, mutually facilitative give and take between affective and cognitive processes. Thus, in social interactions one is constantly making attributions about the other's thoughts and feelings that are based either on one's own inner states or on cultural norms and scripts. Although limited, these attributions generally lead to expectations about others that are sufficiently correct for most purposes due to the similarity in organizational structure between actor and model. At the same time, one is also responding with empathic affect, which allows for a high degree of sensitivity to nonverbal cues and may thus help alert one to the fact that the other person is aroused, provide one with a rough approximation of the particular affect aroused, and at times alert one to the possibility of deception. When one acts on the basis of incorrect attributions, one often receives corrective feedback. This stimulates cognitive operations that result in adjustments in the attributions and also help one zero in and identify the other person's affect more precisely than can the affective response to nonverbal cues alone.

Social cognition and social cognitive development are thus abstractions from what is essentially a matrix of interacting cognitive and affective processes. To return to our initial question, social objects may seem unpredictable from the standpoint of the detached observer who confines his analysis to the cognitive processes involved. From the standpoint of an adult or child actually engaged in social interaction and subject to the affective-cognitive interplay, however, other people may seem quite predictable and understandable – certainly to a greater degree than a piece of machinery that provides few if any cues about its principles of operation.

Finally, it may be worth noting that this argument is entirely consistent with a sociobiological perspective (Hoffman, 1977, 1981). The argument, briefly, is as follows: (1) The limbic system, which mediates affect, hence also presumably motivation, evolved prior to the cerebral cortex; (2) there is reason to believe that the limbic system mediates vicarious or empathic affect as well as direct affect (e.g., MacLean, 1973); and (3) there is agreement among evolutionists that humans evolved not alone but in interaction with others. It seems reasonable to conclude that the predisposition to certain social responses was selected according to affective and behavioral, rather than primarily cognitive criteria. That is, these social responses proved to be adaptive in terms of their affective and behavioral consequences. It follows that humans must be equipped biologically to function effectively in many social situations without undue reliance on cognitive processes. A similar argument for the primacy of affect is made by Zajonc (1980). According to Zajonc, the processing of affective stimuli is independent of, and possibly more efficient than the processing of purely cognitive stimuli. Affective stimuli are remembered longer than cognitive stimuli, for example, sometimes even when the time of exposure to the affective stimuli is relative short. Zajonc is talking about direct affect but the same may be true of empathic affect, as suggested here.

Summary

Because people are more complex and unpredictable than things, one would expect a developmental lag between social cognition and cognition in the physical domain. There appears to be no evidence for such a lag and I have suggested several reasons for this. First, people compensate for their complexity and unpredictability by providing continuous feedback, which allows the actor to reassess and correct the interpretations he makes of their behavior and inner states. Second, the actor and the model have the same organizational structure and are therefore apt to respond to events in similar ways. Consequently, even in the absence of feedback, when action is based on hurriedly made egocentric attributions, shared belief systems, and scripts, it will generally be adaptive.

Third, there is evidence for a natural tendency in humans to respond vicariously or empathically through involuntary, minimally cognitive mechanisms like conditioning and mimicry. The resulting empathic affect provides nonverbal, physiologically based cues, linked to the actor's own past experiences, that alert him to the fact that the model is having an affective experience and may also provide initial information as to what that affect is. The role of social cognition may then be to fine tune the actor's assessment of the other's feeling. Social cognition may thus gain a valuable assist from empathy and this may compensate for the complexity and unpredictability of its subject matter.

An obvious conclusion to be drawn from this argument is that social cognition cannot be divorced from affect. Piaget and other cognitive psychologists have always acknowledged that affect is crucial in human behavior, indeed that it is the driving force behind all cognitive activity. But they have also operated on the assumption that once cognitive processes are set in motion they can be studied without recourse to affect. That may be true of cognition in the physical domain but it is apparently not true in the social domain, in which affect appears to be not only the driving force but also a source of crucial information.

Note

1 The empathic response may not only be a cue to the other's state but it may also serve as a potential stimulus to feelings of guilt in the actor (Hoffman, in press).

References

Aronfreed, J., & Paskal, V. *The development of sympathetic behavior in children.* Unpublished manuscript, University of Pennsylvania, 1966.
Bell, S. M. The development of the concept of the object as related to infant-mother attachment. *Child Development,* 1970, *41,* 291–311.
Borke, H. Chandler and Greenspan's "Ersatz ego-centrism": A rejoinder. *Developmental Psychology,* 1972, *7,* 107–9.
Easterbrook, J. A. The effect of emotion on cue utilization and the organization of behavior. *Psychological Review,* 1959, *66,* 183–201.
Ekman, P., & Friesen, W. V. Detecting deception from the body or face. *Journal of Personality and Social Psychology,* 1974, *29,* 188–98.
Erwin, J., & Kuhn, D. Development of children's understanding of the multiple determination underlying human behavior. *Developmental Psychology,* 1979, *15,* 352–3.
Fein, D. A. Judgment of causality to physical and social picture sequences. *Developmental Psychology,* 1972, *8,* 147.

Gellhorn, E. Motion and emotion: The role of proprioception in the physiology and pathology of the emotions. *Psychological Review*, 1964, *71*, 457–72.

Glick, J. Cognition and social cognition: An introduction. In J. Glick and K. A. Clarke-Stewart (Eds.), *The development of social understanding*. New York: Gardner Press, Inc., 1978.

Hoffman, M. L. Developmental synthesis of affect and cognition and its implications for altruistic motivation. *Developmental Psychology*, 1975, *11*, 607–22.

Empathy, its development and prosocial implications. In C. B. Keasey (Ed.), *Nebraska symposium on motivation* (Vol. 25), University of Nebraska Press, 1977.

Is altruism part of human nature? *Journal of Personality and Social Psychology*, 1981, in press.

Empathy, guilt, and social cognition. In W. Overton and J. Gallagher (Eds.), *Knowledge and development*. New York: Plenum, in press.

Isen, A. M., Shalker, T. E., Clarke, M., & Karp, L. Affect, accessibility of material in memory, and behavior: A cognitive loop? *Journal of Personality and Social Psychology*, 1978, *36*, 1–12.

Izard, C. E. *The face of emotion*. New York: Appleton-Century Crofts, 1971.

Jackson, E., Campos, J. J., & Fischer, K. W. The question of decalage between object permanence and person permanence. *Developmental Psychology*, 1978, *14*, 1–10.

Kahneman, D. *Attention and effort*. Englewood Cliffs, N.J.: Prentice-Hall, 1973.

Kuhn, D., & Ho, V. The development of schemes for recognizing additive and alternative effects in a "natural experiment" context. *Developmental Psychology*, 1977, *13*, 515–16.

Laird, J. D. Self-attribution of emotion: The effects of expressive behavior on the quality of emotional experience. *Journal of Personality and Social Psychology*, 1974, *29*, 475–86.

Lempers, J. D., Flavell, E. R., & Flavell, J. H. The development in very young children of tacit knowledge concerning visual perception. *Genetic Psychology Monographs*, 1977, *95*, 3–53.

Littlepage, G. E., & Pineault, M. H. Detection of deceptive factual statements from the body and the face. *Personality and Social Psychology Bulletin*, 1979, *5*, 325–8

MacLean, P. D. *A triune concept of the brain and behavior*. Toronto: University of Toronto Press, 1973.

Mueller, J. H. Anxiety and encoding processes in memory. *Personality and Social Psychology Bulletin*, 1979, *5*, 288–94.

Piaget, J. *The psychology of intelligence*. New York: International Universities Press, 1963.

Winnicott, D. W. Theory of the parent-infant relationship. *International Journal of Psychoanalysis*, 1960, *41*, 585–95.

Van der Lee, H. & Oppenheimer, L. *Development of temporal ordering of social events*. Unpublished manuscript, Psychologisch Laboratorium, Universiteit van Nijmegen, 1979.

Zajonc, R. B. Feeling and thinking: Preferences need no inferences. *American Psychologist*, 1980, *35*, 151–75.

4 "Concrete thinking" and the development of social cognition

Stephen M. Kosslyn and Jerome Kagan

The term "social cognition" usually refers to two kinds of cognition – that about people, groups, and social events and that colored by feelings, motives, attitudes, and emotional states. In this chapter we consider the implications of a research program on mental imagery for the study of social cognition. If social concepts are abstract and images concrete, one might wonder what relevance the study of mental imagery has to social cognition. We will provide two answers to this question in this chapter. First, the use of mental imagery may provide strategies for empirical assessment of social cognition and its development. To illustrate this point, we suggest a few examples in which methodologies used to investigate imagery can also be used to study social cognition. Second, much of social cognition may be mediated by thinking about particular instances, and we consider how imagery might be used in this context and how this use of imagery might change over age.

Overview of the imagery research program

The present research program has been summarized in a number of places (e.g., Kosslyn, 1978a, 1978b) and has been explicated at length recently (Kosslyn, 1980). Thus, we only touch on the most relevant points here.

The imagery research program had two distinct phases. The goal of the first phase was to delineate the class of theories that would allow one to account for basic phenomena in mental-image processing. The research program was initiated with the idea that images are like spatial displays on a cathode-ray tube screen generated by a computer program (plus data). This scheme led to a number of questions about the functional capacities that underlie imagery. That is, an account of imagery will specify the ways the brain can represent and process information, and the present imagery research program is an attempt to delineate these "functional capacities." In the first phase of the research program, these questions were explored in sets of converging experiments. The first set of experiments was conducted to discover whether images depict spatial extent in an analogue way. Four classes of results supported the inference that mental images do in fact represent information "pictorially." First, it was found that the further one had to scan a mental image to "see" some target, the longer were the scan times (in fact, scan times increased linearly with distance scanned–see Kosslyn 1973; Kosslyn, Ball, & Reiser, 1978). Second, people required more time to examine subjectively smaller images when "looking" for a named part. Subjects reported having to "zoom in" to "see" a named part if the imaged object was seemingly small. This was not necessary if the imaged object was pictured at a larger subjective size (Kosslyn, 1975). Moreover, smaller parts per se required more time to "see" on an image than did larger ones–even when the smaller parts were in fact more highly associated with the object in question than were the larger ones, and in fact were verified as appropriate more quickly when imagery was not used (Kosslyn, 1976a.) Third, Kosslyn (1978c) reasoned that if images are indeed spatial representations that occur in a spatial medium, then it makes sense that that medium would be spatially bounded. Thus, experiments were conducted to demonstrate that the subjective size at which an object may be imaged was bounded by a constant value, as would be expected if the medium per se were limiting the size, and a measure of the "visual angle of the mind's eye" was obtained. In these experiments it was demonstrated that larger objects seem to "overflow" at further subjective distances in one's image, and that the "visual angle" obtained from the estimated distances and object sizes was consistent with estimates obtained from other techniques. In one of these techniques, the amount of time required for a group of subjects to scan each degree of arc along a set of imaged lines was measured. The subjects were also asked to image a line as long as possible without either end overflowing, and to scan this image. Using the estimates of scanning time per degree, it was easy to estimate the "size" of this longest possible, non-overflowing line. The angle obtained in this instance was virtually identical with that obtained by asking different subjects to estimate the apparent distance at which an imaged ruler seemed to overflow. Interestingly, however, the absolute size of the angle depended on the criterion of "overflow" that the subject adopted (see Kosslyn, 1978c). Fourth, in another set of experiments people imaged objects at different subjective sizes. Given that smaller images are more difficult to inspect because parts are less resolved, one would expect people to have more difficulty in recalling objects that were imaged at subjectively small sizes than those imaged at larger sizes. And this prediction was confirmed, using an incidental memory paradigm in which subjects did not intentionally attempt to encode the objects (Kosslyn & Alper, 1977).

Having gathered data that implied that images do in fact "depict" objects in a spatial medium, it then made sense to ask how these representations arise. The results of a series of experiments demonstrated that images are not simply stored intact in long-term memory and later simply activated into awareness. If images were simply activated wholistically, there is no reason to expect that subjectively larger images would require more time to form than smaller ones, nor to expect images of more detailed objects to require more time to form than images of less detailed ones – both of which were found (Kosslyn, 1975; Kosslyn, Reiser, Farah, & Fliegel, submitted). If images may be constructed from individually stored parts, the results obtained make perfect sense: People place more parts on larger images (where the locations of the parts are clearly discernible) and on objects for which one has encoded more parts. Another experiment was conducted to consider the possibility that the foregoing results were not simply a consequence of the overall amount of material encoded into long-term memory. In this experiment, the same geometric shapes could be described as having been formed by combining relatively few overlapping shapes or by juxtaposing relatively many adjacent forms. For example, the Star of David could be described as two overlapping triangles or as a hexagon with six small triangles placed around it. Although the same figures were imaged, people required less time to form the images if they had been described (and presumably encoded) in terms of fewer instead of many units. Furthermore, the effects of number of units were not due to subjects simply retrieving an image, scanning it, and lingering longer over the more detailed images before responding that the image was fully present. In another experiment, the same configuration was parsed into different numbers of units by presenting drawings on different numbers of separate pages; here, subjects required more time to image objects initially presented on more pages, even though the final configuration was identical in all cases. In addition, it was found that no more time was required to form an image of a pair of objects at two different distances – although more time was later required to scan between them when they were relatively far apart. If the effects of amount of detail were an artifact of postretrieval scanning, we would have expected effects of distance on image formation time in this experiment. Thus, the results were taken to show that an image in active memory can be generated on the basis of information initially stored in separate units.

The first phase of the imagery research program concluded with the question of whether images were formed solely on the basis of "perceptual" information stored in long-term memory (which allows one to reexperience "seeing" an object in a mental image) or whether more abstract "descriptive" information can be used in conjuction with perceptual information when one generates mental images from long-term memory. The fact that descriptive information can be used in generating images was demonstrated in several experiments. In one, people were asked to arrange objects into scenes in accordance with descriptions indicating their relative positions. Not only was this reported to .be an easy task, but, after generating these images, subjects required more time to scan between pairs of objects that should have been relatively far apart than those that should have been in closer proximity – providing an independent source of evidence that the image was in fact generated in accordance with the description. Substantially different results were obtained in a control experiment, where people memorized and recalled the verbal descriptions per se. In an additional experiment (see Kosslyn, 1978b), people were shown a matrix of letters, it was removed, and then described in one of two ways (e.g., three rows of six vs. six columns of three). More time was later required to image the matrix if it was described in terms of more units, demonstrating that the conceptual information was in fact used in forming the image. Thus, at the conclusion of Phase I we knew that images represent information by depicting an object or scene's appearance, that images need not be stored intact in long-term memory, that an image may be generated on the basis of information stored in multiple underlying units, and that abstract "descriptive" information can be used to mentally arrange the parts of an image.

Although the foregoing experiments were conducted to distinguish between different alternative "functional capacities" of the cognitive system, they also are of intrinsic interest. That is, the methodologies invented to investigate internal representations and the processes that operate on them can be applied directly to the study of how particular information is represented and processed. Specifically, we can use these methodologies to examine the qualities of particular images an adult or child may form, which may be an index of deeper attitudes, feelings, and/or beliefs. Thus, in the following section we will examine some applications of the methodologies and experimental techniques to problems in the development of social cognition. These applications are direct, and make only the most minimal theoretical assumptions about imagery (e.g., images depict spatial extent).

Using the experimental techniques to study the development of social cognition

The present methodologies could be applied to problems in social cognition and its development. We offer a few suggestions simply to convey the flavor of these kinds of experiments. Obviously, when dealing with phenomena as complicated as those of social cognition, more controls would be required than will be noted before one could draw strong inferences. Nonetheless, the basic ideas sketched in this brief suggestion seem to have some promise of developing into new, more subtle "diagnostic" tests.

Perhaps the most useful methodology developed in the imagery research is the mental-image-scanning technique (see Kosslyn, Ball, & Reiser, 1978). This technique could be used to discover how a person implicitly regards others and how he or she regards relationships between different people and/or classes of people. For example, suppose the investigator wanted to know if a child or adult created an image of the father as larger than the mother. The subject could be asked to image the father at a specified distance, and then be asked to "mentally focus" on the feet of the imaged person. The subject could then be asked to scan the image until reaching the top of the head, and then to respond. The amount of time necessary to scan the image would presumably reflect the extent scanned over, and thus would index relative size. It would also be interesting to conduct this experiment without requiring that both parents be imaged at the same "distance." One might find that subjects seem to image one parent closer than the other (and thus have a greater visual arc to scan); the relative distance could reflect something about one's feelings about that person.

The scanning technique could also be used to investigate more subtle questions. Suppose the investigator wanted to know how close the child normally conceived of two people, be they father and mother, two brothers, or a black and white child. It is possible that subjects will literally image pairs of people closer together in an image if these people are thought of as being "closer" along a more abstract "psychological" dimension. To test this idea, one would first use neutral stimuli to determine how long a given subject required to scan different degrees of visual arc. Next, the child would be asked to image pairs of people standing together, and would be asked to scan between them. This scanning time would be used as an index of relative "distance."

Next consider how these methodologies could be used to investigate a person's values. One could ask a child to imagine a peer or famous adult who is "good at" a number of things ranging from intellectual abilities, athletic prowess, social skills and so on, and again ask the child to scan the lengths of these images. It would be interesting if children systematically varied the size of their image of a "typical person" who excels at each class of performance. It does not seem unreasonable that people who are thought to excel at more valued skills are imaged as "larger."

There is another phenomenon that might be useful for present purposes, called the "congruity effect," which was used to study when imagery is used in answering questions (see Kosslyn, Murphy, Bemesderfer, & Feinstein, 1977). This effect occurs when one is asked to compare two things from memory. For example, if one is asked which of two normally large things is larger, one responds more quickly than if asked which of the two is smaller – but vice versa if asked about two small things. That is, one is faster at evaluating two things if the question is couched in terms of the pole of the dimension at which they fall (see Potts, Banks, Kosslyn, Riley, & Smith, 1978, for a review). Although Kosslyn et al. (1977) examined this effect in the context of an imagery model, it probably is only peripherally related to image processing per se (it occurs, for example, even when people judge which of two digits stands for the larger or smaller quantity). Thus, it would not be surprising if the congruity effect could be used to study other topics.

In the present case, a child's attitudes about two classes of people, or two individuals, could be evaluated by asking him or her to image two instances side by side, and then decide which was more happy, sad, clean, "better," and so on. If the child is asked to evaluate each pair a number of times, each pole of the dimension being used equally often in the question (e.g., happy versus sad, clean versus dirty), the difference in times for the two adjectives would presumably reflect the way in which the child conceived of that class or pair of people. If a child had an unhappy home life, for example, he or she might require relatively less time to decide which parent was the "meaner" than which was the "nicer." Furthermore, it is known that the closer two things are along the probed dimension, the more time is required (e.g., more time is taken to decide whether a mouse is larger than a hamster than whether a mouse is larger than an elephant). Thus, the disparity in the child's relative feelings about two individuals or "typical instances" of some class could be indexed using this technique.

In each of the foregoing kinds of experiments one would want to obtain more conventional measures of the independent variable in order to validate the imagery techniques. For example, in the experiment on relative values, the child could simply be asked to rank various skills in terms of importance; presumably this ranking should correlate highly with the ranking in scan times, if the size of the image is a reflection of value. The advantage of using imagery techniques is that they circumvent a whole host of output variables that normally intervene between one's conception and one's response. If the imagery techniques were valid, they could be used with children who have difficulty in expressing themselves directly, and in cases where some people might be loath to discuss (or think about) highly charged topics concerning people.

Imagery and the development of social cognition

The data described earlier were collected with the intention of constraining the class of viable models of imagery processing. The model that was based on these data is described in depth by Kosslyn (1980), but the details are not of direct relevance here. The important features of the imagery model for issues in social cognition are straightforward. First, there is a distinction between a "surface image," which is a short-term memory representation that gives rise to the experience of seeing something in its absence, and a "deep image representation," which is a long-term memory representation of the object's appearance. The deep image representation encodes information about how an object looked, not what it looked like. These representations encode the "literal" appearance in an analogue way; they are literal in that they are "true to," not simply "true of" the represented object(s) in the way that a tape recording can be "true to" a voice whereas a written transcript cannot. Second, there is a distinction between both of these kinds of image representations and languagelike "propositional" representations. Whereas images depict, propositions describe. They are "true of," and not "true to." Importantly, image representations are concrete, they cannot represent information about classes, and are tied to a particular sensory modality. Propositions, on the other hand, are abstract; they can represent information about classes directly and are amodal.

The development of representation over age

The main assumptions about development of representation are rather simple: First, with increasing experience, it becomes more likely that one will encode a particular piece of information in a propositional format (see Kosslyn, 1976b, 1978a). Consider the following question: What color is a bee's head? (please answer). Most people report having to mentally picture the insect's head, and having to "look" on their image to "see" the color. But note what happens when you answer the question a second time. Or a third time. By now people invariably report that they no longer need to have recourse to imagery in order to answer the question. Now the information is encoded in a more languagelike way, as well as in an imagery form. Presumably as children access information more often it becomes more likely that the information will be encoded in an abstract "propositional" code (in addition to an imagery format) via "reflection," to use Locke's term. Furthermore, much learning is via language, and thus as children grow they come to rely on the vicarious experience of others in learning, especially after they learn to read. These factors would result in an increasingly large proportion of information being encoded into a more abstract, nonimaginal form over the course of development.

In addition to the influence of experience on how information is represented in memory, we can suppose that some maturational factors also influence the frequency with which imagery is used at different ages. In particular, let us consider some implications of the fact that the amount of information one is able to process at a given time tends to increase with age. To explain this, we need only suppose two things. First, children become able to locate and activate an encoding in memory more quickly as they grow older (perhaps due to development of appropriate neural "hardware," such as increasing mylenization of the axons). In addition, we can posit that activated material starts to decay as soon as activation ceases (either due to fading away or competition from other competing input – see Reitman, 1971; Shiffrin, 1973). If so, then material must be repeatedly reactivated to be kept available for further use in on-line computation. Thus, one can think about the limits of "memory capacity" by analogy to juggling. The faster one can move one's hands, the more "balls can be kept in the air" at once. If children are simply less adept at moving their hands quickly, as it were, their memory capacities would appear smaller – which they do. This basic notion might help us explain why deduction generally becomes easier with age. In order to decide that a bee has muscles, for example, the Kosslyn & Shwartz (1977, 1978) computer simulation of imagery processing first searches the propositional encodings directly associated with "bee," looking for an explicit encoding of this fact. This failing, it then looks up the superordinate (insect) and searches the propositions associated with this category; failing to find it here, the simulation repeats the operation of looking up the superordinate and searching the associated propositions and so on, all the while remembering that it is searching for a particular encoding relevant to bees. This operation requires a person to perform considerable "juggling" in order to keep the requisite information available at the same time. Thus, if young children cannot hold in mind the information about how to perform the deduction, about what to look for in the different sets of propositions, about what the queried object is and so on, they will have trouble in performing deductions – even if they are explicitly taught how to do so (cf. Kendler & Kendler, 1962; Smedslund, 1961).

Discovering one's attitudes and beliefs at different ages

In order to explain any of the imagery results, we do not need to posit that information about general classes is abstracted and stored as such. Instead, we need only assume that information about particulars is stored. Let us consider where this assumption leads us in regard to issues of social cognition. First, this putative reliance on information about exemplars has some interesting implications for how one decides what one thinks or believes about some class. Consider, for example, the reader's attitudes about astronauts as a class. At first, one may simply shrug and claim not to have a particular attitude toward such people. But if pressed, either by the demands of circumstances or those of a persistent experimenter, one will come up with something. How? The first author first reviewed the information he knew about a number of particular astronauts (e.g., the ones he could remember had short hair and stiff backs, but at least one of them came back full of mystical ideas and another became an airline president), and then formed an attitude on the basis of this information. One interesting question about representation is: In what way is the information stored that is later retrieved? Is it stored in a languagelike format, or implicit in imagistic or other kinds of representations? In the case of astronauts, visual images of particular instances seemed to have been consulted (and the haircuts were noted) and some remarks one astronaut made were recalled. Most of the information the first author used in forming an attitude about astronauts seemed to be embedded in encodings about particular astronauts. Only a few generalizations seemed to be stored directly (e.g., most had military backgrounds).

Now let us consider the most straightforward extension of these notions of representational development to social cognition. With age, more information is stored in a languagelike form. Thus, one might expect that adults would less often have to compute their attitudes and so on at the time of query, and would tend to have stored directly information about many of their beliefs. For many frequently encountered domains – such as race, family, country, and so on – adults may have "codified" their beliefs and attitudes and stored them explicitly as entries in a list of facts about themselves. In addition, even when adults use exemplars, they may not access imagery as often as younger children. If children often compute attitudes and beliefs on the basis of imagery, we would expect visible attributes of the exemplars to exert a strong influence on what generalizations are drawn.

In addition, if children tend to use imagery in representing information in memory, it should be more difficult for them to represent abstract concepts as such. Thus, although children appear to use abstract terms like "good" appropriately, it could be that their use of this term is based on particular "concrete" exemplars, and is not based on an abstract principle. The mere fact that these terms can be extended beyond the original cases does not implicate abstract representations per se: Children could be responding on the basis of "similarity" to stored exemplars. As one encounters more examples of "good" and "bad," for example, one will be able to generalize to a wider range of new instances. Genuine ability to apply an abstract principle may not emerge until numerous exemplars can be considered at once along specifiable dimensions – which may in part depend on maturational factors.

Consider some further extrapolations from these basic ideas: If, in fact, people sometimes infer their attitudes from encodings about particular exemplars, as opposed to simply accessing abstract generalizations, it becomes important to know which particular encodings about exemplars will be retrieved. This question is of some interest from the point of view of the kind of theory we have been developing. Many theories of adult cognition stress the role of "prototypes" (e.g., Rosch, 1978); that is, when one thinks of astronauts, one might consider a prototypical one (e.g., John Glenn) and use him to induce generalizations. This kind of procedure would be more efficient than retrieving and comparing numerous exemplars, if one has a prototypical instance clearly identified. But consider what is required to identify – or "construct" – a prototype. One must consider similarities and dissimilarities among all (or a reasonable subset) of the exemplars of a class, computing which exemplar is the most "central" of the class. This would involve, in the Kosslyn and Shwartz simulation model, essentially comparing each exemplar with each other one, keeping a running account of which exemplar was on the average most "similar" (in regard to specified dimensions) to other ones. If children perform search and comparison operations more slowly than adults, it seems unlikely that they will sample sufficiently to derive a prototype or set of prototypical exemplars at the time they are asked to generalize about a category.

In addition to the problem of sampling enough exemplars to compute a prototype, one must attend only to those aspects of each exemplar judged to be relevant for the generalization at hand; thus, the nature of "similarity" will vary depending on the purpose of making a comparison (see Goodman, 1972). If one is trying to derive the prototype astronaut for purposes of guessing which of three people on a quiz show is the real astronaut, characteristics like facial features may not be relevant, whereas general size might be. But, in contrast, if one is trying to decide which of two people is the prototypical politician, facial features may very well be something one would weigh heavily when making a decision. Given the literature on selective attention in children (see Gibson, 1969), it would not be surprising if children were not very good at attending to only the relevant aspects of exemplars when computing a prototype. Thus, if the present view is correct, we might expect young children to have a tendency to base generalizations unduly on recent encounters (if "availability" is often a consequence of recency of exposure); furthermore, children would base generalizations on irrelevant characteristics of these exemplars more often than would adults.[1]

Thus far we have considered the notion that young children are more likely to represent information solely in an imagistic form than are older people. If so, then it makes sense that young children will not often have an attitude, a belief, or social concept explicitly represented, available to be "looked up" and reported. Instead, they may often infer their attitudes and beliefs by using information about stored exemplars, represented in an imagistic way. In contrast, there is a greater probability that in adults a given attitude or belief is stored in a propositional form, either because they have had enough occasion to express it to ensure that it is recoded or because it is implied by other attitudes (and hence, by analogy to the "bee's muscles" example used earlier, is deducible from them). Thus, it may be relatively rare in adults that beliefs and feelings are actually computed at the time of query. (It took some thinking to produce the astronaut example used earlier; most adults do not report similar experiences when they are asked to talk about their attitudes about family, race, work, religion, and other common topics.) And when adults do compute their attitudes and beliefs, they may base inductive generalizations on "prototypical" instances, whereas young children may not.

But the analogy between reporting one's attitudes and/or beliefs and answering questions about properties of common objects can be stretched too far – especially in the case of social cognition in general. Let us now turn to some reasons to be chary of the foregoing hypotheses.

The role of affect in altering information processing

So far we have been treating social cognition as simply another form of information processing. But some forms of social cognition seem to have a special status: Thoughts about people and their actions often evoke emotional responses. And the affect associated with a stimulus may alter not only how information about it is stored and later used, but may affect other ongoing information processing as well. In "hot" social cognition we may sometimes find a reverse developmental trend with certain kinds of material. Adults may tend to encode in rich imagery various sorts of stimuli – such as sex symbols, Rolls Royces, diamonds, and sumptuous feasts – to which children give only passing attention. Intuitively, the more laden with positive affect a stimulus is, the more one will tend to linger over it. And perhaps the more one will tend to encode a representation allowing one to re-present the stimulus to oneself in its absence, allowing one to linger again (albeit momentarily) over its image. Thus, the conception of Kosslyn (1978a) may be too simple, ignoring the probable influence of the subject matter at hand.

Moreover, in "hot" cognition we do not necessarily expect differences between adults and children in "processing capacity." If one is very agitated or aroused, one may drop a few balls, as it were. That is, it is precisely in cases where one is emotionally aroused that adult processing may become disrupted – perhaps because numerous associations are called up, almost involuntarily, and these compete with other processing occurring at the same time. The fact that people seem to "regress" to earlier strategies when under pressure has been reported (e.g., see White, 1965), and this may reflect disruption of allocation of capacity – forcing one to rely on more simple ways of reasoning (i.e., involving less inference and deduction).

If adults are agitated, they too may fail to compute typical exemplars, should the need arise. But will this necessarily occur? In fact, if Tversky & Kahneman's (1974) work can be generalized slightly, adults often do not make the effort to consider the "representativeness" of an exemplar, but use availability as a heuristic in drawing generalizations. We would expect this to be especially the case, however, when adults are asked about some highly emotionally charged issue. In this case, the first few exemplars recalled may receive so much attention (because of associations called up and so on) that processing terminates relatively quickly. In addition, even if exemplars are sampled judiciously, if the material is highly charged emotionally, even adults may not attend to only the information about an exemplar that is relevant to the task at hand. Consider one's beliefs about how good most Ku Klux Klan members are as parents, for example. In this case, not only may many adults not carefully compute a typical instance along some relevant dimension, but when an adult does make a generalization about a member of the KKK, it may not be based on careful consideration of only the relevant dimensions – even if a reasonable number of exemplars were sampled. Here, then, the two sorts of social cognition, about people and their actions, and affect-associated cognition, come together. It is thought about social circumstances that is likely to be affect-laden, and such thought processes may look quite different than less emotion-ridden ones. At least some of the changes over age in social cognition may not be changes in the kind of processing, per se, but may be largely matters of which sorts of information are emotion-laden, which sorts of information will engender particular modes of processing.

Conclusion

We have tried to sketch out how research on mental imagery can be applied to social cognition. In so doing, we have advocated using methodologies developed for other purposes to study questions about social cognition. In addition, we have emphasized the usefulness of asking questions within a theoretical framework that was not developed with social cognition in mind, but provides a ready means for thinking about how some forms of social cognition might operate. One moral of our sojourn was that the kind of material being processed may be critical in determining processing at different ages. The only firm developmental trend we posit is that one will have increasing numbers of options as one grows older and has more experience. Whereas children may use imagery largely by necessity – not having any other alternative – adults may use it partly by preference or as one of several alternatives. The theoretical framework outlined here leads one to examine when exemplars will be consulted in drawing generalizations by people at different ages, and how various emotional states affect this sort of processing – and, indeed, processing in general. In particular, it would be of interest to discover whether one stores increasingly more of one's attitudes, beliefs, and social concepts in an explicit languagelike form as one grows older, and whether young children do tend to use imagery in social reasoning more than do adults. If so, then the constraints of the imagery-processing system may have profound effects on the kinds of social thinking in which young children can engage.

Note

1 This is not to say that children do not evince "typicality effects" in verifying words or pictures, however: These effects can simply reflect differences in the child's familiarity with different exemplars, more typical ones being encountered (including in books and movies) more often (cf. Rosch, 1973).

References

Gibson, E. J. *Principles of perceptual learning and development.* New York: Appleton-Century-Crofts, 1969.

Goodman, N. Seven strictures on similarity. In N. Goodman, *Problems and projects.* Indianapolis: Bobbs-Merrill, 1972.

Kendler, T. S., & Kendler, H. H. Inferential behavior in children as a function of age and subgoal constancy. *Journal of Experimental Psychology*, 1962, *64*, 460 – 6.

Kosslyn, S. M. Scanning visual images: some structural implications. *Perception and Psychophysics*, 1973, *14*, 90 – 4.

Information representation in visual images. *Cognitive Psychology*, 1975, *7*, 341 – 70.

Can imagery be distinguished from other forms of internal representation? Evidence from studies of information retrieval time. *Memory and Cognition*, 1976a, *4*, 291 – 7.

Using imagery to retrieve semantic information: a developmental study. *Child Development*, 1976b, *47*, 434 – 44.

Imagery and cognitive development: a teleological approach. In R. Siegler (Ed.), *Children's Thinking: What Develops?* Hillsdale, N.J.: Lawrence Erlbaum Associates, 1978a.

Imagery and internal representation. In E. Rosch & B. B. Lloyd (Eds.), *Cognition and Categorization.* Hillsdale, N.J.: Lawrence Erlbaum Associates, 1978b.

Measuring the visual angle of the mind's eye. *Cognitive Psychology*, 1978c, *10*, 356 – 89.

Image and Mind. Cambridge, Mass.: Harvard University Press, 1980.

Kosslyn, S. M., & Alper, S. N. On the pictorial properties of visual images: effects of image size on memory for words. *Canadian Journal of Psychology*, 1977, *31*, 32 – 40.

Kosslyn, S. M., Ball, T. M., & Reiser, B. J. Visual images preserve metric spatial information: evidence from studies of image scanning. *Journal of Experimental Psychology: Human Perception and Performance*, 1978, *4*, 47 – 60.

Kosslyn, S. M., Murphy, G. L., Bemesderfer, M. E., & Feinstein, K. J. Category and continuum in mental comparisons. *Journal of Experimental Psychology: General*, 1977, *106*, 341 – 75.

Kosslyn, S. M., Reiser, B. J., Farah, M. J., & Fliegel, S. L. *Generating visual images.* Manuscript submitted for publication.

Kosslyn, S. M., & Shwartz, S. P. A simulation of visual imagery. *Cognitive Science*, 1977, *1*, 265 – 95.

Visual images as spatial representations in active memory. In E. M. Riseman & A. R. Hanson (Eds.), *Computer vision systems.* New York: Academic Press, 1978.

Potts, G. R., Banks, W. P., Kosslyn, S. M., Moyer, R. S., Riley, C. A., & Smith, K. H. Encoding and Retrieval in Comparative Judgments. In N. J. Castellan & F. Restle (Eds.), *Cognitive Theory* (Vol. 3). Hillsdale, N.J.: Lawrence Erlbaum Associates, 1978.

Reitman, J. S. Mechanisms of forgetting in short-term memory. *Cognitive Psychology*, 1971, *2*, 185 – 95.

Rosch, E. H. On the internal structure of perceptual and semantic categories. In T. E. Moore (Ed.), *Cognitive Development and the Acquisition of Language.* New York: Academic Press, 1973.

Principles of categorization. In E. Rosch and B. B. Lloyd (Eds.), *Cognition and Categorization*. Hillsdale, N.J.: Lawrence Erlbaum Associates, 1978.

Shiffrin, R. M. Information persistence in short-term memory. *Journal of Experimental Psychology*, 1973, *100*, 39–49.

Smedslund, J. The acquisition of conservation of substance and weight in children: II. External reinforcement of conservation of weight and the operations of additions and subtractions. *Scandinavian Journal of Psychology*, 1961, *2*, 71–84.

Tversky, A., & Kahneman, D. Judgment under uncertainty: Heuristics and biases. *Science*, 1974, *184*, 1124–31.

White, S. H. Evidence for a hierarchical arrangement of learning processes. In L. P. Lipsitt & C. C. Spiker (Eds.), *Advances in child development and behavior*. New York: Academic Press, 1965.

5 Social cognition in a script framework

Katherine Nelson

Social cognition is the process of representing knowledge about people and their relationships. Theorists have usually described such knowledge in terms of static structural models. However, these models cannot account for the fact that our knowledge of the social world is acquired through participation in ongoing dynamic interactive activities. Moreover, although abstract knowledge about social relationships is hard to find prior to the school years, writers such as Halliday (1978) and Trevarthen (1978) have emphasized that the construction of social meanings is an interactive process that begins at birth. It is clear from the observation of children as young as one year of age that much has been learned about reciprocity relations in social interactions, as well as about expected social routines (Bruner, 1975, 1978; Nelson, 1978). Although the infant has much to learn about kinship relations and gender roles, the beginnings of understanding of mother roles and child roles are established in well-practiced caretaking and play routines. It is on this mundane knowledge base that children, in partnership with parents, build conversational models (Snow, 1977) and patterns of social play and dialogue with peers (Garvey, 1977; Nelson & Gruendel, 1979).

Taken together, these observations point to three challenges to an adequate theory of the development of social cognition. The first is to find a way to describe the acquisition of knowledge within these active participatory frameworks. A second challenge is to represent adequately the dynamic relationships that are both the source and outcome of such knowledge. Although the child experiences a world of ongoing activity, most models of developing knowledge systems are static and structural,

The research reported in this paper was supported by National Science Foundation Grant No. BNS 78-25810. I would like to thank Janice Gruendel, whose collaboration in developing the ideas and the research described has been invaluable; and Maryl Gearhart and Lee Ross for detailed and helpful comments on an earlier version of this paper.

97

representing abstract categorical knowledge. The standard cognitive developmental position (e.g., Kohlberg, 1969) requires that children be able to abstract general categories (such as male and female) in order to act in accordance with their role requirements. Observations of young children in everyday interactions and play reveal a surprising social cognitive competence in activity before they can verbalize or manipulate abstract categorical knowledge. The third challenge, then, is to explain the basis for this competence in action and relate it to later categorical knowledge.

This chapter will expand on these considerations and will outline a framework for taking them into account in building a more adequate theory of the development of social cognition. Such a theory is not yet in place. What I hope to achieve here is to suggest how one should proceed and what sort of research may be required to construct it adequately in order to account for the interactive source of knowledge, the dynamic relationships involved, and the display of competence prior to understanding. Unlike most discussions of social cognitive development, the emphasis here will be on the early years of childhood, where it all begins, in accord with the general developmental principle that unless we understand the source we will misunderstand the outcome.

Schema theories

The theoretical stance developed in this chapter falls within the general class of schema theories that have recently become influential within branches of cognitive psychology, social psychology, cognitive anthropology, and artificial intelligence (e.g. Bartlett, 1932; Bransford & Franks, 1971; Goffman, 1974; Mandler, 1979, Minsky, 1975; Rumelhart & Ortony, 1977; Schank & Abelson, 1977). Traditional theories of cognition have relied on representational schemes that relate like elements in linear fashion at different levels of a hierarchy, specified in terms of features or attributes that give rise to coordinate, subordinate, and superordinate relations in taxonomic or paradigmatic schemes (Miller, 1969). Although such analytic models have served well to describe certain aspects of knowledge, it has become clear that they cannot account for many kinds of natural knowledge systems. Knowledge in such areas as spatial layouts, story structures, games, and everyday routines appears not to be taxonomic in any sense, but rather schematic, relating diverse elements in a holistic structure by means of different types of relationships. The holistic nature of a schema is probably its most important characteristic. A schema specifies particular essential elements in specific relations to one another, while other elements may be optional. Some elements may be specified in terms of default values that are called up when specific values are not specified. For example, a living room schema specifies essentially four walls, a door, and windows (related in terms of angles, parallel planes, and so on). It may have as an optional value a fireplace and may specify default values in terms of furniture such as a sofa, chairs, lamps, and a rug. However, if the room is unoccupied, as in a house for sale, these values may go unfilled without destroying the living room schema. How do we know such things? This is one of the problems that schema theorists are concerned with. Unlike taxonomic categories such as "animal: cow, horse, dog" the elements of a schema do not imply their superstructure. It is possible to conceive of a sofa without implying a living room; nor is it appropriate to designate a sofa as a living room (as one can designate a cow as an animal). The converse is partially true, however; living room does imply, unless otherwise specified, a sofa as one element within it. A schema can be thought of, then, as a whole consisting of parts.

Rumelhart and Ortony (1977) have identified four essential features of schemata: (1) Schemata have variables. As in the living room example, there may be both obligatory and optional variables to be filled in, and default values may be specified for each. (2) Schemata may be embedded within one another. Just as we have a house schema, we have a living room schema, and we also may have a sofa schema, specifying parts in relation to each other. (3) Schemata are generic concepts that vary in their level of abstraction. The living room schema can be seen to be generic (it applies to any and not to any specific living room), but thus far we have not considered different levels of abstraction. It is clear, however, even within the spatial framework we have been using, that the schema for room is necessarily more abstract than that for living room, and it will become clear later that this is a powerful characteristic of schemata of different types. (4) Schemata represent knowledge rather than definitions. This characteristic does not need to be dwelt on here, except to point out that the categorical approach to knowledge has generally been pursued in the effort to determine what features are necessary to define a structure, abstracting away from those attributes of a structure that are known to be characteristic but not necessary. Schemata are used to characterize what we know – what is generally true as well as what is only occasionally true. (It should be noted that recent theories of category structure such as those in Rosch and Lloyd [1978] also take characteristic, nondefining features into account.)

Thus far the notion of a schema has been discussed primarily in terms of a static structure, in particular the spatial schema of a living room. The great appeal of the notion, however, has been its capability of being extended to structures that are composed in terms of temporal and causal relations as well as spatial ones. Bartlett (1932) used it initially to talk about story schemas, a use that has been revitalized in recent years. Others have referred to planning schemas and problem-solving schemas. In all cases the essential notions of the whole implying related variables and encompassing embedded schematic parts applies although the specific relations and variables may be very different.

It is worth noting that this use of the schema notion departs from its typical use in developmental psychology taken from Piaget. In Piaget's sense a schema derives from an action that can be applied to a range of phenomena in the world, for example, initially sucking and grasping and later in the sensory-motor stage, pulling, pushing, and so on. At the end of the sensory-motor period the child has at his command a set of action schemas that form the foundation for the development of representational thought, but are not themselves representational. Piaget also extends the term to highly abstract structures such as the schema of the permanent object, the number schema, and the operational schemata of the various conservations (Piaget, 1971). These abstractions, although based in the subject's actions, are very different from the use of schemata that has been set forth here.

The present use is more akin to Piaget's figurative knowledge; in this view the schema is essentially representational. It is not constrained to represent the subject's own activities, although it may include them. For example, the child of one year may give good evidence of having a "bath schema" (or script – see the discussion in the following section) as evidenced by his or her anticipation of the sequence of bath activities carried out in partnership with mother (see Church, 1966; Nelson, 1978). Piaget's description of the same situation would likely be in terms of particular component generalized object schemata, or in terms of such abstractions as means-end relations, permanent objects, and so on. The particular level of knowledge about the world, particularly the social world, that the current use of schemata is meant to capture, is neglected in Piaget's conception, for the very reason that Piaget is concerned with the child's construction of a logically consistent knowledge system, and such a system does not well describe the social relationships that the child is engaging in (see Kessen & Nelson, 1978; Nelson, 1979). The primary point to be emphasized is that the use of schema in this account is quite different from its use in Piagetian terminology.

Event Representation: The Script

In order to account for the development of an understanding of social relationships within a participatory framework we need a model of event representations that can specify what the child knows about the routine events that he or she engages in, such as the bath sequence referred to earlier. Such a model has been set forth by Schank and Abelson (1977) in their theory of scripts, a variation on the schema notion, in this case a schema that specifies a sequence of actions related temporally and causally.

In applying the Schank and Abelson model it is important to bear in mind that it was devised initially as a model for a computer understanding system, one that permits appropriate inferences to be made in the course of story or discourse understanding. The description is therefore couched in the terms of this type of model. In their theory the script is a basic level of knowledge representation in a hierarchy of representations that reaches upward through plans to goals and themes. We will be concerned here primarily with the script level, although the other levels are of major importance to adult functioning, and recently both Schank (1979) and Abelson (1979) have indicated modifications and extensions to different types of both more general and more specific memory-organizing packets (MOPS). Scripts are not only concrete and well specified in contrast to the abstract levels of goals and themes, but they are also less problematic than the plan level where problem solving takes place. Their basic concrete nature makes them appear particularly appropriate to the description of the beginnings of children's social knowledge representation.

The script is a general event representation derived from and applied to social contexts.[1] It is basically an ordered sequence of actions appropriate to a particular spatial–temporal context, organized around a goal. The script is made up of slots and requirements on what can fill those slots. That is, the script specifies roles and props and defines obligatory and optional actions. For each of these slots there are default values that are assumed if the person, object, or action is not specified when the script is instantiated in a particular context. For example, in a restaurant script a waiter or waitress is assumed, as are a menu, food, a bill, and a tip. Persons hearing a story about a restaurant can easily fill in these items from their general script knowledge.

To illustrate this concept more concretely consider the following example of a restaurant script constructed from the customer's point of view, based on Schank and Abelson's account.

Script: Restaurant (this is termed the script Header)
Roles: customer, waitress, chef, cashier
Goal: to obtain food to eat (of course other goals may enter in, such as being
    sociable)
Subscript 1: Entering
    move self into restaurant
    look for empty tables
    decide where to sit
    move to table
    sit down
Subscript 2: Ordering
    receive menu
    read menu
    decide what you want
    give order to waitress
Subscript 3: Eating
    receive food
    ingest food
Subscript 4: Exiting
    ask for check
    receive check
    give tip to waitress
    move self to cashier
    move self out of restaurant

At this level the script model is simply a description of what we all know about typical events, knowledge that we can use to make predictions and inferences. Its organization in terms of goals, roles, and hierarchically arranged subscripts is merely a convenience. If this organization represents how such information is organized in memory we should expect certain consequences, such as agreement among adults on necessary elements, and inferences based on the script organization when subjects are asked to recall script-based stories. Bower, Black, and Turner (1979) have recently presented such evidence from experiments with adults.

If young children's knowledge system is script-based, the following implications should follow:

1. Recall or report of an event by a child should contain similar elements in a similar sequence at different recall times.
2. Recall should follow a specific sequence that maps the sequence of events in real life.
3. Because scripts are based on common experience, reports should be similar across children.
4. The report should reveal indications of implicit underlying structure, such as reference to elements that have not been explicitly identified.
5. The report should be couched in general rather than specific episodic terms.

In a number of related studies with children ranging in age from three to eight years, we have found these predictions to hold. In most studies we have used an interview format in which we ask the child to tell "what happens when . . ." he or she engages in a familiar activity such as eating dinner at home, having lunch at the day-care center, going to a restaurant, going grocery shopping, and so on. This format has been supplemented with acting out with props, puppet shows, picture arranging, and story recall. Our general conclusion is that script knowledge in young children is general in form, temporally organized, consistent over time and socially accurate.

As an illustration of the type of data we have in hand, it is of interest to compare the following examples of elicited restaurant scripts with Schank and Abelson's prototype.

1. Well, you eat and then go somewhere. (Boy aged 3; 1)
2. Okay. Now, first we go to restaurants at nighttime and we, um, we, and we go and wait for a little while, and then the waiter comes and gives us the little stuff with the dinners on it, and then we wait for a little bit, a half an hour or a few minutes or something, and, um, then our pizza comes or anything, and, um, (interruption) . . .
   [So then your food comes . . .]
   Then we eat it, and, um, then when we're finished eating the salad that we order we get to eat our pizza when it's done, because we get the salad before the pizza's ready. So then when we're finished with all the pizza and all our salad, we just leave. (Girl 4; 10)
3. First one calls and makes reservations.
   Then you drive there and you get there and the hostess meets
   you and you say you have reservations.
   Then you are seated and given menus.
   Then you discuss around what to eat.
   The food is brought.
   There is a lot of talking.
   Then one lingers over coffee.
   And pays.
   And leaves. (Girl 17; 0)

It is clear that these scripts adhere in major form to the prototype. The youngest child specifies subscripts 3 and 4 including what Schank and Abelson term the MAINCON, "you eat." The four-year-old describes each of the component subscripts – entering, ordering, eating, and exiting – although her script varies from the prototype in its particulars. Note that paying is not a salient part of her script. The seventeen-year-old has a nice skeletal script appropriate to somewhat more cosmopolitan settings than the prototype, and it includes entering, parts of the ordering scene but not ordering itself, the condition for the eating subscript but not eating (!), and the exiting subscript.

In our research we have attempted to probe for specific characteristics of children's event knowledge by interviewing children between the ages of three and eight and asking them to tell us what they know about a number of different particular events. The events we have queried vary in terms of their familiarity to young children, in their novelty, in the degree of their conventionality and the arbitrariness of their sequences, and no doubt in other ways as well. We have found in general that children do organize their script knowledge in terms of a temporal sequence that reflects the actual sequence of events with great veridicality as the restaurant examples illustrate. Although when recounting events the script is told from the child's point of view, there is additional evidence that the child has coded knowledge about others' roles and is able to utilize that knowledge appropriately.

Perhaps the most striking thing that has emerged from this research on children's scripts is their generality. The general account of "what happens" is distinctly different from a narrative account of a particular episode. Even the youngest children that we have tested (young threes) typically respond to our questions with a general skeletal account of a sequence of actions, usually appropriately employing the general "you" and almost always the general tenseless verb (as in the first example of the restaurant script). Responses of this kind have led us to the conclusion that indeed children's script knowledge is generalized, although context-bound, knowledge, structured in such a way as to allow for variations within a frame. Certain acts seem to be obligatory as indicated by their necessary inclusion; there may also be optional slots that can be filled with appropriate values, and there are default values that are assumed for unspecified slot fillers, in much the way that Schank and Abelson describe. Apparently through participation in a routine event the child constructs an expected sequence, in which those actions, roles, and props that vary from one instance to the next take on a general character.

What our investigations have demonstrated most forcefully is that our questions make sense to young children, indicating that they do indeed have knowledge of this form, and that it is understood to be general knowledge, not knowledge about specific happenings. Script descriptions differ from narratives and young children understand this, although specific narratives may be reported when they depart from script expectations in some way. Moreover, the accessibility of this knowledge indicates that it is not simply implicit but is available for social evaluation.

One problem that is apparent in the restaurant script examples is interpreting the significance of missing components in elicited scripts. Because much of our research to date has been based on such elicitation, this problem is worth considering here briefly. When components are omitted it may be an indication that they are missing from the script (as one assumes in the first and second examples) or it may be an indication that they are implicit elements and therefore are easily overlooked in the recounting (as one assumes in the third example). At present there is no certain way to distinguish between these two contradictory explanations in any given case. One aim of our research is to establish general developmental principles with respect to this problem, however. Supplementing verbal accounts with specific probe questions and with acting out are two methods that we have used toward this end.

The script model is not meant to characterize all of social knowledge – indeed it cannot. As noted previously, Schank and Abelson (1977) describe more abstract knowledge schemes, themes that run through much of social interaction, and plans that are more abstract and general than scripts and that are constructed in problem-solving situations. There has thus far been little concern with how scripts and plans are acquired and change with development or how representations of mundane reality such as scripts are related developmentally to abstract categories such as gender roles, belief systems, and attitudes. One aim of this chapter is to consider these questions.

In subsequent sections we will consider three interrelated problems suggested by this model: the acquisition of scripts, their application, and their utility in the formation of more abstract levels of knowledge.

Script acquisition

As we have shown, even young children have script knowledge that is accessible to recounting. If not *the* knowledge organization for the young child it at least seems to be a very important one. However, it seems obvious that children are not born with such knowledge; it is somehow acquired from experience. It is in fact a kind of map or model of experience. It should be emphasized, however, that it is not a particularized, episodic model; rather, children seem to build up generalizations about experience from the beginning. Their scripts are about what usually happens, not about what happened last week, although what happened last week may serve as the basis for their expectation of what will happen next time. In general terms, we can state that the child builds up an event representation from the experience of an event that is structured in specific ways. For example, the component acts of an event are linked temporally and may be linked causally as well. An accurate representation of the event must include these structural relations. Two developmental questions may be asked with respect to this type of structure: Do children understand and accurately code such relations from the beginning, or do they only gradually come to understand them, and, in the acquisition of a particular event representation, do children encode one type of relation first, or is their acquisition of the script more or less haphazard? In either case, under what conditions are scripts acquired? Are some experiences more easily "scripted" than others?

As we noted at the outset, knowledge of social relationships is acquired from social interactions, and some facility in participating in social interactions is present very early in life (Schaffer, 1977; Stern, 1977; Trevarthen 1978). Infants seem predisposed to enter into social exchanges, and these exchanges involve both temporal ordering and role reciprocity. However, although such general "exchange structures" may be important precursors of later social interaction sequences and may even be prerequisites for more precise constructions, they cannot in themselves explain how scripts applicable to specific social contexts are acquired.

Although at this point we have little systematic data, there is considerable evidence that young children's scripts are initially acquired within contexts that are highly structured for them by adults. In this regard, it is of interest to note that although organization around a goal is considered by Schank and Abelson to be an important characteristic of scripts, it may not be central for young children. Most of the script reports we have gathered do include what they describe as the MAIN-CON or central goal act, for example, eating. However, one of the salient facts about the social events that children participate in is that they are most often directed by adults and that the goals involved are the goals of others. Thus children's parts in the interactions are determined for them. What they need to learn is precisely the *script* and their part in it. Adults provide directions for the activities, and often even supply the lines. Consider two very common scripts that we have a good deal of data on: eating dinner at home and having lunch at the day-care center. The presumed goal activity in both cases is eating, and is so specified by the adults involved. However, the children involved do not have any part in planning these activities or anything that goes into them; they simply experience them. In child terms the goal may be pleasing mother or avoiding conflict or getting dessert or any number of other goals, together or separately. But children must nonetheless learn the dinner and lunch scripts from participating in them and being directed in the parts they are to learn to play. This type of learning can be termed *participatory interaction*. Although this is not the only type of learning that leads to script knowledge, it is clearly a very important type. Although adults direct the action and set the goals, they do not necessarily provide direct tuition for the child; rather they provide conditions under which the child fills in the expected role activity.

The knowledge that results from the child's participatory interaction may be quite different from the structure of the event as viewed by the adult. For example, although the child may learn the reciprocal roles of others through learning his or her own part in the event, that knowledge may be distorted or incomplete. For example, paying may not be represented in the child's restaurant script because it is a role activity in which the child plays no part. In the same way, although their understanding of the sequence of activities may be correct from their own point of view, that point of view may be deficient in terms of understanding the logic of a sequence. This deficiency may then be reflected in distortions in the child's account of the event. For example, as we have found, children usually do not understand the sequence of activities that leads to the provision of lunch in their preschool (Nelson, 1978).

Recent research verifies that adults typically structure events in such a way that children can learn their parts. Of course different adults, parents and teachers, may do this more or less consciously and more or less effectively. Bruner (1975; 1978) has reported detailed observations of mothers engaging children in give-and-take games, and later in structuring request sequences in which the child's part is gradually more demanding. Also, recent analyses of preschool interactions (Dore, Gearhart, & Newman, 1978) reflect the conscious structuring of situations by teachers and the directing of children's activities within an overall school script. Indeed, in many day-care centers and nursery schools, very little of the day-to-day activity needs to be negotiated afresh. Each participant knows his or her part in the script. Although adults in family and school are usually aware to some degree of structuring situations for children, they seem rarely to reflect on what the child's event representations of those situations are and how these representations may change with experience.

One natural source of information about children's scripts is their application in fantasy and role play. Routines such as pretending to drive a car are frequently observed in children as young as eighteen months (e.g., Church, 1966). In play it is clear also that although scripts are constructed and (as in our examples) are related from the point of view of the experiencer, even young children give evidence of knowledge of the roles of others. Examples abound (see Garvey, 1977); one in particular from our research, in which two four-year-olds were recorded while carrying on a pretend telephone conversation, follows:

Gay: Hi.
Daniel: Hi.
Gay: How are you?
Daniel: Fine.

Gay: Who am I speaking to?
Daniel: Daniel. This is your daddy, I need to speak to you.
Gay: All right.
Daniel: When I come tonight, we're gonna have . . . peanut butter and jelly
    sandwich, uh, at dinner time.
Gay: Uhmmm. Where're we going at dinner time?
Daniel: Nowhere. But we're just gonna have dinner at 11 o'clock.
Gay: Well, I made a plan of going out tonight.
Daniel: Well, that's what we're gonna do.
Gay: We're going out.
Daniel: The plan, it's gonna be, that's gonna be, we're going to McDonald's.
Gay: Yeah, we're going to McDonald's. And, ah, ah, ah, what they have for
    dinner tonight is hamburger.
Daniel: Hamburger is coming. Okay, well, good-bye.
Gay: Bye. [Nelson & Gruendel, 1979, p. 76]

These two four-year-olds clearly have command of a "mother and daddy dinner planning script"; they act out their roles quite realistically, although of course they have never personally taken part in such a situation. This highlights the fact that observation as well as participation must be an important source of script knowledge. Stories and television also become significant sources at some point. What differences in structure and application different learning conditions may involve are at present unknown but can be fruitfully addressed by future research efforts.

One way in which scripts differ structurally is in terms of the links between acts. Some events are more tightly bound in terms of invariant, temporal, spatial, or causal relations than are others, where the elements can be rearranged without destroying the coherence of the whole. Young children appear to be sensitive to these aspects of structure; they more readily link acts in invariant sequences in their reports, and they use temporal terms to link acts that are invariant or causal before they apply these terms to more loosely structured sequences (Nelson, 1979). It is possible that different learning conditions will be reflected in the child's understanding of causal and temporal links.

The application of scripts

We have seen that scripts are acquired through participation in or observation of their application. Once acquired, what is the range and utility of their application? Basically, scripts serve as a guide to routine encounters with the world. They enable the individual to predict what will happen next in a familiar situation, to infer unstated propositions in a given context, and when well established, to run through a sequence of actions and interactions more or less automatically. In other words, scripts tell people what to do in familiar situations, thus freeing them from constantly attending to the ongoing action. The cognitive space so gained can be used in the consideration of elements of the situations that are problematic – variations from the routine, obstacles to the completion of a goal, negotiations between individuals engaged in an activity together, problem-solving activities of all kinds. Although a great deal of emphasis has recently been put on the construction of plans and the negotiation of a problem space within a task framework, this emphasis plays down the very large amount of context-dependent knowledge that individuals bring to familiar encounters.

Consider the person who does not have a script for a particular event context. This might be a child beginning school, a young person in a new job, a novice gambler in a Las Vegas casino. Every encounter is problematic. There are no predictive rules, no way of understanding the signs and signals. With luck a teacher or co-worker will provide the structure and the interpretations. The second day requires less concentration on what happens when, and by the second week the routine has become the background against which each day's special activities stand out. A well-learned script is really very boring, but it is also very helpful; without it we are quite literally lost. And although we may find our way by guidance or by trial and error this process takes mental effort that is not required once the representation is in place. As adults we encounter relatively few unscripted situations. In fact we import our expectations from well-known scripts onto novel situations, sometimes (as in foreign cultures) leading to misunderstandings. However, young children begin with few scripts; much of their ongoing cognizing space must be spent in building new ones and differentiating the old. Correspondingly they will be more preoccupied with the details of activities than an adult and are likely to be less accurate in identifying the crucial as opposed to the incidental script components. By grade school years, children are script experts; they readily divide up their day into well-defined events (such as recess, math lesson) and can articulate the rules for each event (Clement, 1979).

While scripts enable the individual to concentrate on the novel or problematic in a new situation, they also serve social encounters crucially by providing a shared knowledge base within which interactions take place. Although some negotiation between participants usually is necessary, without shared scripts every social act would need to be negotiated afresh, effectively prohibiting action. Indeed, one can think of script knowledge as precisely cultural knowledge that enables people within a given culture to operate effectively together. It is the lack of shared scripts and the conflict between scripts within a given situation that produces cultural conflict. The acquisition of scripts is in this sense basic to the acquisition of culture itself.

It appears that in any interaction, the individual draws on a script that may be more or less appropriate to that context. Individual scripts may be expected to vary as a function of prior experience with similar contexts, and also as a function of the person's general level of cognitive development. In particular cases the script may be inappropriate in a number of ways. It may be appropriate to a different context; it may not specify important elements – roles, actions, props; it may specify these incorrectly. Thus an important factor to consider with respect to the activation of scripts in the real world is the potential for matching and mismatching; this may occur in two ways. On the one hand, the individual's script may fit the event structure in the real world, or it may err in some way, for reasons deriving either from deviant prior experience or from distortions in the script itself. On the other hand, the individual's script may match or mismatch the scripts of others in the situation. Because all participants come to the interaction with their own scripts based on their own prior experience there is always the possibility that they may mismatch in some way, and negotiation may become necessary.

There is a very nice illustration of matching and mismatching in one of the dialogues from our research. Here two four-year-old girls are comparing their "snack scripts." Note how important agreement on the structure of snacks appears to be to them. Not only does it occupy an extensive portion of their conversation, but when they come to places where their scripts apparently do not match, they find it necessary to discuss these and find some common ground for agreement. Note that for details, variable fillers (e.g., what one has for snacks, who comes), there does not need to be the same kind of agreement. For example, they recognize without concern that they may know different children.

G-1: And also, at night time, it's supper time.
G-2: Yeah, at night time it's supper time. It is.
G-1: It's morning.
G-2: At morning, it's lunch time!
G-1: At morning, we already had breakfast. Because at morning, it's lunch time!
G-2: RIGHT!
G-1: Yeah, at morning, it's lunch time.
G-2: At morning it's lunch time.
G-1: But, *first* comes snack, then comes lunch.
G-2: Right . . . Just in school, right?
G-1: Yeah, right, just in school.
G-2: Not at home.
G-1: Well, sometimes we have snacks at home.

G-2: Sometimes.
G-1: Sometimes I have a snack at home.
G-2: Sometimes I have a snack at my home, too.
G-1: Uh-hum. Because when special children come to visit us, we sometimes have snack. Like, like, hotdogs, or crackers, or cookies or, something like that.
G-2: Yeah, something. Maybe cake. (Laughs)
G-1: Cake.
G-2: Cake. Yeah, maybe cake.
G-1: Or maybe, uh, maybe, hotdog.
G-2: Maybe hotdog.
G-1: But, but, but, Jill and Michael don't like hotdog. Don't you know, but, do you know Michael or Jill?
G-2: I know another Michael.
G-1: I know, I know another Michael.
G-2: No, I know just one Michael. I just know one Michael.
G-1: Do you know Flora?
G-2: No! But you know what? It's a, it's it's one, it's somebody's bro . . . it's somebody's brother.
G-1: Are you eating your dinner? (Laughs) But not for real.
G-2: Not for real.
G-1: Because at morning, it's lunch time.
G-2: Right, at morning it is lunch time.
G-1: Right, at morning it is lunch time.
G-2: Yeah.
G-1: I think . . . I'll have . . . lunch. [Nelson & Gruendel, 1979, pp. 80–81]

Shared scripts may become social customs or conventions. It is interesting that even our most private routines, such as dressing in the morning, are subject to established scripts common to a given culture. Not surprisingly, the preschoolers whom we interviewed share common scripts for getting dressed in the morning as well as for social situations such as going to a restaurant. There is a classic sketch in one of the episodes of the television comedy "All in the Family" in which Archie Bunker and his son-in-law engage in a heated discussion about whether it is "correct" to follow the sequence sock-shoe, sock-shoe or sock-sock, shoe-shoe. It is obvious that "correct" scripts are the hallmark of the "cultured" person in any society. And as the example of the snack exchange shows, young children strive to agree on script knowledge in an apparent convergence on the cultural "truth."

As noted previously, in most instances the real-life scripts in which children engage are directed by adults. Although our interviews have revealed extensive knowledge about these situations by young children, it is in play that one can observe this knowledge most completely and naturally. When children "play house" or "school" they are not directed by adults and must rely on their own scripts to direct the action, determine role content, and so on. In some of our studies we have used props (a school house, a McDonald's model, and so on) and have found that in enactive play the children include more information about roles and props than they do in verbal recall. When children engage in cooperative imaginative play the extent of their script knowledge is revealed as in the telephone dialogue quoted previously. Here the two four-year-olds have simultaneously invoked a telephone script, a dinner script, and a restaurant script, and although some of the details are faulty (for example, the dinner hour), the structure is not, and the role play of father and mother is strikingly true to life.

In both the snack conversation and the telephone conversation, it is clear that talk between peers as young as four can be cooperative and can sustain a topic over a large number of turns, where each turn is linked to those preceding it. In other words, a high capacity to sustain dialogue is evident in these examples. Yet prior work (beginning with Piaget, 1926) indicates that four-year-olds appear to be quite egocentric in their discussions with peers. We have suggested (Nelson & Gruendel, 1979) that when dialogue is organized around shared script knowledge as it is in the examples given here, children will reveal a high level of competence in exchanging information and keeping a conversation "on target," that is, sustaining a topic over many turns. On the other hand, when there is no shared script, when the situation is novel, when one or both participants lack script knowledge, or when a script is not invoked (as in play with blocks or artwork), then the conversational support of the shared script will be lacking and "egocentric" speech may result. Young children do not appear to be very skilled negotiators of uncharted social territory. A fruitful area for further investigation is the specification of how they begin to deal cooperatively with problems and plans when scripts are lacking.

The importance of shared script knowledge to the development of play and conversation with peers is a natural extension of its presumed importance to the beginnings of conversation in mother-child dyads. Analysis of such exchanges has only begun but it appears that children begin to take their part in contexts that are well structured and well understood in script terms. When the context is not so structured, the child is likely to falter, to misunderstand, or to contribute irrelevantly.

At the other end of the spectrum, the talk of adults may also appear egocentric when shared scripts are absent. This will most often happen when the individuals are not aware of the discrepancy; when there is awareness, adults, unlike young children, are usually capable of repairing, explaining, and thereby establishing a shared perspective.

These examples of the knowledge displayed by young children bring out an important point – children and adults alike often act competently in a structured routine situation without either tacit or articulated knowledge of the script as viewed from another's point of view and without full knowledge of the rules and goals involved. Knowing one's part does not necessarily involve knowing how the play is constructed – the perspective of the playwright is not shared by the bit player. Quinn's (1976) research on the litigation system of the Mfantse people of Ghana illustrates this point nicely. She notes: " . . . apprentices may operate for relatively long periods of time with erroneous or partial understandings of the litigation system. They can correct their models of the system . . . only by attending to new cases which come along, searching for regularities in the settlement of these cases" (Quinn, p. 347). Quinn sees this as a basic and pervasive method of learning natural systems. It is not simply that people cannot talk about what they know, but often that they do *not* know but can act anyway on the basis of partial knowledge, incomplete rules, and appropriate cues. Action without comprehension is, we believe, the typical situation of the young child, whose confidence in the face of ignorance is truly impressive.

Abstracting from script representations

Script knowledge, although generalized, remains close to the structure of real world events. The ideal script is one that is just skeletal enough to include all the reliable and expected components, but open and flexible enough to include slots for all possible acceptable tokens. Scripts specify acceptable tokens that may fill their open slots, but cannot account for how more abstract categories, for example, knowledge of appropriate role behaviors in different contexts, are built up. That is, scripts are a first level of approximation to the real world; they constitute a basic but limited level of social cognition. The problem then is to account for how more abstract categories of knowledge are related to the mundane level of script knowledge. Thus far our research has not really addressed this problem; we have been concerned instead to describe the form that the young child's knowledge takes, and it seems clear that the script form serves its purpose of representing dynamic relationships from experience and providing a framework within which the child may competently play out a role in a familiar setting without understanding role relations in themselves.

Before many years, however, children are able to articulate knowledge about what is and is not true *in general* and not only in specific situations. They can talk about the general categories of good and bad, truth and falsehood, men and women, brothers and sisters. Somehow this knowledge too is built up without direct tuition. The most reasonable assumption is that it is abstracted from the script level of knowledge representation. That is, categorical knowledge is derived from script knowledge rather than directly from experience.

There is a parallel here with language that may be helpful. We have spoken of script knowledge as a type of schematic knowledge. It may also be characterized in terms of syntagmatic relations as compared to paradigmatic relations. In linguistics these two types of relations are pervasive and they seem to be applicable to the problem at hand. As Lyons (1969) states: "By virtue of its potentiality of occurrence in a certain context a linguistic unit enters into relations of two different kinds. It enters into *paradigmatic* relations with all the units which can also occur in the same context . . . ; and it enters into *syntagmatic* relations with the other units of the same level with which it occurs and which constitute its context" (p. 73). Probably the most familiar usage of this concept in psychology is in terms of paradigmatic and syntagmatic word association responses (see, for example, Ervin, 1961; Nelson, 1977). Words that can occur in the context of one another in sentences (for example "high mountain") are considered to be related syntagmatically, whereas words that can occur in the same sentence context (for example, "mountain, hill") are said to be related paradigmatically. More generally, instances of word classes such as noun or verb are related paradigmatically while these classes are related to one another syntagmatically. It is a well-established finding that in general younger children give more syntagmatic responses on word association tests than do older children and adults, whose responses, especially to nouns, are very largely paradigmatic (but see Nelson, 1977 and Petrey, 1977 for alternative explanations of this phenomenon).

Consider in this regard the script context. Relations between elements within a single script are syntagmatic whereas relations between elements occupying the same slot in a script are paradigmatic. For example, we can schematize the child's typical "lunch at the day-care center" (from Nelson, 1979) as shown in the diagram.

Here we have certain acts, people, and objects in syntagmatic relations with one another at different levels. In some cases there are no open slots (the cots are always the same for example), while in others there is an open class of slot fillers (children, toys, teachers, foods) the members of which stand in paradigmatic relation to each other. These classes may be the beginnings of the child's categories; indeed, such slot-filler groupings may constitute those first early categories found in the vocabularies of two-year-olds (Nelson, Rescorla, Gruendel, & Benedict, 1978).

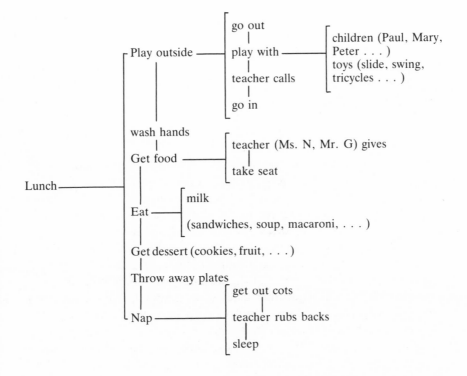

Beyond the categories established from a single script, however, lie those that are established on the basis of similar roles in a number of different scripts. For example, the teacher role is played out in a variety of schoolday scripts, and knowledge of his or her general role is based on the accumulation of evidence across these domains. But research reported by Clement (1978) supports the assumption that building up role knowledge from the event knowledge base is a slow process and proceeds first in terms of syntagmatic relations and later in terms of more abstract paradigmatic relations. When presented with words specifying school roles (e.g. teacher, principal) kindergarten children (five–six years) give activity definitions whereas older children (twelve–thirteen years) give relational responses such as nice or mean. The first type of response appears to be based directly on script knowledge, whereas the latter is an abstraction from it, the result of comparing and contrasting roles in different scripts for the same and different people, that is, relating paradigmatically. Incidentally, Clement (1978) also presents evidence that this result is experience-dependent and not solely age-dependent in that family/kin responses were more abstractly represented by both age groups, suggesting that it was not age per se but years of experience with family roles that produced the categorical types of structures.

The general argument here is that the child's experiential knowledge is structured in a way that contains both syntagmatic and paradigmatic relations; and that the child first has access to syntagmatic relations of rather specific sorts. These syntagmatic relations may next be generalized from different contexts; categories may be established on this basis; and finally relations between the abstract paradigmatically based categories may be defined.

It is worth noting that a recent theory of language development (Maratsos & Chalkley, 1980) suggests a similar progression of syntactic knowledge in which knowledge of word classes is presumed to be an outcome of relational analysis of sentences rather than an a priori of grammatical construction as earlier theories presupposed. In both cases the essential steps in development are seen as being from a rather direct representation of dynamically experienced relationships to an increasingly more general, abstract, and therefore more static and categorical representation.

In addition to role and other categorical knowledge, there are other types of schematic structures that seem to have their basis in scripts, although exactly how has yet to be spelled out. For example, plans are more abstract than scripts. We are currently investigating how children may use scripts in planning functions. It seems likely that scripts that are organized around the child's own goals may be more amenable to entering into plans than those that are organized around adult's goals. In addition, the relations between scripts and stories needs to be established. Clearly both children and adults call up scripts when hearing or reading a story. What is not clear is whether a story schema is simply an elaborated script or whether even for young children the two are essentially different. Certainly young children tend to tell script-based stories, as Gruendel's (1980) research has shown. However, this may be a production difficulty associated with the lack of a well-established story schema. Again this possibility deserves direct investigation.

In summary, it seems clear that children's knowledge of the social world is script based and may remain at that level for many years. Although this level enables the child to enter competently into social relationships, it does not represent a very sophisticated categorical structure. It is general but concrete. To understand the development of the child's knowledge one must begin at this level. In many cases one may not need to go very much beyond it. Indeed, it seems a fair speculation that most of us operate at this level much of the time as Schank (1976) and Abelson (1977) originally suggested.

Note

1 Strictly speaking a script can be asocial and individual, applicable to situations such as getting dressed in the morning or making preparations for and going through the motions of writing a paper. However, even these routines are heavily loaded with cultural meaning and probably derive from social experiences.

References

Abelson, R. P. Script processing in attitude formation and decision making. In J. S. Carroll and J. W. Payne (Eds.), *Cognition and Social Behavior*. Hillsdale, N.J.: Lawrence Erlbaum Associates 1976.

The interaction of feelings and goals. Talk presented at SSRC Workshop on the Representation of Cultural Knowledge, August 12, 1979.

Bartlett, F. C. *Remembering: A study in experimental and social psychology.* Cambridge: Cambridge University Press, 1932.

Bower, G. H., Black, J. B., and Turner, T. J. Scripts in memory for text. *Cognitive Psychology,* 1979, *11,* 177–220.

Bransford, J. D., & Franks, J. J. The abstraction of linguistic ideas. *Cognitive Psychology,* 1971, *2,* 331–50.

Bruner, J. From communication to language – a psychological perspective. *Cognition,* 1975, *3,* 255–87.

Acquiring the uses of language. The Berlyne Memorial Lecture, Toronto, March 1978.

Church, J. (Ed.). *Three Babies.* New York: Random House, 1966.

Clement, D. C. *Children's understanding of school roles and school people.* Paper presented at American Anthropological Association Meeting, Los Angeles, California, November 18, 1978.

Dore, J., Gearhart, M., and Newman, D. The structure of nursery school conversation. In K. E. Nelson (Ed.), *Children's Language* (Vol. 1). New York: Gardner Press, 1978.

Ervin, S. M. Changes with age in the verbal determinants of word association. *American Journal of Psychology,* 1961, *74,* 361–72.

Garvey, K. *Play.* Cambridge, Mass.: Harvard University Press, 1977.

Goffman, E. *Frame Analysis.* New York: Harper & Row, 1974.

Gruendel, J. M. *Children's memory for real-life events.* Doctoral dissertation, Yale University, 1980.

Halliday, M. A. K. Meaning and the construction of reality in early childhood. In H. L. Pick, Jr. & E. Saltzman (Eds.), *Modes of perceiving and processing information.* Hillsdale, N.J.: Lawrence Erlbaum Associates, 1978.

Kohlberg, L. Stage and sequence: the cognitive-developmental approach to socialization. In D. A. Goslin (Ed.), *The Handbook of Socialization, Theory, and Research.* Chicago: Rand McNally, 1969.

Lyons, J. *Introduction to theoretical linguistics.* Cambridge: Cambridge University Press, 1969.

Mandler, J. *Categorical and schematic organization in memory.* Paper presented at Society for Research in Child Development. San Francisco, March 1979.

Maratsos, M. P., and Chalkley, M. A. The internal language of children's syntax: the ontogenesis and representation of synthetic categories. In K. E. Nelson (Ed.), *Children's Language* (Vol. II). New York: Gardner Press, 1980.

Miller, G. A. The organization of lexical memory: Are word associations sufficient? In G. A. Talland & N. C. Waugh (Eds.), *The pathology of memory.* New York: Academic Press, 1969.

Minsky, M. A framework for representing knowledge. In P. H. Winston (Ed.), *The psychology of computer vision.* New York: McGraw Hill, 1975.

Nelson, K. The syntagmatic-paradigmatic shift revisited: a review of research and theory. *Psychological Bulletin,* 1977, *84,* 93–116.

How young children organize knowledge of the world in and out of language. In R. Siegel (Ed.), *Children's Thinking: what develops?* Hillsdale, N.J.: Lawrence Erlbaum Associates, 1978.

Time and space in children's event descriptions. Talk presented to the New York Child Language Group, May 11, 1979.

Nelson, K., and Gruendel, J. At morning it's lunchtime: A scriptal view of children's dialogues. *Discourse Processes,* 1979, *2,* 73–94.

Nelson, K., Rescorla, L., Gruendel, J., and Benedict, H. Early lexicons: what do they mean? *Child Development,* 1978, *49,* 960–8.

Petrey, S. Word associations and the development of lexical memory. *Cognition,* 1977, *5,* 57–72.

Piaget, J. *The language and thought of the child.* New York: Harcourt Brace, 1926.

Biology and knowledge. Chicago: University of Chicago Press, 1971.

Quinn, N. A natural system used in Mfantse litigation settlement. *American Ethnologist,* 1976, *3:2,* 331–51.

Rosch, E., and Lloyd, B. B. (Eds.), *Cognition and Categorization.* Hillsdale, N.J.: Lawrence Erlbaum Associates, 1978.

Rumelhart, D. E., and Ortony, A. The representation of knowledge in memory. In R. C. Anderson, R. J. Spiro, & W. E. Montague, *Schooling and the acquisition of knowledge.* Hillsdale, N.J.: Lawrence Erlbaum Associates, 1977.

Schaffer, H. R. Acquiring the concept of dialogue. In M. H. Bornstein & W. Kessen (Eds.), *Psychological development in infancy: from image to interaction.* Hillsdale, N.J.: Lawrence Erlbaum Associates, 1979.

Schank, R. C. The structure of episodes in memory. In D. G. Bobrow and A. Collins (Eds.), *Representation and understanding.* New York: Academic Press, 1975.

Language and memory. Talk presented at La Jolla conference on Cognitive Science, August 15, 1979.

Schank, R. C., and Abelson, R. *Scripts, plans, goals and understanding.* Hillsdale, N.J.: Lawrence Erlbaum Associates, 1977.

Snow, C. E. Mother's speech research: from input to interaction. In C. E. Snow & C. Ferguson (Eds.), *Talking to Children.* Cambridge: Cambridge University Press, 1977.

Stern, D. N. Mother and infant at play; the dyadic interaction involving facial, vocal and gaze behavior. In M. Lewis and L. Rosenblum (Eds.), *The effect of the infant on its caretaker.* New York: Wiley, 1974.

Trevarthen, C. Modes of perceiving and modes of acting. In H. L. Pick, Jr. & E. Saltzman, *Modes of perceiving and processing information.* Hillsdale, N.J.: Lawrence Erlbaum Associates, 1978.

6 Role taking and social judgment: alternative developmental perspectives and processes

E. Tory Higgins

Man is essentially the role-taking animal. Charles Morris

Social cognition, and its development, has increasingly become a focus of interest to psychologists in recent years (cf. Carroll & Payne, 1976; Damon, 1978; Higgins, Herman, & Zanna, in press; Howe & Keasey, 1978). In developmental psychology, there has been both a theoretical concern with how children's understanding of the social world develops and a practical concern with training and improving social skills. Whether the concern has been theoretical or practical, the psychological construct that has received the greatest emphasis and attention is role taking (cf. Chandler, 1979; Shantz, 1975). What is role taking? How does role taking develop? What is the relation between role taking and social judgment in general, and social inference in particular? The answers to these questions depend upon the processes one posits as underlying role taking. Although various perspectives on role taking have been presented in the literature, no attempt has been made to relate these perspectives to one another in terms of the processes they explicitly or implicitly presuppose. The purpose of this chapter is to examine some of the most influential role-taking proposals, analyze the various types of role-taking processes implicated in these proposals, compare these processes to each other as well as to alternative non–role-taking processes, and consider the implications of these processes for social judgment and its development.

Dimensions underlying role-taking development

Role taking is frequently described metaphorically as "seeing the world through another's eyes" or "putting yourself in another's shoes." There is general agreement in the literature that role taking involves taking into consideration another's viewpoint when making judgments or planning

119

one's behavior, and, thus, role taking has been contrasted with egocentrism in which a person is embedded in his or her own point of view (Piaget, 1926). There is also general agreement that role taking becomes increasingly complex with age. The nature of the dimensions underlying this development, however, is different for different role-taking proposals. This section will review and critically examine these various dimensions and consider their implications.

Independence from stimulus input

Role taking requires that a person "go beyond the information given" in making judgments of another. According to Sarbin (1954), Flavell (Flavell, Botkin, Fry, Wright, & Jarvis, 1968; Flavell, 1974), and others, role taking is a process whereby one apprehends or determines certain attributes of another person. Moreover, with development the attributes become primarily inferential (e.g., another's needs, intentions, etc.) rather than directly perceptible (e.g., another's appearance). In most role-taking proposals, a judgment based on information directly available in the immediate context is not considered to involve role taking. However, simply categorizing a person as tall or young involves "going beyond the information given" to some extent; categorization involves recognizing that the particular instance observed is a member of a specific class, thus accessing information about the class that is not directly available in the instance (cf. Huttenlocher & Higgins, 1978).

What may be critical for role taking, therefore, is not simply whether the judgment "goes beyond the information given" but whether the judgment is an inference about, rather than just a description of, another person. In many cases, of course, it is difficult to know whether or not a judgment involves inference. For example, when someone observes another person smiling and judges that the person is happy, it is unclear whether inference is involved. If smiling is considered to be part of feeling happy, then the judgment would follow directly from the categorization of smiling as "happy behavior." In Piaget's (1958) terms, smiling would be an "index" of the state of happiness (i.e., part of the whole) and, thus, no inference would be necessary to judge the person as happy. In contrast, an inference is likely to be involved in the judgment that a person who gave money to a poor, elderly neighbor is charitable.

Content of judgments

Role taking has been described as increasing in complexity as the mental elements involved in role taking and the judgments resulting from role taking become more "psychological" or abstract. Miller, Kessel, and Flavell (1970), for example, suggest that one aspect of role-taking development is the development from a consideration of others' actions to a considerations of others' thoughts. Chandler (1979) compares the difficulty of different role-taking tasks, and suggests that the tasks require more complex role taking when they involve "second-order" concepts; that is, concepts that were acquired from inferences or mental operations. Role taking has also been considered to increase in complexity as the judgments that result from the role taking become more "psychological" (cf. Livesley & Bromley, 1973). This perspective is based, at least in part, on the empirical evidence suggesting a general development from judgments primarily referring to others' concrete, overt characteristics, such as appearance and behavior, to judgments primarily referring to others' covert, "psychological" characteristics, such as feelings, thoughts, and personality traits (cf. Shantz, 1975). Moreover, because the internal characteristics of others are generally less accessible to observation than the external characteristics of others, and knowledge about internal characteristics is generally acquired later in development, young children's judgments about internal characteristics are more likely to require inferential processes than their judgments about external characteristics. Nevertheless, a general developmental change in the content of judgments does not necessarily reflect a developmental change in the process of role taking (i.e., how the judgment is derived).

A developmental change in the content of judgments could, for example, reflect a developmental change in non-role-taking processes used to make judgments, or it could reflect a developmental change in the kinds of judgments that are emphasized or considered most useful for maximizing goal attainment.[1] Even if the developmental change in the content of judgments reflected some general change in role-taking processes, the type of judgment or mental element involved in role taking is not an adequate criterion for distinguishing levels of role taking. First, a judgment concerning an internal characteristic need not involve an inference (e.g., someone could judge that a person is selfish after being told by various people that they think the person is selfish), and a judgment concerning an external characteristic may involve an inference (e.g., someone could judge that another person is tall when told that the person bumped his/her head on a door lintel). Second, role taking can be just as complex when it involves external characteristics as when it involves internal characteristics. For example, predicting that a child will not eat a ripe apple hanging from the branch of a tree six feet off the ground is more complex when based on the information that the child is only three feet tall (an external characteristic) than when based on the information that the child hates apples (an internal characteristic). Only in the former case must the judge take into consideration both the child's characteristics and the situation's characteristics (i.e., the height of the apple).

Thus, there is no simple correspondence between the content of a role-taking process and its complexity, nor between the content of a judgment and whether role taking is required to make the judgment. In many cases, activation of a category is sufficient to call to mind information that can be directly used to make a judgment without an inference being necessary. Even if the information called to mind through categorization is itself very complex and/or abstract, the judgmental process itself can be relatively simple and not require inference. This is true even when the category information was itself previously acquired through a complex, inferential process (e.g., an abstract proposition derived from a complex series of logical deductions).[2] The emphasis, therefore, should be on the nature of the judgmental process and not the content of the judgment or the elements involved in making the judgment.

Interrelating multiple elements

As role taking develops, the number of mental elements involved in the judgmental process increases and there is increasing consideration of the relations among elements. Previous accounts of role-taking development can be described in terms of this increase. Flavell et al. (1968) and Miller et al. (1970) describe the development of role taking from responses to another person's characteristics (a minimum of one mental element), to responses to another person's responses to another person's characteristics (a minimum of two mental elements), to responses to another person's responses to another person's responses to another person's characteristics (a minimum of three mental elements), and so on. This development requires that the judge simultaneously maintain in active memory an increasing number of mental elements. Moreover, when the judgmental process includes consideration of how each person's response is affected by or depends on the other person's response, this development requires simultaneous consideration of an increasing number of interdependent relations. Similarly, there is a progressive increase in the number of elements and relations that must be kept in mind in Selman and Byrne's (1974) proposed development from Level 1 role taking in which children cannot relate self and other's perspective (subjective role taking), to Level 2 role taking in which children can reflect on self from another person's viewpoint (self-reflective role taking), to Level 3 role taking, in which children can consider the relation between their viewpoint of another person and this other person's viewpoint of them (mutual role taking).

It is also possible to conceptualize Feffer's (1970) three levels of role-taking in terms of a progressive increase in the number of elements and relations considered. Feffer (1970) measured three levels of roletaking through a role-taking task in which subjects were asked to make up an initial story to an ambiguous scene and then retell the story from the viewpoint of each of the characters or roles in the story. At the initial level, a subject in Role 2 considers only Role 2 and does not coordinate with Role 1, and, thus, only one mental element is involved. At the next level, a subject in Role 2 considers Role 2's response in relation to Role 1's response, and, thus, there are two mental elements involved (i.e., Role 2/Role 1) as well as a coordinating relation between them. At the next level, a subject in Role 2 considers Role 2's response in relation to Role 1's viewpoint concerning Role 2, and, thus, there are three mental elements involved (i.e., Role 2/Role 1:Role 2) and separate coordinating relations.[3]

The development of other kinds of social judgments (e.g., moral judgments, attributions of attitudes) may also be reinterpreted in terms of a developmental increase in the number of elements that are considered and interrelated. The traditional emphasis in the moral judgment literature, for example, has been on the development from judgments based predominantly on outcome or consequences to judgments based predominantly on motives or intentions (cf. Piaget, 1965), an age-related change in the content of the elements considered in making the judgment. In naturalistic settings this content development would reflect the development from categorization to social inference because information about outcome is typically directly available whereas information about motives typically requires an inference. Most experimental studies of moral judgment, however, have directly provided subjects with information about both outcome and motives, and, therefore, neither type of information has required an inference in order to be available for consideration. Thus, moral judgments based only on outcome and moral judgments based only on motives would both involve consideration of only a single factor, with the development simply consisting of a change in which type of information is most salient or given greater weight.

When the value and salience of outcome and motives are systematically varied, there is evidence that the development of moral judgment may involve an increase in the number of elements considered rather than the type of element considered. Feldman, Klosson, Parsons, Rholes, and Ruble (1976) presented children aged four–five and eight–nine with

stories in which the motive or intent information was given either before
or after the outcome or consequence information, and the stories varied
systematically in whether the intent was positive or negative and whether
the consequence was positive or negative. The moral judgments of four-
to five-year-olds were based on the evaluative tone of whichever information came last in the story, regardless of whether it was intent or consequence information; that is, their judgments were based solely on the
most recent or most salient information. Although the moral judgments
of the eight- to nine-year-olds were also affected by the salience manipulation (i.e., the information given last had the greatest impact), their
judgments were determined by *both* types of information; that is, regardless of information order, both the intent and consequence information
were considered in their judgments. These results suggest that the critical
developmental change involved the number of elements considered when
making the judgment rather than the type of information considered.

Other kinds of developmental changes in social judgment can also be
interpreted in terms of an increase in the number of elements considered
and coordinated. Karniol and Ross (1976) had kindergarteners, first-
graders, second-graders, and college students listen·to stories about one
child character who freely chose to play with a particular toy, and another
child character who was either ordered to play or was rewarded for playing with the same toy by his or her mother. Kindergarteners' judgments
of which child really wanted (or really liked) to play with the chosen toy
appeared generally to reflect the use of an additive principle (i.e., mother
approval increased attributions of wanting or liking), whereas older children's and adult's judgments appeared generally to reflect the use of a
discounting principle (i.e., mother approval decreased attributions of
wanting or liking). Karniol and Ross suggest that this developmental
change in judgments cannot be explained in terms of "decentration"
because even the kindergarteners considered both the child's behavior
and the mother's behavior in making their judgments. Nevertheless, the
development could be due to an increase in the number of elements
considered. Karniol and Ross suggest that the kindergarteners' judgments
were based directly on the child's choosing the toy and the mother's
positive response to this choice. In contrast, the older children's and
adult's judgments, they suggest, were based on the child's choosing the
toy and their inference that the mother must believe the toy is less enjoy-
able because she orders or rewards the child in order to get the child to
play with it. Because this inference involves additional assumptions or
factors, the older children's and adult's judgments require consideration
of a greater number of elements.[4]

In a developmental study of achievement-related predictions, Kun, Parsons, and Ruble (1974) also found that even the six-year-olds used both the ability and effort information in making their judgments of performance (i.e., they did not "center" on only one cue). However, whereas the six-year-olds appeared to simply combine the independent value of the effort information with the independent value of the ability information in making their performance predictions (i.e., an additive principle), the ten-year-olds and adults appeared to consider not only the independent values of the effort and ability but also the relation between these two values. In particular, the ten-year-olds and adults appeared to assume that differences in ability have a greater effect on performance when effort is high than when effort is low and vice versa. Thus, once again, the results suggest a developmental increase in the number of elements or factors considered when making the judgment.

These studies provide evidence in different spheres of social judgment that suggests a development from considering one factor to considering two factors and a development from considering two factors to considering more than two factors. A study by Collins, Berndt, and Hess (1974) provides evidence in the same social judgment sphere suggesting a development from considering one factor to considering two factors to considering three factors. Kindergarteners, second-graders, fifth-graders, and eighth graders were shown a television program depicting aggression and were asked to evaluate the aggressor. In a detailed analysis of the children's comprehension of the program, Collins et al. found that approximately 70 percent of the kindergarteners mentioned only the aggressive behavior when recounting the plot, approximately 70 percent of the second-graders mentioned both the aggressive behavior and consequences, approximately 40 percent of the fifth-graders mentioned both the aggressive behavior and consequences and another 35 percent of the fifth-graders mentioned motives as well as the aggressive behavior and consequences, and approximately 50 percent of the eighth-graders mentioned motives as well as the aggressive behavior and consequences. Thus, there was a development from considering one factor (behavior) to considering two factors (behavior and consequences) to considering three factors (motives, behavior, and consequences) when recounting the plot. Moreover, although the kindergarteners and second-graders did not differ in the externality of the factors they considered (i.e., behavior and consequences are both external), they did differ in the number of factors they considered.

The proposed development in the number of elements or factors considered in making social judgments is similar in some respects to the general development proposed in recent neo-Piagetian or information processing models (cf. Case, 1978; Pascual-Leone, 1970). Pascual-Leone has suggested that the maximum number of schemas or units of thought that a person's psychological system is capable of simultaneously activating increases linearly with age. The results of the studies described in this chapter are certainly consistent with this proposal. However, a developmental increase in the number of factors considered when making social judgments would not necessarily require a developmental increase in maximum mental effort (Pascual-Leone's M-power). It could be that by routinizing previously acquired schemas and acquiring organizing principles and higher-order schemas (cf. Case, 1978; Miller, 1956; Shatz, 1978) children can increase the number of factors they consider without increasing their mental effort. Thus, we are suggesting that role-taking development consists of a developmental increase in the ability to consider and interrelate multiple factors, and not necessarily a developmental increase in maximum mental effort or attentional capacity.

Controlling the self

Children become progressively better at preventing other viewpoints (in particular, their own viewpoint) from interfering with their judgment of a target person's viewpoint. Piaget's (1932) description of development from a stage when children do not differentiate their own viewpoint from the viewpoint of others to a stage when children differentiate their own viewpoint from others' viewpoint and can take the viewpoint of others is the role-taking development most emphasized in the literature (cf. Chandler, 1969; DeVries, 1970; Flavell et al., 1968; Rubin, 1973; Selman, 1971; Shantz, 1975). According to Piaget, a nonegocentric judgment does not simply or necessarily mean an accurate social judgment but, rather, implies having taken into account another's viewpoint precisely when the viewpoint is different from the judge's own viewpoint (cf. Chandler, 1979). That is, role taking requires controlling one's own viewpoint when making judgments of others.[5]

Controlling one's own viewpoint when making judgments of others can vary in difficulty. It is difficult to recognize that another person may have a different response than oneself because the person is in different circumstances. It is even more difficult, however, to recognize that another person's response may be different even though the person is in the same circumstances. Controlling the self is more difficult when comparing the characteristics of another person to one's own characteristics than when simply judging another person's characteristics. It is still more difficult to judge one's own characteristics from the standpoint of another person. Each of these levels of difficulty in controlling the self is considered in this section.

"Situational" versus "individual" viewpoints. In considering the ability to control competing viewpoints when making judgments of others, a distinction should be made between two different kinds of competing viewpoints – "situational" viewpoints and "individual" viewpoints. The viewpoints of judge and target person may be different either because the judge and target person are in different situations or circumstances (a difference in situational viewpoints) or because the judge and target person have different individual characteristics, such as different personality traits, different abilities, different beliefs or attitudes, and so on (a difference in individual viewpoints). This distinction between situational role taking and individual role taking is reflected in Selman's (1971) distinction between Level C and Level D role taking. According to Selman (1971), children at both levels are able to put themselves in the different situation of another person and differentiate their present viewpoint from the other person's viewpoint. At Level C, however, children assume that the other person's thinking would be similar to their own thinking in the same situation, whereas at Level D children do not make this assumption. Basically, children at Level C judge the other's viewpoint by asking themselves, "What would I do, think, feel, see, etc. if I were in that situation?" (i.e., situational role taking).

Role-taking tasks vary in whether they require situational role taking or individual role taking or both (cf. Higgins, 1977), although it is often difficult to judge which type of role taking is involved. In Piaget's classic "three mountains" task (Piaget & Inhelder, 1956), for example, a child views a scale model of three mountains and must imagine or represent the mountains' visual appearance from the viewpoint of another person whose position relative to the model is different from the child's own position. This task requires situational rather than individual role taking, as the child can solve the task by asking, "If I were sitting in that position, what would I see?" In Krauss and Glucksberg's (1967) referential communication task, the speaker must describe each stimulus in an array of stimuli so that the listener can select the same stimulus from among an identical array of stimuli. This task also requires situational rather than individual role taking, as the child can solve the task by asking, "What information about this stimulus would I need if I had to select it from among this array of stimuli?" On the other hand, Flavell et al.'s (1968) communication Task IIA requires individual role taking, as subjects have to tell a story to a younger child so that the child can understand it, thus requiring subjects to take into account that the younger child's abilities are different from their own.

Children become progressively better at considering their own character- istics and viewpoint in relation to those of others without permitting their own to intrude upon and dominate their judgments. An initial aspect of this development is the ability to take into account differences in individual characteristics and viewpoints rather than simply differences in situational viewpoints. Once individual role taking is achieved, there is a further development of the ability to compare and relate one's own characteristics and viewpoint to those of others, and the ability to judge one's own charac- teristics and viewpoint from the standpoint of others. Each of these devel- opments will be considered in turn.

Situational role taking. Situational role taking may be easier than individ- ual role taking for a number of reasons. First, in situational role taking children can base their judgments on their own personal experiences in the same situation or circumstances, whereas in individual role taking children cannot use their own experiences as a basis for judgment because the target person's experiences in the same situation or circumstances are not assumed to be the same. Second, in situational role taking only the implications of the situation or circumstances need to be considered, whereas in individual role taking the implications of both the circum- stances and the target person's characteristics and viewpoint need to be considered. Both of these kinds of role taking, however, can vary in difficulty depending on the task requirements with respect to inhibiting competing information. Situational role taking is more difficult, for ex- ample, when children's present circumstances directly compete with their judgment or response. For instance, Huttenlocher and Presson (1973) report that children find it much easier to judge the view of a target stimulus from a position different from the position in which they initially viewed the target if they are permitted to actually move to the new position before giving their judgment than if they have to remain in their original position. (In each condition, the target is hidden after subjects have viewed it from their original position.) Thus, even if children judge another person's view of a target (e.g., Piaget's "three mountains") by asking themselves, "What would I see if I were in his position?" such situational role taking would be more difficult if the children must remain in their own position than if they are allowed to actually move to the other person's position. To take another example, in Flavell et al.'s Task IIB, the referential communication task was immediately preceded by a task requiring communicators to describe the target in detail (so someone could draw it exactly). Under these circumstances, it is very difficult for communicators to include only the discriminating information in their referential messages and inhibit or ignore the nondiscriminating information because the nondiscriminating information has recently been made salient. Thus, this referential communication task would involve more difficult situational role taking than Krauss and Glucksberg's (1967) task where the nondiscriminating attributes of the target are not made salient.[6]

Individual role taking. Individual role taking can also vary in difficulty depending on the extent to which competing information relating to one's own characteristics and viewpoint is accessible or salient. For example, children's own feelings are more likely to interfere with predicting how a man feels having his pet python draped around his arm when they suffer from snake phobia (especially when they are asked to make this judgment while actually observing the event). To take another example, older children's personal knowledge of a game is more likely to lead to "egocentric" errors when they are asked to explain it to a younger child than when they are asked simply to predict the extent of a younger child's knowledge of the game. Only when explaining the game is the older child's own knowledge of the game, including its special terminology, an integral part of the task and, thus, likely to intrude.

1. *"Target-only" judgments and "comparison" judgments.* Differences in the difficulty of individual role taking are also involved in the development of role taking. The first level of difficulty is to correctly judge others whose characteristics and viewpoint are different from one's own even when they are in the same situation or circumstances. The next level of difficulty is to compare and relate one's own characteristics and viewpoint to the characteristics and viewpoint of others. In the former "target-only" judgment, children can avoid having their own characteristics and viewpoint intrude upon their judgment by totally inhibiting them or directing their attention away from them. In fact, in some cases the children's own characteristics and viewpoint may be sufficiently nonsalient that there is little need for control. In the latter "comparison" judgment, however, children must keep their own characeristics and viewpoint in mind and pay attention to them in order to compare and relate them to the target person's characteristics and viewpoint. Yet the children must not allow their own characteristics and viewpoint to interfere with or become confused with their judgment of the target person's characteristics and viewpoint. Thus, in comparison judgments children must control their characteristics and viewpoint during the judgmental process while being unable to ignore them.

Target-only judgments and comparison judgments have not been clearly distinguished in the role-taking literature, and this has sometimes led to children's performances being interpreted as reflecting comparison judgments when the performance requires no more than target-only judgments. For example, Borke (1971) found that children as young as three years of age will select different faces for the characters depicted in different situations (e.g., a "happy" face for a child eating a favorite snack; a "sad" face for a child who lost a toy). Borke (1971; 1972) interpreted these results as indicating that even very young children are aware that other people have feelings that are different from their own. That is, Borke interpreted the children's selections as reflecting comparison judgments. However, the children's selections required, at most, target-only judgments.[7] More generally, there is a need to distinguish between children's ability to infer another person's response based on an awareness of the differences between themselves and the other person, which requires a comparison judgment, and children's ability simply to infer another person's response that is different from their own response in the same situation, which does not require a comparison judgment.

2. *"Self-as-object" judgments.* A further level of difficulty in individual role taking is the ability to consider one's own characteristics and viewpoint from the viewpoint of others – "self-as-object" judgments. According to Mead (1934), role taking involves becoming an object to oneself by taking the viewpoint of others toward oneself, and role-taking development consists of acquiring the viewpoint of the group (the "generalized other") rather than the viewpoint of particular other individuals. Alternative perspectives on role-taking development, however, argue that children do not initially have the ability to judge themselves from the viewpoint of a particular other and that the acquisition of this ability is a major step in role-taking development. In Selman and Byrne's (1974) model, for example, the development from Level 1 (subjective role taking) to Level 2 (self-reflective role taking) involves a development of the ability to judge oneself from another person's viewpoint. DeVries (1970) suggests that children are able to take account of another's viewpoint before they are able to take account of another person's taking account of their viewpoint. Flavell et al. (1968) suggest that at any given level of the role-taking hierarchy, operations in which the judge's viewpoint is an object of another's viewpoint have a higher maturity status than operations not including the judge as an object of another's thought.

It is not surprising that self-as-object judgments would be even more difficult than comparison judgments. In both cases, both self and other need to be considered. In the comparison judgment, however, children can take their own standpoint (cf. Turner, 1956) when considering their self, whereas in the self-as-object judgment children must take another person's standpoint when considering their self. Moreover, the self is the specific focus of the judgment for self-as-object judgments, which should make it especially difficult for children to prevent their own standpoint from intruding in the judgment.

An integrated perspective on role-taking development

This review of possible dimensions underlying role-taking development suggests the following conceptualization of role taking and its development. First, role taking involves inferences (rather than just categorization), and role taking can vary in the level of reasoning that is required. Second, role taking involves interrelating two or more mental elements, and role taking can vary in complexity as the number of mental elements and relations increase. Third, role taking involves controlling and, when necessary, inhibiting information competing with the judgment, and role taking can vary in difficulty depending on the salience of the competing information.

The latter two features of role taking reflect a development away from two major characteristics of preoperational thought as described by Piaget (cf. Flavell, 1963) – "centration" and "egocentrism." The ability to interrelate two or more mental elements in active memory reflects a development away from centration, and suggests that such "decentration" is a continuous dimension involving the ability to interrelate an increasing number of mental elements. The ability to prevent the "self" from intruding or dominating judgment reflects a development away from egocentrism, and suggests that such "non-egocentrism" is a continuous dimension involving the ability to control the self under conditions of increasing salience of the self. The differential nature of development along these two dimensions points up the value of maintaining the conceptual distinction between decentration and non-egocentrism. The distinction is also of value when comparing different role-taking tasks because the principal requirement of some tasks is decentration (e.g., coordinating the perspectives of two or three different story characters), whereas the principal requirement of other tasks is non-egocentrism (e.g., communicating to a dissimilar other). In fact, differences among role-taking tasks in whether the principal requirement is decentration (i.e., interrelating multiple elements) or non-egocentrism (i.e., controlling the self) could account for the relatively weak and inconsistent correlations typically found in studies comparing role-taking tasks (cf. Chandler, 1979; Glucksberg, Krauss, & Higgins, 1975; Shantz, 1975). Moreover, the continuous nature of each of these dimensions suggests that the development of these role-taking abilities continues well beyond childhood.

The features of role taking (type of judgment; number of mental elements and relations; controlling competing information) are not specific to role taking but are involved in various areas of cognitive development. For example, there is evidence from problem-solving tasks that the number of items subjects can hold in working memory increases with age (cf. Case, 1978). In addition, the ability to inhibit competing information is an important aspect of development in many cognitive domains (cf. White, 1965). A more unique feature of role taking and, perhaps, the essence of role taking, is the need to prevent one's own personal characteristics and viewpoint (i.e., the self) from intruding upon and interfering with one's inferences about others.

The role of the self in social inferences, however, is often difficult to determine. In many cases, it is difficult to know whether a judgment involved controlling the self or the self simply did not intrude. For example, a target person's behavior and/or circumstances may be so salient or gripping that all of a judge's attention is drawn to it, removing any need for the self to be actively controlled. Another problem is that controlling the self is not an all or nothing process. It is possible for one aspect of a child's self to be inhibited while another aspect intrudes. For example, in a developmental study of moral judgment, Costanzo, Coie, Grumet, and Farnill (1973) found that when a target child's behavior had negative consequences, kindergarteners thought an adult judge would rate the target more positively when the target's intentions had been positive, even though the kindergarteners' own ratings of the target were not affected by whether the target's intentions were positive or negative. These results suggest that the kindergarteners inhibited their own standpoint when predicting the judgment of the adult. However, because the procedure of the study gave the kindergarteners, but *not* the adult, information about the target's intentions, the kindergarteners failed to inhibit their privileged information about the target's intentions when predicting the adult's judgments.

It is also difficult to know whether differentiation of judgments for self and others reflects an actual recognition that one's own characteristics and viewpoint differ from the characteristics and viewpoint of others. A child could successively make different judgments for self and other without ever engaging in a comparison process where self and other are compared together. In addition, if the differentiation involves categorization processes, it would not necessitate any inhibition of self. For example, inhibition of self would not be necessary for a boy to judge that another child is a girl, or, if the proposition "all girls are crybabies" is contained within his "girl" category, to judge that this other child is a "crybaby."

Still another problem of interpretation arises when the judge and the target person have similar characteristics and the judge gives the same judgment for self and other. In such cases, it is unclear whether the judgment of the target person is a result of an inference based on the target person's behavior and/or characteristics, is the result of the judge recognizing the similarity in characteristics and then inferring a similarity in viewpoint, or is a result of the judge's own viewpoint intruding into and overwhelming his judgment of the target person's viewpoint without there being any consideration of the target person's characteristics.

It is evident from these problems of interpretation that it is not always possible to know whether role taking underlies a particular judgment. For this reason, one needs to consider what kind of judgment is especially likely to involve role taking:

Judgments involve role taking when there is an inference about a target's viewpoint (or response) under circumstances where the judge's own viewpoint is salient and different from the target's.

This characterization of role taking has a number of implications. First, it emphasizes that role taking is an inferential process in which a conclusion is drawn by relating separate pieces of information (i.e., consideration of multiple elements). Not only does this rule out judgments based solely on categorization rather than inference, it is consistent with other proposed features of role taking. It is consistent with the notion that role taking involves "going beyond the information given" to make judgments that are not directly evident from observation. It is also consistent with the notion that role taking involves avoiding egocentric errors in judging the viewpoint of others. Categorization involves a one-step process in which a category instance (the stimulus input) activates the category information required to make the judgment. Intrusion of self is relatively unlikely both because one's attention is focused on the stimulus input and because any false judgment from self intrusion would be directly contradicted by the stimulus input. Inference, on the other hand, involves a multistep process in which the final judgment is relatively far removed from the stimulus input. Thus, self intrusion is more likely because one's attention is not so fixed on the stimulus input, false judgments are not directly contradicted by the stimulus input, and there are more steps in the process during which self intrusions could occur. Inference, therefore, requires greater inhibition of self to avoid egocentric errors than does categorization.

This characterization of role taking also emphasizes the ability to judge another person's viewpoint even when it is different from one's own viewpoint and one's own viewpoint is salient or active. If one's own viewpoint were the same as the target's viewpoint, it would not be necessary to take the target's attributes into account. If one's own viewpoint were not salient, inferences about social objects would be no more susceptible to egocentric errors than inferences about nonsocial objects (e.g., a car). However, because social inference is often distinguished from nonsocial inference in terms of the likelihood of such errors, it is important that the conceptualization of role taking include a feature (i.e., salience of the judge's own viewpoint) that assures the possibility of such "egocentric" errors.

An interesting and important question, of course, is how do people inhibit their own viewpoint when judging others? Is there a development in the strategies and operations available for inhibiting one's own viewpoint that is comparable to the development of strategies and operations in other domains (e.g., memory)? Are different strategies used under different conditions? Is there a development in children's awareness of the need to inhibit their own viewpoint or in their knowledge of which strategies are useful (i.e., a development in meta–role taking)? These questions need to be addressed in future research.

A final feature of role taking implicit in this characterization is the notion that role taking requires a recognition that one's own viewpoint can differ from the target person's viewpoint. A number of approaches to role taking suggest that differentiation of judgments for self and others is an initial step in role-taking development (e.g., Elkind, 1967; Flavell et al., 1968; Rubin, 1973). As discussed earlier, however, differentiation of judgments for self and others per se does not require recognition that one's own viewpoint is different from the viewpoint of others, and it is the recognition of potential or actual differences – Flavell's (1974) "Existence 2" – that would seem to be the important initial step in role taking. When the target person's viewpoint is different from one's own viewpoint and one's own viewpoint is salient, recognition of potential or actual self–other differences becomes necessary. Such recognition may develop from a recognition that self–other differences in circumstances can cause self–other differences in viewpoint (required for situational role taking) to a recognition that self–other differences in personal characteristics can cause self–other differences in viewpoint even in the same circumstances (required for individual role taking). Recognition of individual self–other differences in turn may often require some self inhibition in order for the differences to be noticed in the first place. Thus, learning how to inhibit intrusions of personal characteristics may facilitate the development from situational to individual role taking. On the other hand, the increasing recognition of self–other individual differences is likely to increase children's awareness of the need to inhibit intrusions of their personal characteristics. That is, if a child is unaware of self–other individual differences in a particular domain (e.g., responses to large dogs), the child is unlikely to inhibit self intrusions when making judgments in that domain even though the child inhibits self intrusions in other domains (e.g., responses to meals).

Interpreting performance on role-taking tasks

This perspective on role taking and its development suggests the need to reconsider previous interpretations of performance on role-taking tasks. Is role taking sufficient, or even necessary, for successful performance on traditional "role-taking" tasks? When role taking is required for successful performance on a task, are there alternative role-taking processes that could underlie accurate judgments? When children inaccurately use their own viewpoint in judging the viewpoint of others, does this necessarily reflect an absence of role taking? These issues of interpretation are examined in this section.

Role taking as neither sufficient nor necessary for performance

The role of role taking in children's performance on previous "role-taking" tasks has frequently been overinterpreted. That is, performance has been interpreted in terms of role taking both when the task requires much more than role taking for successful performance (i.e., role taking is not sufficient) and when the task does not require role taking for successful performance (i.e., role taking is not necessary).

When role taking is not sufficient. Successful performance on some traditional "role-taking" tasks has been interpreted in terms of role taking and its development when a necessary, and sometimes defining, requirement of the task has been the ability to employ some additional non-role taking process. For example, in describing the levels of role taking involved in visual role taking (what is the other seeing?), Flavell (1974) proposes a Level 3, which consists of the ability to infer another's exact retinal-image percept, in contrast to Level 2, which consists of the ability to infer another's visual perspective (how the stimulus appears in the other's location). The development from Level 2 to Level 3 would seem to require not so much an increase in role-taking ability per se as it requires the acquisiton of a rather complex cognitive operation for forming exact retinal images.

It has also frequently been suggested that role playing (e.g., a child assuming the role of an adult) requires role taking (cf. Kelley, Osborne, & Hendrick, 1975; Mead, 1932), where role playing (as distinct from role enactment) is the symbolic representation of the behavior of others in one's own behavior. Role taking has been considered to be the basic process underlying role playing, in part because role taking and role playing have both been considered to be symbolic processes (cf., Blumer, 1962; Mead, 1934; Sarbin & Allen, 1969). However, the role taker's response does *not* designate the response of the other and is, therefore, not symbolic, whereas role playing is symbolic (cf. Huttenlocher & Higgins, 1978). Thus, the critical ability underlying role playing is not the ability to role take but the ability to symbolically represent others' behavior in one's own behavior.

When role taking is not necessary. Successful performance on many traditional "role taking" tasks does not necessarily require role taking. Some referential communication tasks, for example, require communicators to describe the referent in the context of different nonreferents, where the discriminating property (or properties) of the referent varies depending on the nonreferent context (cf. Ford & Olson, 1973; Harris, 1978; Higgins & Akst, 1975) The children could vary their descriptions because the salient property (or properties) of the referent varies in different contexts (i.e., a "context" effect on judgment), so that role taking may not even be necessary for successful performance. There are other communication tasks for which role taking may not be necessary for successful performance. For example, Shatz and Gelman (1973) have found that four-year-olds' descriptions of how to play with a toy are shorter and simpler when their listener is a two-year-old than when their listener is an adult. It is possible that even young children learn that a particular speech style is appropriate when talking to a very young child, or, indeed, to any small object (e.g., a dog, a cat, a doll). In fact, Sachs and Devin (1976) found that young children's speech was also relatively short and simple when talking to a doll. Thus, categorization of the listener as a small child or childlike object may activate rules for appropriate speech style without role taking being required. Recently, there has been an increasing concern with the extent to which role taking is necessary for successful performance on communication tasks (cf. Chandler, Greenspan, & Barenboim, 1974; Higgins, 1976; Shantz, in press).

Other tasks have also been interpreted as involving role taking even though successful performance on such tasks would not require role taking. Feffer (1970), for example, argues that role taking is involved in social interaction when the actions of the participants are different and complementary, and are executed simultaneously and with reference to each other, such as when two boys carry a log together. However, each of these conditions can be met when two ants work together to carry a large seed to their nest, and certainly such interaction does not require the participants to inhibit their own viewpoint while inferring the viewpoint of the other. As mentioned previously, Borke (1971; 1972) interpreted successful performance on "empathy" tasks as reflecting an initial level of role taking. There are a variety of processes, however, that do not involve role taking that are sufficient for successful performance on such tasks (cf. Chandler & Greenspan, 1972; Shantz, 1975). The situation of the target person could directly elicit an emotional response in the judge, which is then projected on to the target. Alternatively, the situation of the target person could remind the judge of a previous personal experience in which he/she felt a particular emotion in a similar situation, with this emotion then being projected on to the target. It is also possible that the situation of the target person could be categorized by the judge as being an instance of a particular type of situation, with a particular emotion being part of such situations.

Successful prediction of a target person or target group's abilities or preferences has also been interpreted in terms of role taking, although role taking need not be involved. For example, findings that five–six-year-olds will select different and appropriate gifts for their mother, father, and an opposite-sex peer (Zahn-Waxler, Radke-Yarrow, & Brady-Smith, 1977) and four–five-year-olds will select different and appropriate gifts for a peer and a two-year-old (Shatz, 1978) have been interpreted as reflecting social inference or role taking. In interpreting the results of another study on preference prediction, Higgins, Feldman, and Ruble (in press) suggest an alternative, non–role-taking process that could underlie social prediction – "social category knowledge."

Higgins et al. (in press) presented four–five-year-olds, eight–nine-year-olds, and undergraduates with separate arrays of snacks, meals, and activities depicted on cards and, for each array, asked subjects to select the item they liked best, the item they thought other persons their own age (i.e., peers) would like best, the item they thought "grown-ups" (i.e., older nonpeers) would like best, and the item they thought "two-year-olds" (i.e., younger nonpeers) would like best. All age groups, including four–five-year-olds, significantly differentiated their selections for peers, older nonpeers, and younger nonpeers, and there was no developmental difference in the extent of differentiation. Subjects in each age group selected their own personal preference significantly more often for peers than nonpeers. In addition, in every age group the amount of agreement in selecting the most preferred item in an array for each target group was substantially and significantly greater than chance. Thus, the differentiation of selection for different target groups was not a result of either random selection or an implicit demand to select a different item on each trial. However, the accuracy of selections for grown-ups (as determined by comparing a subject's selection for grown-ups with the actual selections of a group of thirty–fifty-year-olds obtained from the same community as the subjects) was significantly greater for eight–nine-year-olds than for four–five-year-olds, and was significantly greater for undergraduates than for eight–nine-year-olds.

Interpreting these results in terms of "social category knowledge," Higgins et al. (in press) suggest that a subject could retrieve stored information about the category of people whose preferences are to be predicted. For example, when predicting activity preferences for grown-ups, an older child may retrieve the information that "grown-ups love to read." This information may have been acquired from the person's own observations of grown-ups, from statements about grown-ups' activity preferences provided by others, and so on. Social category knowledge could have been used by each age group in our study, resulting in differentiated predictions for the different target groups. Moreover, both the accuracy of the social category knowledge and the ability to apply it could increase with age because social experience increases with age, thus accounting for the developmental increase in accuracy. The use of social category knowledge to make preference predictions does not require social inference or role taking because the information is stored within the category (i.e., part of the whole) and is activated when the category is activated.

In sum, role taking is neither sufficient nor necessary for successful performance on many "role-taking" tasks. This could also help explain why studies comparing different "role-taking" tasks and measures have typically found relatively weak and inconsistent correlations, especially when age is partialled out (cf. Chandler, 1979; Glucksberg et al., 1975; Shantz, 1975).

Social reference and social deduction as alternative role-taking processes

Social judgment through role taking can involve either inductive or deductive inference. Developmental differences in preference prediction have been interpreted in terms of both of these types of role taking. Higgins et al. (in press) suggest an inductive inference process, "social reference," as another possible explanation for their results. They suggest that a person could retrieve information about a salient or typical member of the target group and assume that the group's preferences are the same as that member's. Rosch (1975) has suggested that natural categories (e.g., colors, line orientations) have reference point stimuli (i.e., focal colors, vertical and horizontal lines) in relation to which other stimuli of the category are judged. Analogously, social categories (e.g., grown-ups) may have prototypic or especially salient members (e.g., parents, grandparents) who serve as reference points for predicting the motives, attitudes, responses, and the like of other members of the same social category. These prototypic or salient members can be used to predict the responses of other individual members of the category and the group or category as a whole. Sarbin, Taft, and Bailey (1960) suggest that people will sometimes infer a characteristic of a group or individual member of the group by analogy with a significant member of the group. In addition, there is evidence that people will assume that even very small samples are representative of the population from which they are drawn (Nisbett & Borgida, 1975; Tversky & Kahneman, 1971). Another variation of social reference that occurs when making judgments of individuals is to predict the responses or characteristics of the target person on the basis of one's knowledge of a salient person (or "significant other") who the target person resembles in some way (cf. Sarbin et al., 1960; Higgins & King, in press). For example, a woman may judge a target male to be "domineering" and "belittling" because he reminds her of her father or a high school teacher who was domineering and belittling.

The factors underlying the relative salience or accessibility of a person, and thus the likelihood the person will be used in social reference, also need to be examined. A number of factors are known to affect accessibility, such as frequency and importance (cf. Higgins & King, in press), but it is unclear how activation of the social reference leads to the prediction. It is possible that once the social reference is activated the judge searches for those behaviors or responses of the social reference that are relevant to the judge's task (e.g., searching for the activities of his/her mother), and whichever behavior is remembered first (i.e., is most accessible) is assumed to be most important to the social reference. Alternatively, the judge may search for those behaviors that the social reference has previously emphasized or paid special attention to when the judge was present (e.g., mothers showing their children how to make their beds), and these behaviors are assumed to be most important to the social reference.[8] It is also possible that a judge will attempt to calculate the actual frequency of different behaviors of the social reference and assume that high-frequency behaviors are most important to the social reference. A judge may even have heard the social reference state his/her preference and use this statement as the basis for prediction. Which of these strategies, if any, are actually used, and whether there are developmental differences in which strategies are used, are unexplored questions.

Social reference could also have been used by each age group in the Higgins et al. (1977) study, resulting in differentiated predictions for the different target groups. The developmental increase in accuracy could then be due to a number of factors. It may be that the types of people serving as social references change developmentally, and that the social references used by older children and adults are more representative or typical of their social category than the social references used by young children. For example, in some pilot studies we found that four–five-year-olds almost always use their parents when predicting for grown-ups whereas older children and adults frequently use salient people in the media (e.g., television newscasters, political figures, etc.). It may be that salient people in the media are projected to be relatively representative of their social category.

It is also possible that older children, and especially adults, are more likely to use a two-stage judgmental process in which they reject a highly salient or accessible group member if they decide that he/she is not representative of the target group. For example, there was some evidence in our pilot studies that some older children first thought of one of their parents when asked to select for grown-ups, but then decided their parent was "not like other grown-ups" and selected the preference of another grown-up (e.g., their best friend's mother or a grown-up living next door) who they thought was "more like other grown-ups." If the use of such a two-stage social-reference process increases with age, then one would expect social-reference judgments to increase in accuracy with age, provided, of course, that people perform at better than chance levels when determining representativeness. This expectation raises the interesting questions of how people determine representativeness or select representative examplars and whether these operations or strategies change developmentally. For example, children may be more inclined than adults to use popularity as a measure of representativeness and, thus, select a popular recording star or athlete or a popular teacher as the social reference for grown-ups.

As mentioned previously, the use of social reference to make preference predictions involves inductive inference, but it is also possible to make preference predictions through the use of deductive inference. Shatz (1978), for example, reports that one of the children in her study defended his choice of a pull toy for the two-year-old target by arguing that the sewing cards were "too hard for little hands." Shatz (1978) suggests that the children in her study based their preference predictions on an analysis of the implications of the general characteristics (e.g., abilities) of two-year-olds for playing with each toy given its characteristics (e.g., task demands) – a deductive inference strategy. It seems likely, however, that a deductive inference strategy would be used only when simpler strategies, such as social category knowledge or social inference, are not available. This may be the case for certain social predictions. For example, when five-year-old children in a study by Markham (1973) were asked to guess how many balls of a particular size a two-year-old could hold in one hand, a primitive type of deductive inference strategy may have been used, as the children were unlikely to have relevant social category or social reference information to draw upon. Of course, other strategies could have been used, such as assuming that the number of balls would be less than the children themselves could hold. In any case, it may be rare that a person needs to use deductive inference in order to predict the responses of others. It seems likely that people would first use social category knowledge to predict others' responses when the necessary social category information is available, and, when it is not, they would use social reference to make their judgments, with social deduction only being used when neither of these strategies is available. Because adults are more capable of using deductive inference but also have more social category and social reference information available to use, the development of the use of social deduction may not be as evident in how often it is used as when it is used (i.e., in those cases when it is the only possible strategy or is clearly the best strategy).

Self-reference (inferred similarity) versus egocentrism

The discussion thus far has been restricted to the case where people make judgments of target persons whose viewpoint or characteristics are different from their own (i.e., dissimilar others), because this case most clearly reveals whether or not role taking is involved in the judgment. However, people often make judgments of target persons whose viewpoints or characteristics are similar to their own (i.e., similar others). It is important to consider whether role taking is involved in accurate judgments of similar others. It is also important to consider whether inaccurate judgments of similar others necessarily reflect an absence of role taking.

How to unambiguously interpret the processes underlying accurate prediction when judges make predictions for similar others has been an issue for many years (cf. Cronbach, 1955; Hastorf, Bender, & Weintraub, 1955). In both the adult and developmental literatures, it has been suggested that accurate prediction of similar others could be based on an "assumed similarity" set. By "assumed similarity," the developmental literature has meant an egocentric judgment where the judge does not differentiate self from others, or, at least, does not adequately inhibit self when judging others (cf. Flavell et al., 1968). It is not clear in the adult literature whether assumed similarity refers to an egocentric judgment or to "inferred similarity" where the judge infers that because the target person has similar characteristics he/she is also likely to have similar responses (cf. Bronfenbrenner, Harding, & Gallwey, 1958; Bender & Hastorf, 1953; Gage & Cronbach, 1955; Heider, 1958; Tagiuri, 1969). Certainly, inferred similarity is a common judgmental strategy. Situational role taking, where people infer that another person's response would be the same as their own in the same circumstances, is an example of one type of inferred similarity. Using oneself as the basis for making judgments about similar others is another type of inferred similarity that can be used when making judgments of target groups as well as target persons. For example, in the Higgins et al. (in press) study subjects may infer that a target group's preference is similar to their own because they believe they are typical or representative of (i.e., similar to) the target group. Such "self-reference" would be a social-reference strategy where one uses oneself to make predictions of others.

Another purpose of the Higgins et al. (in press) study was to examine whether assuming similarity when judging similar others (specifically, selecting one's own preferences when predicting similar others' preferences) increases with age and whether assuming similarity is associated with egocentrism as some developmental models would predict. In order to examine this issue, subjects were asked to select the item they liked best, second best, third best, and so on in each array. In every age group, subjects' predictions of the preferences of similar others (i.e., peers) were more similar to their own preferences than their predictions of dissimilar others (i.e., nonpeers). In every age group, however, subjects differentiated their predictions of dissimilar others' preferences from their own preferences. These results suggest that the process underlying subjects' selection of their own preferences when predicting similar others' preferences was inferred similarity and not egocentrism. In particular, self-reference as an inductive inferential strategy may have been used. In sum, just as one should be careful not to assume that accuracy in judging similar others necessarily reflects role taking, one should also be careful not to assume that selecting one's own response when judging similar others necessarily reflects egocentrism.

An interesting variation in the use of self-reference could contribute to an increase in judgmental accuracy with age. One strategy when predicting the responses of target persons or groups younger than oneself might be to remember one's own responses (e.g., preferences) when one was the same age as the target and predict the same response for the target. In fact, even when people do not consider themselves to be typical of their present peer group, they may, nevertheless, consider themselves to have been typical of their peer group in the past. Such "retroactive self-reference" would be a particularly interesting strategy for it would simultaneously involve self-reference *and* the ability to distinguish one's present response from the target's response (assuming one's responses have changed over time). In another study by Higgins et al. (in press) using the same basic procedure as described earlier, four–five-year-olds and eight–nine-year-olds predicted the preferences of peers and grown-ups (i.e., nonpeers), and college students predicted the preferences of peers and four–five-year-olds (i.e., nonpeers). Only the college students were as accurate in predicting nonpeers' preferences as peers' preferences, and this may be due, at least in part, to the fact that only the college students could have used a retroactive self-reference strategy when predicting the preferences of nonpeers. Shatz (1978) found that four-year-olds' selections of a gift for a two-year-old became less accurate when irrelevant gifts suitable for infants or suitable for school children were added to the array of gifts suitable for two-year-olds. This may have been partly because four-year-olds can use self-reference and retroactive self-reference to distinguish four-year-old and two-year-old gifts but not to distinguish gifts for school children or gifts for infants (because they cannot remember their own infant preferences).

Finally, it should be pointed out that egocentrism and the use of self-reference are not the only factors that could result in predictions of similar others' responses being the same as the judge's own responses. People may base their predictions for a target group on those group members they have known, and biased sampling factors (e.g., selective interpersonal association) may lead to greater experience with those members of the target group most similar to the judge (Ross, Green, & House, 1977). The salient group member used in social reference may also be more similar to the judge than the group members as a whole. Finally, rather than predicting similar others' responses on the basis of their own responses, people may select their own responses to be consistent with what they believe to be the responses of similar others. Perhaps, even when there is little developmental difference in the tendency for predictions of similar others to match the judge's own responses, there are developmental differences in the processes that determine whether a match occurs.

Summary and implications

Previous accounts of role-taking development have generally described a development away from two major characteristics of preoperational thought. Many proposals have embodied the general notion that role-taking development involves acquiring the ability to simultaneously consider an increasing number of factors (e.g., Feffer, 1970; Flavell et al., 1968; Selman & Byrne, 1974), a notion that reflects Piaget's proposed development from "centration" to "decentration." In addition, many proposals have embodied the general notion that role-taking development involves acquiring the ability to prevent the self from intruding upon the judgmental process under conditions of increasing salience of self (e.g., Chandler, 1979; De Vries, 1970; Flavell et al., 1968; Selman & Byrne, 1974), a notion that reflects Piaget's proposed development from "egocentrism" to "nonegocentrism." Previous role-taking proposals, however, have not explicitly distinguished between these two dimensions of role-taking development nor have they emphasized their continuous nature. Instead, role-taking development has frequently been described as a series of levels in which each level differs from the previous level on one or both of these dimensions (e.g., Selman & Byrne, 1974), with the shift to the next level often requiring development along a different dimension at different points in the series. In contrast, the perspective on role-taking development presented here emphasizes the distinct and continuous nature of these dimensions and suggests the need to examine their development independently.[9]

Distinguishing between the ability "to interrelate multiple factors" and the ability "to control the self" has both theoretical and practical implications. As mentioned previously, the relatively low correlations between performance levels on different "role-taking" tasks could be because the critical ability for effective performance varies for different tasks.[10] It could be that the pattern of development for the two abilities is quite different, with the period of most rapid development occurring at different points for the two abilities. An attempt should be made in future research to chart the development of each of these abilities separately, using tasks and measures that, as much as possible, independently tap these two developmental dimensions. This, in turn, may provide a clearer picture of how role-taking development relates to other aspects of intellectual and social development. For example, it may be that the development of conservation is more closely related to the development of the ability "to interrelate multiple factors" than the development of the ability "to control the self," whereas the reverse is true of the development of altruism, and the development of cooperative interaction is closely related to the development of both abilities.

Individual differences in the development of these two abilities should also be examined. It may be that some children develop the ability "to interrelate multiple factors" relatively quickly but lag behind in their ability "to control the self," and vice versa. The presence of such individual differences would be an important factor to take into account when developing programs for training social skills. That is, the training of social skills is likely to be more effective and efficient if these two role-taking abilities are taught and assessed independently.

The approach to role taking taken in this chapter also emphasizes that children must learn to control the self rather than simply inhibit the self because various role-taking processees, such as comparison and self-reference processes, require that the self be actively incorporated into the judgmental process. A major issue for future research is how and what do people learn to prevent the self from intruding on judgments of others, especially when information about the self is highly accessible or salient. Are there systematic developmental changes in the ability to prevent self-intrusion as the accessibility or salience of the self is increased?

One possible way to examine these issues would be to measure the impact on judgments of others when the accessibility of self-information is experimentally increased. The increased accessibility of self-information could be accomplished by a variety of methods, including methods whereby the processes involved would be relatively automatic and passive (cf. Higgins & King, in press). For example, one could vary whether children were or were not asked to introduce themselves prior to the judgment task. Introducing oneself should activate information about the self. This activation in turn should temporarily increase the accessibility of self-information in the subsequent judgment task because recent activation of a construct automatically increases the accessibility of the construct and closely associated constructs (cf. Collins & Loftus,

1975; Higgins & King, in press; Warren, 1972). One could then compare the impact of such increased accessibility of self-information on judgments of others by different age groups (using such measures as overall accuracy and number of self-intrusions). Stronger manipulations of self-accessibility could be used, but the possibility of introducing demand effects would also increase.

The impact of the self on judgments of others could also be investigated through either task variability or individual variability in self-accessibility. One could systematically examine the extent of self-intrusion as the salience of self-information increases from target-only tasks to comparison tasks to self-as-object tasks. Because there are individual differences in the accessibility of different social constructs (cf. Higgins & King, in press; Kelly, 1955; Markus, 1977), one could also select subjects and tasks such that the required judgment involves constructs that have high accessibility for some subjects but low accessibility for other subjects. In future developmental comparisons of the amount of self-intrusion in judgments of others, it is important to ensure that the task selected involves judgmental constructs that are equally accessible to the different age groups. This has not been done in previous research and may in part account for the developmental differences found.

Another difference between the perspective on role-taking development proposed here and some previous proposals is that the present proposal does not consider changes in judgmental content to be a crucial part of role-taking development. Content differences per se do not necessarily reflect differences in underlying role-taking processes. Moreover, because any particular content could be directly stored as part of a social category, role taking may not even be required to activate such content. This latter point reflects a distinction emphasized in the present proposal that has received relatively little attention in most previous proposals; namely, the distinction between role-taking development and the acquisition of social category knowledge.

It was argued that making a judgment of a stimulus person on the basis of inductive or deductive inferences (i.e., role taking) should be distinguished from making a judgment on the basis of information activated when categorizing the stimulus person. It may be that the age-related changes in social judgment described in the literature reflect, in large part, age-related changes in social category knowledge (or, more generally, social knowledge structures) rather than the development of role taking per se. That is, an important aspect of social development consists of increasing one's knowledge about the social world (through direct observation, communicated information, etc.). Age-related changes in social knowledge need to be examined independently of the development of role-taking abilities. Moreover, the relation between these two kinds of social development needs to be studied (cf. Higgins & Parsons, in press). For example, the information that is considered and interrelated when making social judgments may be retrieved from stored knowledge structures. Thus, a child may have both the ability "to interrelate multiple elements" and the ability "to control the self" but, nevertheless, make inaccurate judgments if the child's stored knowledge is inaccurate. Some children may have relatively developed role-taking abilities but relatively underdeveloped social knowledge structures, and vice versa.

There may also be individual and developmental differences in the extent to which social category knowledge is used and how it is used when making social judgments. For example, there may be a point in development when judges decide not to consider all possible factors relevant to the judgment, but, instead, select those factors that are the best predictors or meet a certain threshold of predictive power because consideration of additional factors with less predictive power would lower the overall predictive accuracy (assuming an averaging model of predictive accuracy). In any case, it is necessary for judges to decide which factors to consider and how much weight to assign to each factor, and there could be both developmental and individual differences in which factors are considered and what weights are assigned to them.

Furthermore, judges must decide whether to use role taking at all. It may be that the savings in mental effort from using social category knowledge and not engaging in role-taking processes more than compensate for any reduction in judgmental accuracy. Thus, drawing inferences by interrelating multiple factors may be done relatively infrequently even in cases where such inferences would increase judgmental accuracy. Moreover, even when judges do role take, they may consider a limited set of factors if the small increase in judgmental accuracy from considering additional factors does not sufficiently justify the great increase in mental effort required to include additional factors. Similarly, judges may decide that the amount of mental effort required "to inhibit self-intrusion" is not justified by the increase in predictive accuracy, especially the amount of mental effort required to inhibit "individual" aspects of the self. Possible developmental and individual differences in such decision making and resource allocation should be included as a central issue in future investigations of role taking. In addition, an attempt should be made to relate decision making in this domain of development to decision making in other domains, such as interpersonal communication (cf. Higgins, Fondacaro, & McCann, in press).

A final comment: It is useful to consider the scope and boundaries of the term "role taking" in order that its application in social development be sufficiently restricted to permit a meaningful examination of the antecedents, consequences, and acquisition of the general skills that it designates. Nevertheless, it is less important to evolve a precise definition of this particular construct than to begin to analyze and investigate the various processes and factors underlying the age-related changes in social judgment that have been described in the role-taking literature. This will not be easy. It will be difficult to distinguish operationally and experimentally among such processes as social deduction, induction from social referents, and application of social category knowledge, or between interrelating multiple elements and controlling the self. It will also be difficult to know when a conceptual or phenomenological difference has significant developmental or behavioral implications. By meeting this challenge, researchers in social cognitive development could open new vistas on social development generally.

Notes

1 In fact, the goals themselves may also change developmentally (cf. Higgins, Fondacaro, & McCann, in press; Higgins & Parsons, in press), and different judgments may be necessary to attain different goals.

2 Implicit in some proposals is the notion that information derived from an inference or operation is itself an inference or operation (cf. Chandler, 1979). However, although mode of acquisition has implications for the accessibility and use of stored information (cf. Higgins, Kuiper, & Olson, in press), there is no necessary correspondence between the nature of stored information and the nature of its acquisition. For example, stored information is not itself symbolic simply because it was acquired through symbolic means (Huttenlocher & Higgins, 1978).

3 The critical difference between these levels, therefore, may be that they require consideration of a different number of elements rather than, as Feffer (1970) suggests, that they involve a shift from "sequential" to "simultaneous" decentering per se. In fact, both levels in Feffer's study involved simultaneous processing, with the shift being from simultaneous coordination of responses to simultaneous coordination of viewpoints. Other evidence of a development from "sequential" to "simultaneous" decentering (e.g., Urberg & Docherty, 1976) can also be interpreted in terms of an increase in the number of elements considered and interrelated together. In any case, because a person can simultaneously consider events that occurred sequentially (as in Feffer's study) and sequentially consider events that occurred simultaneously, there is no simple one-to-one correspondence between information input (as in a story) and judgmental process.

4 The older children and adults could also have reasoned that the intrinsic value of the chosen toy need not have been greater than the intrinsic value of the unchosen toy, and could even have been less, because the mother's order or reward provided extrinsic reasons for choosing the toy. Such reasoning would also increase the number of elements to be considered.

5 In some role-taking models, however, what is critical for role taking is the ability to inhibit a competing viewpoint, regardless of whether the viewpoint is the judge's own

viewpoint or another person's viewpoint. For example, in Feffer's (1970) role-taking task, the subject must not let the viewpoint of the first story character interfere with, or persevere as, the viewpoint of the second story character. That is, the viewpoint of the first story character must be coordinated with but not substituted for the viewpoint of the second story character.

6 In some studies involving this task, it is doubtful that role-taking is even involved. For example, when speakers learn from observing a model (Whitehurst, in press) or from being questioned by the listener (Patterson, in press) that the purpose of the task is to describe the target's criterial or discriminating properties, it is not necessary for them to consider the listener's needs in producing their message (i.e., there is no need for them to infer that the listener needs criterial information).

7 In fact, as Shantz (1975) suggests, the children's selections could derive from their knowledge of which expressions are associated with which situations (see also Chandler & Greenspan, 1972). If so, this would require only situational categorization, and, thus, role taking would not even be involved. This issue is discussed in a later section.

8 I am grateful to Judy Smetana for suggesting this alternative.

9 This is not to say that these two dimensions are totally independent. For example, in order to recognize that there are differences between self and others (nonegocentrism), one must be capable of comparing self and others, which requires considering and interrelating multiple elements (i.e., decentration).

10 In fact, in Rubin's (1973) study all the tasks required consideration of multiple elements except for the private speech task, which was also the most direct measure of the ability to control the self. It is, therefore, interesting that this was the only measure that did not correlate with the other measures.

References

Bem, D. J. Self-perception theory. In L. Berkowitz (Ed.), *Advances in experimental social psychology* (Vol. 6). New York: Academic Press, 1972.

Bender, I. E., & Hastorf, A. H. On measuring generalized empathic ability (social sensitivity). *Journal of Abnormal and Social Psychology,* 1953, *48,* 503–6.

Blumer, H. Society as symbolic interaction. In A. M. Rose (Ed.), *Human behavior and social processes.* London: Routledge & Kegan Paul, 1962.

Borke, H. Interpersonal perception of young children: Egocentrism or empathy? *Developmental Psychology,* 1971, *5,* 263–9.

    Chandler and Greenspan's "Ersatz egocentrism": A rejoinder. *Developmental Psychology,* 1972, *7,* 107–9.

Bronfenbrenner, U., Harding, J., & Gallwey, M. The measurement of skill in social perception. In D. C. McClelland, A. L. Baldwin, U. Bronfenbrenner, & F. L. Strodtbeck (Eds.), *Talent and society.* Princeton: Van Nostrand, 1958.

Carroll, J. S., & Payne, I. W. (Eds.), *Cognition and social behavior.* Hillsdale, N.J.: Lawrence Erlbaum Associates, 1976.

Case, R. Intellectual development from birth to adulthood: A neo-Piagetian interpretation. In R. S. Siegler (Ed.), *Children's thinking: What develops?* Hillsdale, N.J.: Lawrence Erlbaum Associates, 1978.

Chandler, M. J. *Social cognition: A selective review of current research.* Unpublished manuscript, 1979.

Chandler, M. J., & Greenspan, S. Ersatz egocentrism: A reply to H. Borke. *Developmental Psychology,* 1972, *7,* 104–6.

Chandler, M. J., Greenspan, S., & Barenboim, C. Judgments of intentionality in response to videotaped and verbally presented moral dilemmas: The medium is the message. *Child Development*, 1973, *44*, 311–20.

Collins, A. M., & Loftus, E. F. A spreading-activation theory of semantic processing. *Psychological Review*, 1975, *82*, 407–28.

Collins, W. A., Berndt, T. J., & Hess, V. L. Observational learning of motives and consequences for television aggression: A developmental study. *Child Development*, 1974, *45*, 799–802.

Costanzo, P. R., Coie, J. D., Grumet, J. F., & Farnill, D. A re-examination of the effects of intent and consequence on children's moral judgment. *Child Development*, 1973, *44*, 154–61.

Cronbach, L. J. Processes affecting scores on "understanding others" and "assumed similarity." *Psychological Bulletin*, 1955, *52*, 177–93.

Damon, W. *The social world of the child*. San Francisco: Jossey-Bass, 1977.

DeVries, R. The development of role-taking as reflected by the behavior of bright, average, and retarded children in a social guessing game. *Child Development*, 1970, *41*, 759–70.

Elkind, D. Egocentrism in adolescence. *Child Development*, 1967, *38*, 1025–34.

Feffer, M. Developmental analysis of interpersonal behavior. *Psychological Review*, 1970, *77*, 197–214.

Feldman, N. S., Klosson, E. C., Parsons, J. E., Rholes, W. S., & Ruble, D. N. Order of information presentation and children's moral judgments. *Child Development*, 1976, *47*, 556–9.

Flavell, J. H. *The developmental psychology of Jean Piaget*. New York: D. Van Nostrand, 1963.

The development of inferences about others. In T. Mischel (Ed.), *Understanding other persons*. Oxford, England: Blackwell, Basil, Mott, 1974.

Flavell, J. H., Botkin, P. I., Fry, C. L., Jr., Wright, J. W., & Jarvis, P. E. *The development of role-taking and communication skills in children*. New York: Wiley, 1968. Reprinted by Krieger, 1975.

Ford, W., & Olson, D. The elaboration of the noun phrase in children's description of objects. *Journal of Experimental Child Psychology*, 1975, *19*, 371–82.

Gage, N. L., & Cronbach, L. J. Conceptual and methodological problems in interpersonal perception. *Psychological Review*, 1955, *62*, 411–22.

Glucksberg, S., Krauss, R., & Higgins, E. T. The development of referential communication skills. In F. D. Horowitz (Ed.), *Review of child development research* (Vol. 4). Chicago: University of Chicago Press, 1975.

Harris, P. L., Macrae, A., & Bassett, E. Disambiguation by young children. *Journal of Child Language*, in press.

Hastorf, A. H., & Bender, I. E. A caution respecting the measurement of empathic ability. *Journal of Abnormal and Social Psychology*, 1952, *47*, 574–6.

Hastorf, A. H., Bender, I. E., & Weintraub, D. J. The influence of response patterns on the "refined empathy scores." *Journal of Abnormal and Social Psychology*, 1955, *51*, 341–3.

Heider, F. *The psychology of interpersonal relations*. New York: Wiley, 1958.

Higgins, E. T. Social class differences in verbal communicative accuracy: A question of "Which question?" *Psychological Bulletin*, 1976, *83*, 695–714.

Communication development as related to channel, incentive, and social class. *Genetic Psychology Monographs*, 1977, *96*, 75–141.

Higgins, E. T., & Akst, L. *Comparison processes in the communication of kindergartners*. Paper presented at meetings of the Society for Research in Child Development, Denver, 1975.

Higgins, E. T., Feldman, N. S., & Ruble, D. N. Accuracy and differentiation in social prediction: A developmental perspective. *Journal of Personality*, in press.

Higgins, E. T., Fondacaro, R., & McCann, D. Rules and roles: The "communication game" and speaker-listener processes. In W. P. Dickson (Ed.), *Children's oral communication skills*. New York: Academic Press, in press.

Higgins, E. T., Herman, C. P., & Zanna, M. P. (Eds.), *Social Cognition: The Ontario Symposium*. Hillsdale, N.J.: Lawrence Erlbaum Associates, in press.

Higgins, E.T., & King, G. Accessibility of social constructs: Information processing consequences of individual and contextual variability. In N. Cantor and J. F. Kihlstrom (Eds.), *Personality, cognition, and social interaction*. Hillsdale, N.J.: Lawrence Erlbaum Associates, in press.

Higgins, E. T., Kuiper, N. A., & Olson, J. Social cognition: A need to get personal. In E. T. Higgins, C. P. Herman, & M. P. Zanna (Eds.), *Social Cognition: The Ontario Symposium*. Hillsdale, N.J.: Lawrence Erlbaum Associates, in press.

Higgins, E. T., & Parsons, J. E. Social cognition and the social life of the child: Stages as subcultures. In E. T. Higgins, D. N. Ruble, & W. W. Hartup (Eds.)*, Social cognition and social behavior: Developmental issues*. New York: Cambridge University Press, in press.

Howe, H. E., Jr., & Keasey, C. B. *Nebraska symposium on motivation, 1977: Social cognitive development*. Lincoln, Neb.: University of Nebraska Press, 1978.

Huttenlocher, J., & Higgins, E. T. Issues in the study of symbolic development. In W. A. Collins (Ed.), *Minnesota symposia on child psychology* (Vol. 11). Hillsdale, N.J.: Lawrence Erlbaum Associates, 1978.

Huttenlocher, J., & Presson, C. C. Mental rotation and the perspective problem. *Cognitive Psychology*, 1973, *4*, 277–99.

Karniol, R., & Ross, M. The development of casual attributions in social perception. *Journal of Personality and Social Psychology*, 1976, *34*, 455–64.

Kelley, R. L., Osborne, W. J., & Hendrick, C. Role-taking and role-playing in human communication. *Human Communication Research*, 1974, *1*, 62–74.

Kelly, G. A. *The psychology of personal constructs*. New York: W. W. Norton, 1955.

Krauss, R. M., & Glucksberg, S. The development of communication: Competence as a function of age. *Child Development*, 1969, *40*, 255–66.

Kun, A., Parsons, J. E., & Ruble, D. N. Development of integration processes using ability and effort information to predict outcome. *Developmental Psychology*, 1974, *10*, 721–32.

Livesley, W. J., & Bromley, D. B. *Person perception in childhood and adolescence*. London: Wiley, 1973.

Markman, E. *Factors affecting the young child's ability to monitor his memory*. Unpublished doctoral dissertation, University of Pennsylvania, 1973.

Markus, H. Self-schemata and processing information about the self. *Journal of Personality and Social Psychology*, 1977, *35*, 63–78.

Mead, G. *Mind, self, and society*. Chicago: University of Chicago Press, 1934.

Miller, G. A. The magical number seven, plus or minus two: Some limits on our capacity for processing information. *Psychological Review*, 1956, 63, 81–97.

Miller, P. H., Kessel, F. S., & Flavell, J. H. Thinking about people thinking about people thinking about. . . :A study of social cognitive development. *Child Development*, 1970, *41*, 613–23.

Nisbett, R. E., & Borgida, E. Attribution and the psychology of prediction. *Journal of Personaltiy and Social Psychology*, 1975, *32*, 932–43.

Pascual-Leone, J. A mathematical model for the transition rule in Piaget's developmental stages. *Acta Psychologica*, 1970, *63*, 301–45.

Patterson, C. J., & Kister, M. C. The development of listener skills for referential communication. In W. P. Dickson (Ed.), *Children's oral communication skills*. New York: Academic Press, in press.

Piaget, J. *The language and thought of the child*. New York: Harcourt, Brace, 1926.

   Play, dreams and imitation in childhood. New York: Norton, 1951.

   The moral judgment of the child. New York: Free Press, 1965 (original transl. London: Kegan Paul, 1932).

   Piaget's theory. In P. H. Mussen (Ed.), *Carmichael's manual of child psychology* (Vol. 1). New York: Wiley, 1970.

Piaget, J., & Inhelder, B. *The child's conception of space*. London: Routledge & Kegan Paul, 1956.

Rosch, E. Cognitive reference points. *Cognitive Psychology*, 1975, *7*, 532–47.

Ross, L., Greene, D., & House, P. The "false consensus effect": An egocentric bias in social perception and attribution processes. *Journal of Experimental Social Psychology*, 1977, *13*, 279–301.

Rubin, K. H. Egocentrism in childhood: A unitary construct? *Child Development*, 1973, *44*, 102–10.

Sachs, J., & Devin, J. Young children's use of age-appropriate speech styles in social interaction and role-playing. *Journal of Child Language*, 1976, *3*, 81–98.

Sarbin, T. R. Role theory. In G. Lindzey (Ed.), *Handbook of social psychology*. Cambridge, Mass.: Addison-Wesley Publishing Co., Inc., 1954.

Sarbin, T. R., & Allen, V. L. Role theory. In G. Lindzey and E. Aronson (Eds.). *Handbook of social psychology* (Vol. 1). Reading, Mass.: Addison-Wesley, 1969.

Sarbin, T. R., Taft, R., & Bailey, D. E. *Clinical inference and cognitive theory*. New York: Holt, Rinehart, & Winston, 1960.

Selman, R. L. Taking another's perspective: Role-taking development in early childhood. *Child Development*, 1971, *42*, 1721–34.

Selman, R. L., & Byrne, D. F. A structural-developmental analysis of levels of role-taking in middle childhood. *Child Development*, 1974, *45*, 803–6.

Shantz, C. U. The development of social cognition. In E. M. Hetherington (Ed.), *Review of child development research* (Vol. 5). Chicago: University of Chicago Press, 1975.

   The role of role-taking in children's referential communication. In W. P. Dickson's (Ed.), *Children's oral communication skills*. New York. Academic Press, in press.

Shatz, M. The relationship between cognitive processes and the development of communication skills. In H. E. Howe, Jr., & C. B. Keasey (Eds.), *Nebraska symposium on motivation, 1977: Social cognitive development*. Lincoln, Neb.: University of Nebraska Press, 1978.

Shatz, M., & Gelman, R. The development of communication skills: Modifications in the speech of young children as a function of listener. *Monographs of the Society for Research in Child Development*, 1973, *38* (5, Serial No. 152.).

Tagiuri, R. Person perception. In G. Lindzey, & E. Aronson (Eds.), *Handbook of social psychology* (Vol. 3). Reading, Mass.: Addison-Wesley, 1969.

Turner, R. H. Role-taking, role standpoint, and reference-group behavior. *American Journal of Sociology*, 1956, *61*, 316–28.

Tversky, A., & Kahneman, D. Belief in the law of small numbers. *Psychological Bulletin*, 1971 *76*, 105–10.

Urberg, K. A., & Docherty, E. M. Development of role-taking skills in young children. *Developmental Psychology*, 1976, *12*, 198–203.

Warren, R. E. Stimulus encoding and memory. *Journal of Experimental Psychology*, 1972, *94*, 90–100.

White, S. H. Evidence for a hierarchical arrangement of learning processes. In L. P. Lipsitt

& C. C. Spiker (Eds.), *Advances in child development and behavior* (Vol. 2). New York: Academic Press, 1966.

Whitehurst, G. The development of communication: Changes with age and modeling. *Child Development*, 1976, *47*, 473–82.

Zahn-Waxler, C., Radke-Yarrow, M., & Brady-Smith, I. Perspective-taking and prosocial behavior. *Developmental Psychology*, 1977, *13*, 87–88.

7 Exploring children's social cognition on two fronts

William Damon

In most psychological research, the study of cognition has focused on subjects' laboratory-tested comprehension of the physical world. Almost without fail, researchers have operationalized human cognition by presenting physical, logical, or scientific tasks individually to subjects in a laboratory setting. Perhaps in reaction to this dominant experimental paradigm, two new approaches to studying cognition have begun to infiltrate the psychological literature. Each of these approaches may be called "social cognitive" in nature, although the two are somewhat different from one another in methodology and in substance.

The first of the two approaches retains the individualized laboratory paradigm of most cognitive research, but tests subjects for conceptions of social rather than physical reality. Like many groundbreaking studies of cognition before it, this approach relies on problem-solving tasks, interview questions, story telling, dilemmas, and other verbally administered procedures: In this case, however, these procedures are structured around social issues and concerns. This approach to social cognition has become particularly popular as a means of establishing age trends in children's social understanding. For example, already this line of research has provided some initial accounts of how children at different ages reason about other people (Livesley & Bromley, 1973); about the self (Keller, Ford, & Meacham, 1978; Broughton, 1978; Montemayor & Eisen, 1977); about social relations, such as friendship and authority (Damon, 1977; Bigelow, 1977); about interpersonal transactions, such as kind and hostile acts (Baldwin & Baldwin, 1970; Youniss, 1975); about social and moral regulation (Turiel, 1978; Damon, 1977; Berndt, 1977); and about societal institutions, such as money, politics, and government (Connell, 1971; Furth,

I am grateful to John Flavell, Bernard Kaplan, Lee Ross, Elliot Turiel, and James Youniss for their comments on an earlier draft of this chapter. The current research described in this chapter has been supported (in part) by a grant from Carnegie Corporation of New York.

154

1978). Generally those following this approach have attempted to describe the major qualitative changes associated with age in children's social understanding, often employing stage (or similarly sequential models) of development as the means to express these qualitative changes.

The second type of social cognitive study differs more radically from traditional cognitive research, at least methodologically. This approach focuses on cognition during actual social interaction, rather than simply on subject's thinking about things social; and, in some cases, removes itself from the laboratory altogether. Because the focus of this approach is on thinking during actual social interaction, its method of study is observational and more or less naturalistic. From observations of children in either natural or semistructured settings, the researcher draws inferences about children's social cognitive abilities without the exclusive aid of children's responses to verbally administered tasks or to probing interview questions. It is not surprising that this approach has flourished in the study of infants' social knowledge (Lewis & Brooks, 1975; Lewis & Feiring, 1978; Lewis & Brooks-Gunn, 1979), where interview or other verbal measures would be useless. In addition, other adaptations of this approach with young children have succeeded in revealing the early presence of surprisingly sophisticated social cognitive abilities. Noteworthy in this view are studies of early peer reciprocity (Mueller & Lucas, 1975; Mueller & Brenner, 1977), and of early perspective-taking and referential communication skills (Shatz & Gelman, 1973; Asher, 1978). In general, those following this approach have attempted to confirm the existence of social cognitive skills at one or another age during early childhood, and to relate these skills to the nature of social interchanges at this age. Occasionally there also has been an attempt to describe relatively short-term changes with age in these social cognitive abilities. Within this approach there has not been an effort to characterize major developmental trends in the long-term, year-by-year growth of children's social understanding.

Aside from representing different sorts of reactions away from traditional cognitive research, each of the two social cognitive approaches has had its own particular uses and shortcomings in the investigation of children's developing social cognition. For example, it is not by accident that the first of the approaches has resulted mainly in sequential accounts of social cognitive development across broad age spans, whereas the second has resulted in the discovery of rudimentary social skills and processes among children previously thought to be socially naive, egocentric, and essentially noninteracting. Clearly the strength of structured tasks like interviews and dilemmas is that responses from various subjects (such as those in different age groups) may be compared with one another along a specified dimension of interest (in this case, the quality or mode of social understanding). On the other hand, observations of actual social interaction are less suited for controlled comparisons between the abilities of subjects across broad age spans, but do allow access to types of behavior that may never become manifest in the course of an interview or other tasks, particularly among children too young to adapt easily to psychologists' individualized testing procedures. Hence the past employment of the first approach for charting broad developmental trends in social cognition, and of the second for revealing children's early use of social cognition in their actual social interactions.

In fact, the differences between the two approaches go even deeper when we realize that social cognition means more than one thing, and that the two approaches have often focused on different facets of the social cognitive prcess. This is because social cognition plays several distinct roles in the life of child or adult. Perhaps most obviously, it provides a person with his or her understanding of social situations. This is the conceptual, or organizational, aspect of social knowledge, enabling one to categorize, interpret, and order social reality. Such knowledge structures (or "mediates") social behavior, active as well as verbal. But social cognition also enables a person to impart and to derive messages from ongoing social interactions. This is the communication aspect of social cognition, providing the mechanism for a sharing of ideas and perspectives among persons. It is this aspect of social cognition that enables an individual to be influenced (and thus to benefit from) his or her social experiences. In this sense, social cognition not only organizes one's social experience but also provides the conditions for its own continual change.

Social cognition, therefore, is a many-sided phenomenon, and it is not surprising that neither of the major approaches to its study has succeeded in investigating all of the sides together. It is generally true that in the first approach social cognition tends to be considered the child's developing mode of organizing and understanding social experience and in the second, the child's method of communicating with others, of generating and receiving social information, and of thereby profiting from social experience.

This chapter has two themes. The first is that social cognition, in at least some of its many facets, is sufficiently different from physical cognition to demand its own psychological study. The recent flurry of social cognitive research represents more than a blind reaction away from traditional methods of cognitive study. Rather, the new, social cognitive experimental paradigms are necessary to fill a yawning gap in developmental psychology. This comment applies, in different ways, to both of the approaches outlined. The second theme is that both approaches have essential roles to play in the systematic study of children's social cognitive development. Both approaches to social cognitive study can contribute to the resolution of some broader problems in the field of developmental psychology as a whole – problems such as the origins and nature of cognitive change. For such achievements, however, some integration between the two approaches is necessary. The chapter will close with a description of one such attempt at integration.

Differences between social and physical cognition

As noted previously, social cognition has many aspects. In discussing the relation between social and physical cognition, I shall focus first on the organizational aspect of social cognition, that is, on the basic categories and principles that structure a person's social knowledge and that shape his or her understanding of social reality. It is in these categories and principles that we find the most profound differences between physical and social cognition. We shall, however, return shortly to the "processing" aspect of social cognition, which is responsible for communication and change through social interaction, and which bears important, although often overlooked, connections to the organizational aspect.

Social knowledge is structured according to different categories and principles than physical knowledge because social interactions have unique features that do not pertain to physical interactions. Understanding social interaction, therefore, requires special sorts of knowledge. I must emphasize that the operating word here is "interaction." It is *not* necessarily the case, as has been often suggested, that social objects in themselves are wholly different from physical objects. I have never seen convincing evidence demonstrating that social objects are, to mention a few of the old clichés, more complex, more variable, or more unpredictable than are physical objects. Rather, the undeniable difference crucial to social knowledge is in the potential of social objects for social interaction – a type of interaction having properties nonexistent in the inanimate world. The organization of social knowledge differs, therefore, from that of physical knowledge not so much because the two bear on different kinds of objects, but rather because, in the social case, these objects exist in a special kind of relation to one another and to the cognizing self. The "specialness" of a kind of relation is defined by principles of social interaction; and it is precisely these principles that a child must come to understand.

Coordinated intentions in social interaction

What, then, are the principles unique to social interaction that call for a special kind of knowing? Most significantly, there is the ability of persons *intentionally* to coordinate their actions, thoughts, and perspectives with one another. Persons do not simply react to one another, but do so consciously, purposefully, with mutual intent. This intentional coordination makes possible forms of communication and reciprocal exchanges unimaginable in the inanimate world. In rudimentary ways, even the young infant can participate in such communicative and reciprocal social interactions, as recent work on early mother–child relations has demonstrated (Trevarthen, 1974; Hubley & Trevarthen, 1979; Bretherton & Bates, 1978). Of course the character of the reciprocity changes as the social relation (as well as the participants in it) develop. Mother–infant reciprocity originates with primitive turn taking between mother and child in act and sound (Brazelton, Kowalski, & Main, 1974). In early childhood relations between peers, social reciprocity takes the form of sharing toys, exchanging favors, and even in establishing shared sentiments such as trust and intimacy (Mueller & Lucas, 1975; Damon, 1977; Gottman, in press). But regardless of its form or its relative level of sophistication, the communication and reciprocity at the heart of all social interaction is brought about by persons intentionally coordinating their actions and thoughts with one another.

The focus on coordinated intentions as the distinguishing aspect of social interaction is neither new to this chapter nor mysterious and inaccessible to operational definition. Bruner (1973) has offered a perfectly adequate operational definition: "Intention, viewed behaviorally, has several measurable features; anticipation of the outcome of the act, selection among appropriate means for achievement of an end state, sustained behavior during development of means, a stop order defined by an end state, and finally some sort of substitution rule whereby alternative means can be deployed for correction of deviation or to fit idiosyncratic conditions" (Bruner, 1973, p. 2). (Bruner also notes that "it can be argued from evidence that the capacity for all these is present at birth.") The formulation presented here of the social–physical distinction has already been put to several good uses in both the philosophical and the psychological literatures. For example, it is the basis of Macmurray's philosophical analysis of personal relationships and their genesis: "Even in the most personal of relationships the other person is in fact an object for us. We see his movements and gestures; we hear the sounds he makes; if we did not we could not be aware of him at all. Yet we do not hear mere sounds or see mere movements or gestures. What we apprehend through these are the intentions, the feelings, the thoughts of another person who is in communication with ourselves" (Macmurray, 1961, p. 34). Other versions of this were long ago introduced into the psychological literature by Baldwin (1906) and Mead (1934), both of whom emphasized the uniquely reciprocal and perspective-sharing bases of social interaction. The view of human relations as entailing a continued attempt by participants to coordinate thoughts and actions with one another was also adopted by Sullivan (1953), who called this interactional phenomenon "mutuality."

My own use of this argument is as follows: Unlike all other components of the world, other people have the capacity to establish mutually intentional relations with the subject. Such relations are composed of a series of interactions in the course of which the subject shares perspectives and coordinates actions and reactions with the other. It is this mutuality of conduct and communication that distinguishes social from merely physical events and that engenders (and requires) a special sort of understanding. The developmental study of social cognition is, in part, a study of this understanding as it grows and changes in the child. In primitive form, this understanding begins to develop as soon as the infant experiences the first rudiments of meaningful commerce with a parent or peer (Lewis & Brooks, 1975). This can be seen as early as day 1, when the mother responds to the child's cries. The eventual fruits of this mutuality, in terms of the child's social understanding, are social-relational concepts like friendship, authority, rivalry; social-regulational concepts like fairness, custom, convention; intrapersonal concepts like identity and self; and extrapersonal concepts like other persons and social institutions. One common thread unites all of these conceptual achievements: the gradually constructed, many-stepped grasp of what it means for one voluntarily and intentionally to enter into coordinated social exchanges with individual and collective others.

Types of coordinated social exchanges

These coordinated social exchanges may differ radically in character from one social interaction to another. Coordination in social interaction is not all of one type. Reciprocal activity can be intended to serve many different purposes, and therefore the nature of the reciprocation varies greatly with these purposes. Generally we can group together interactions of similar intentions into units called "social relations," each of which can be seen as serving a distinct social purpose. For example, social relations between peers during childhood are often characteristic of the friendship relation. Here actions and thoughts are coordinated in order to maintain

160

companionship and affection. Adult–child interactions are often characteristic of the authority relation. Here the social purpose of coordinating thoughts and actions is to maintain the parent's leadership and the child's obedience.[1] Serving different purposes, the reciprocal exchanges in the two relations differ greatly. In childhood friendships, there may be an exchange of favors, goods, trust, or play activity; in child–adult authority relations there may be an exchange of the child's submission for the adult's investment of power, experience, knowledge, or caring. Because each relation has its own purpose, intentional acts within the relation are directed in particular ways unique to that relation.

Because social relations, and the interactions that they organize, are varied in nature and purpose, the child faces a complex task in bringing order to the social network into which he or she is born. For successful functioning in a diverse social world, the child must construct a social understanding sufficiently articulated to distinguish among various types of intended social actions and reactions. At the same time, the child's social understanding must be sufficiently coherent to be able to relate one aspect of social experience to another, and to classify and order the self and others according to their various affiliations and social significances to one another. Children must establish in the course of development their own systematically organized understanding of social relations and of the multiple types of interactions (transactions, regulations, communications) that maintain these relations.

In my own work (Damon, 1977), I have begun with the assumption that children's social understanding is indeed organized around relations and their constitutive interactions, each of which is intended to serve identifiable social purposes. I have focused on authority and friendship as two social relations particularly common to childhood; and on fairness and social rules as two types of regulation that serve to maintain these relations. As a psychologist interested in social cognition, I have seen it as my initial task to describe the ways in which children's understanding of these key relations and regulations progressively change as the child develops. For example, as friendship develops it no longer focuses only on sharing toys and playing with whomever is at hand, but extends to the exclusive exchange of psychological intimacies with trusted, long-term compatriots. Authority is no longer legitimized by the leader's unilateral assertion of power or superior ability, but rather is built upon a consensual agreement that one party's voluntary (and temporary) submission to another may be in the mutual interest of both parties. The child's understanding of each relation becomes, with development, increasingly able to deal with the particular purposes of that relation, and to determine the types of social interaction that will best serve those purposes. It is this increasing ability that the developmental psychologist tries to characterize in a model of social cognitive growth.

In this chapter section I have shown: first, that social interactions differ from physical interactions because they are mutually intentional in nature; and second that social interactions are themselves a diverse lot because they represent many different attempts at coordinated thought and action (and thus serve many different social relations). From the standpoint of psychological analysis, both points lead to the same conclusion: If we, as psychologists, are to understand the flexibility, scope, and power of cognitive functioning, we must admit to structural diversity in knowledge. This diversity can be seen at the beginnings of life in the young infant's differential response to animate and inanimate objects; and can be traced along its varied courses in the subsequent development of children's many social and physical conceptions. In this light, the study of children's social cognition certainly has its role to play in developmental psychology, and cannot be derived from, nor reduced to, the study of physical cognition. A social cognitive model requires its own categories and principles of organization, principles that account for the subject's understanding of social interaction's core mutuality in all of its forms. A developmental model of social cognition will, of course, demonstrate how these categories and organizational principles undergo systematic improvement as the child (and the child's social world) changes with the child's age.

As noted earlier in this section, I have discussed the distinction between social and physical cognition with reference to the organizational rather than the processing aspects of cognition. The point that I have emphasized is that knowledge of social interaction must be different than knowledge of nonsocial phenomena, because social interactions are themselves organized in unique ways. This point, however, says nothing about social cognition as a process of generating and receiving social experience: that is, the means by which social influence is communicated and registered, and through which an individual may be led towards cognitive change. The question then arises: Do the processing aspects of social cognition differ from other, "nonsocial" cognitive processes, either in their properties or in their role in children's cognitive growth? I shall examine this question in the following section.

Social cognition as a process

All developmental psychologists would agree that social interaction is essential to a child's intellectual growth. Social interaction provides a

child with an introduction to new ideas as well as with feedback on the
child's own, often inadequate, conceptions. But social interaction can
have no influence on the child's thinking if the child does not actively
participate in, or at least attend to, the interaction. By definition, we call
the intellectual aspect of this participation the social cognition process.
Social cognition in this sense means all of the ways in which the child
exchanges, receives, and processes information from others. These ways
include some general cognitive processes, such as attention and memory
as well as some that are strictly social, such as communication and perspective taking. These social cognitive processes constitute the child's
primary tools for exploiting his or her cultural heritage, for these constitute the cognitive mechanism of social learning.

Social cognitive processes and the acquisition of knowledge

There are a number of hypotheses that account for the specific role of
social cognitive processes in the overall acquisition of knowledge. One is
that social cognitive processes – in particular those that are strictly social,
like communication and perspective taking – are particularly responsible
for the acquisition of social concepts (such as friendship, authority, and so
on). Accordingly, physical concepts (like space, time, weight) could be
derived more from nonsocial cognitive processes such as an individualistic
"figuring out" of the world around one's self. Flavell and Ross have
described this possibility as a "domain X mode of acquisition interaction"
hypothesis: "that is, mechanisms of development entailing social interaction versus those involving solitary activities might contribute more to
social knowledge than to non-social knowledge" (Flavell and Ross, personal communication). I cannot, however, agree with this hypothesis – not
because it suggests too strong a role for social cognition in the acquisition
of social knowledge; but rather because it underplays the social cognitive
role in other areas of intellectual growth.

There can be no distinction between the process of acquiring social
knowledge and that of acquiring other types of knowledge, because, as
Chandler (1977), among others, has argued, all cognition is intrinsically
social in origin and in function. Categories of the world – whether social or
physical – are not derived by the child in social isolation, but are worked
out in the course of innumerable social exchanges. In the course of these
social exchanges, the child's attention is drawn to particular aspects of
subject – object interactions that have special social and cultural meaning
(El Konen, 1972). In this manner, the child's cognitive development is
continually guided by the social context in which all knowledge is pre-

sented and created. Thus it is more accurate to say that knowledge is "co-constructed" by the child in relation to others than that it is simply constructed unilaterally. This is equally true of social and physical knowledge: Mathematical logic is as much a social-cultural construction as is friendship or justice. Each child does not reinvent the number system from scratch when learning to count, add, and multiply: Rather, the child constructs a mathematical knowledge from the information provided him through social as well as nonsocial interactions. We must recognize, therefore, the fundamental similarity in the ways in which knowledge of any type is constructed. The child comes to know all aspects of the world through a similar process of construction imbedded within a specific matrix of social influence. Important features of the matrix (and thus of the concepts acquired) may vary from social setting to social setting, but its presence is universal and essential.

This view of cognition's social origins is by no means new to developmental psychology: The theories of Piaget, Vygotsky, Luria, Bruner, and others all, in their own ways, have recognized the relations between social interaction and cognitive growth. But this relation has often been obscured in psychological studies by the predominance of the traditional experimental paradigm described earlier in this chapter, that is, by the individual testing of children in laboratory settings. Findings and conclusions about cognitive development have been overwhelmingly derived from observations of children in solitary reflection, wrestling with intellectual problems as presented in psychologist-structured testing conditions. This common means of operationalizing cognition has led to narrowly focused models that describe cognition and change as problem-solving activities carried out in relative social isolation.[2]

One good example of this tendency is Piaget's recent descriptions of his equilibration model (Piaget, 1977). (The tendency is apparent as well in other contemporary American cognitive development models, such as those summarized in Flavell, 1977.) On a theoretical level, Piaget's writings yield to no one's in their recognition of the two-way relations between cultural heritage and individual cognitive growth (Piaget, 1961, 1966, 1972). But it seems that the Genevan experimental paradigm has led to a particular emphasis in Piaget's latter-day explanations for children's cognitive progress. Unlike Piaget's early writings (Piaget, 1932), in which social cooperation and conflict were cited as the prime instigators of development, the more recent writings have emphasized the child's active manipulation of the physical world. This is especially clear in Piaget's most recent work on the equilibration process (Piaget, 1977), and reflects, I believe, his empirical shift from phenomena like moral judgment as manifested in real-life settings to phenomena like physical causality and seriation as presented in the laboratory. The social-interaction explanations that permeate Piaget's earlier work are now present in only the most metaphoric sense: No longer do we read of the direct clash of children's ideas, nor of the coordination of children's viewpoints, but rather of a general subject–object feedback system that can rely on physical as easily as social experience. Although Piaget's earliest and later explanations of development may be seen as simply different aspects of his equilibration model, and although the two explantions are by no means self-contradictory, nevertheless when isolated from one another they represent different visions of human development. Because the two have tended to become isolated from one another, in the work of Piaget and his Genevan colleagues as well as in others' interpretations and applications of Piagetian theory, there is now a need to revive the former explanation, long-neglected in forty years of experimental cognitive study. But this will not be possible until cognitive psychologists depart from their individualistic, laboratory-testing model of research and adopt a paradigm that is social cognitive in nature.

I refer, of course, to the second of the two social cognitive paradigms described at the beginning of this chapter: the study of cognition during real-life social interaction. The focus in this research is on the mechanisms of social influence and its relation to subsequent cognitive change. Not only is such research essential for a complete view of mental development; it alone can inform us about the nature of the "socializing" interaction between culture and child. This, then, is the other important role of social cognitive study in developmental psychology.

Some recent experimental work on children's peer learning has, in fact, suggested exactly this potential for in vivo social cognitive studies. A number of conservation training studies have placed children in social interaction with one another (Murray, 1972; Silverman & Geirunger, 1973), or with an adult (Smedslund, 1966; Kuhn, 1972; Brainerd, 1977), as a means of effecting progressive cognitive change. These training attempts generally have been successful, although there has been some debate concerning the type of social interaction that is most stimulating for change. Botvin and Murray (1975), for example, were unable to find differences between children placed in a peer conflict condition and those placed in a modeling condition: Significant numbers of both experimental groups became conservers by the time of a posttest.

The systematic experimental work of Willem Doise and his collaborators (Doise, Mugny, & Perret-Clermont, 1975; Perret-Clermont, Mugny, & Doise, 1976; Mugny & Doise, 1978; Doise & Mugny, 1979) has shed some further light on the relations between cognitive development and children's social-interactional experiences. Doise begins with an assumption that social interactions that engender cognitive conflict are potentially effective for cognitive change: " . . . our hypothesis states that conflicts of cognitive centrations embedded in a social situation are a more powerful factor in cognitive development than a conflict of individual centrations alone" (Doise & Mugny, 1979, p. 2). In his studies, Doise has compared the cognitive performances of children working singly with the performances of children working in social interaction with other children or with adults. Presenting subjects with a spatial perspective-taking task, Doise found that "two children, working together, can successfully perform a task involving spatial coordinations; children of the same age, working alone, are not capable of performing the task" (Doise et al., 1975, p. 367). Even more interesting were the results from a similarly presented conservation-of-quantity task: " . . . subjects who did not possess certain cognitive operations . . . acquire these operations after having actualized them in a social coordination task" (Doise et al., 1975, p. 367). It seems that children in social interaction must restructure their cognitive performances in order to coordinate them with others. Moreover, this act of restructuring may have some direct influence on the organization of each participating child's thinking. This suggests a model of development with social interaction as an intrinsic feature, rather than as an additional, external factor.

Doise's experiments, therefore, demonstrate a particular role for social interaction in children's cognitive development. Doise has shown that progress is achieved through the coordinating of one's perspective and actions with those of another, rather than through the transmission of information and ideas from one participant to another. The mechanisms of change are coordination and social conflict, rather than learning or imitation. Empirically, Doise has been able to support this assertion with some striking findings. In another spatial perspective-taking study, Doise found that "collective performances are structurally superior to those of the group members taken individually" in cases where children were paired with peers *either* less advanced *or* more advanced than themselves (Mugny & Doise, 1978, p. 190). Progress, therefore was not so much a result of imitating another with superior knowledge as it was a result of coordinating one's approach with that of another.

Interestingly, in this and other studies, Doise found that "more progress takes place when children with different cognitive strategies work together than when children with the same strategies do so . . . " (Mugny & Doise, 1978, p. 181). He has even shown this to be true in cases where both children's initial strategies were incorrect (Doise & Mugny, 1979). Thus, to have a significant effect, the act of social coordination must require a child to alter his or her standard way of approaching the problem. That is, coordinations that are successful in leading to a progressive restructuring of children's cognition must consist of an initial social conflict imbedded within a context of cooperation. It should be noted that such developmental social interactions need not be limited to the sphere of child–child relations: Doise has established essentially the same pattern of results in studies of children in social interaction with adults (Doise, Mugny, & Perret-Clermont, 1976).

Doise's studies are an important first step toward an experimental paradigm that does justice to the social foundation of cognitive growth. In observing children working through cognitive problems in the course of social interaction, such a paradigm is capable of examining cognition as a process rather than merely as a product; and Doise's approach has also shown that the organizational aspects of cognition need not be overlooked in the study of developmental process. But Doise's work is only a first of many necessary steps toward a paradigm that is "social" enough to explore the whole process of change through social interaction. What is needed is the addition of truly social cognitive categories to experiments like Doise's.

Although Doise has been able to observe the process of development via social interaction in his laboratory, his measures of development have been limited to the same conceptual domain that has generally monopolized Genevan research in the past forty years: children's physical-world conceptions. Yet the work of Doise virtually calls out for a social-cognitive analysis. The unanswered questions left by Doise's research have to do precisely with how children establish the social interactions that enable them to restructure their own collective and individual cognitive performances. This, of course, is a social-cognitive question, for it entails explaining how children comprehend the thoughts, intentions, and actions of another, as well as how they contribute to the perspective sharing by communicating their own thoughts and actions. In other words, we may interpret Doise's results as one manifestation of the mutuality during childhood discussed earlier in this chapter; but the development of the mutuality itself must be explained, and this is a social cognitive task.

Furthermore, in Doise's findings (as in any set of findings), there is by no means uniformity of results. In none of Doise's many conditions – including the ones arranged most optimally for social conflict and coordination – did all, or even the great majority, of subjects change. That is, developmental progress even in the most optimal conditions for mutuality is limited to certain children. One is therefore led to wonder about the characteristics of these children. Part of the answer surely lies in the initial state of cognitive "readiness," which varies from child to child. Indeed, findings from one study (Perret-Clermont et al., 1976) support this explanation. But even among children at similar initial readiness levels some change positively and some do not. It seems that some children seem particularly able to benefit from their social interactions, whereas others at the same cognitive level (cognitive, that is, in a task-specific sense) are unable to benefit in similar conditions. This variation may well reflect differences among children in social-interaction skills. Such skills, of course, may be expected to derive directly from children's comprehension of other persons, of themselves, and of social relations. To tap such comprehension, one needs to introduce into the experimental paradigm indexes of social cognitive development like perspective-taking ability, communication skills, self-awareness, understanding of other persons, and mode of interpreting interpersonal transactions and relations. Such indexes may be measured directly through naturalistic observations of subjects' ongoing social interactions, or through standard social-reasoning instruments apart from the actual interactions. There are other possible measurement strategies, as well as other social cognitive categories, of potential interest. I shall explore some of these possibilities in the final section of this chapter.

An approach to studying social cognition in the developing child

In the preceding sections of this chapter I have stated that the study of children's social cognition can serve two purposes. First, it can give us an account of how children understand social interaction in all of its variety, including an account of how this understanding changes (and improves) with age. Second, it can show us how children are able to profit intellectually from their social interactions. I also suggested that the former goal is most readily attainable through interview and other testing procedures focusing on social material: In this way, long-term developmental trends may be charted by comparing task responses typical to one age group with task responses typical to another age group. The latter goal is most readily attainable through observations of children's actual social interactions in either natural or structured situations. Through such observations we may isolate the types of interaction patterns that most effectively lead children to progressive cognitive change.

In this chapter I have separated these goals for social cognitive research, partly because they do indeed reflect two different research traditions that are presently forming in this new area of study. Although these goals are clearly distinguishable, however, it should be equally clear that there must be important connections between them. The study of short-term change and the processes responsible for it has very much to do with the study of long-term developmental trends, and vice versa. For example, it has been confirmed in a number of studies that a child's developmental level influences the outcome and conduct of the child's participation in social interaction. In studies of training in physical concepts, Inhelder, Sinclair, and Bovet (1974), Doise et al. (1975), and many others have found that children at transitional levels are most likely to benefit from a training experience. This seems to be true whether the experience be social interaction in the form of adult-administered instruction or in the form of peer conflict. As for the conduct of children's social interactions, I have evidence from my own studies that suggests that children's peer dialogues about issues such as positive justice are strongly influenced by the developmental levels of the participants' justice conceptions. For example, children who reason about justice at higher developmental levels are more likely to arrive at a consensus with peers on a problem in distributive justice (Damon, 1977); and children at higher levels of justice reasoning quickly anticipate "fair" solutions (like equality) that less advanced children arrive at only after lengthy peer debate, if at all (Gerson & Damon, 1978; Damon, in press, b). Finally, the connection between social-interaction processes and the level of children's conceptual development is self-evident, for there can be no doubt that long-term development must ultimately derive from short-term changes, affected (at least in part) through social influence.[3]

A systematic study of social cognition and its role in children's intellectual development must explore not only the structure-of-knowledge and processing aspects of social cognition, but also the connections between these aspects. Such a study should address questions like: How do the developmental levels of children's social understanding affect their social interactions (including not only the nature of communication and conduct within the interaction, but also the extent to which children at various developmental levels are able to benefit from the interaction)? Conversely, how do social interactions affect children's levels of social (and nonsocial) understanding? Are some types of social interaction (for example, adult versus peer centered) more beneficial for progressive cognitive change than others? If this is the case, is it true generally, or only for certain children? That is, is it only children with certain histories, or with certain types of social-interaction styles, that profit more from one or another type of interaction? Or, if some types of social interaction are indeed particularly effective, is this true only for the acquisition of certain concepts? That is, are some concepts best learned through one type of social interaction, and others through different types? (This is a different version of Flavell and Ross's hypothesis noted previously, because it assumes the general necessity of social influence but distinguishes among different forms of its occurrence).

In general, we need to know more about the aspects of children's social understanding that account for the nature of their ongoing social interactions, and more about how children construct a social understanding from their social experience. The goal is to capture, in one coherent model, the knowledge organization as well as the process aspects of social cognition; or, in other words, to convey through the model not only the pattern of children's thinking at various developmental levels, but also the nature of children's growth potential at each of these levels. In effect, such a model relies on stagelike descriptions in order to capture the quality and organization of children's behavior from age to age, but it avoids the static character of traditional stage models by emphasizing the relation between organizational and process aspects of cognition. In this way, the model should be able to explain how a child's pattern of thinking at any time has an underlying coherence and concurrently a dynamic potential for further development.

A model of social interaction among children

Deriving such a model, as I have argued in this chapter, requires the observation of children from various backgrounds and at various developmental levels engaged in diverse social interactions with others, and determining the extent to which the children are capable of benefiting from such interactions. In one such investigation, I engaged children in a peer-group situation that I had used previously for an entirely different purpose (Damon, 1977). Children were asked to make bracelets and then allowed to determine among themselves their own distribution of rewards for performing this task. The heart of this experimental situation is a group debate in which children are encouraged to exchange ideas and arrive at a consensus concerning the "fairest" means of distributing the rewards. In the past I had been interested in relations between children's verbal justice conceptions and their behavior in this actual situation; in this instance, I observed how children influence one another during this encounter and the long-term effect of this peer influence on individual children's conceptions of fairness. Pre- and posttests on positive-justice measures established children's levels of reasoning about fairness before and after the group encounter. (Children in this study ranged in age from five through eight, and represent three basic levels of justice reasoning— 0-B, 1-A, and 1-B.) The children placed in this peer-group situation were compared with children who engaged in a discussion with an adult about identical issues for a similar period of time, as well as with a control group who were simply pre- and posttested on the justice measures.

There were several experimental variations upon the sample of children exposed to the peer encounter. For example, some groups consisted of children who reasoned at the same developmental level on the justice pretest, whereas other groups consisted of subjects at different levels. Some groups consisted entirely of relatively advanced reasoners, others entirely of relatively primitive reasoners. Children from different backgrounds were represented; for example, a middle-class sample versus a lower-class Hispanic-speaking sample were included.

Initial results from this study have shown that children in the peer-group conditions were indeed more likely to change positively in their reasoning about justice than were children in the adult discussion group. Overall, 56 percent of the children in the peer situation showed some progressive change[4] in their reasoning, as opposed to 34 percent of the children in the adult-oriented setting, a statistically significant difference. Results from the control group showed fewer than 20 percent of the children changing positively from pre- to posttest.

As noted previously, the training potential of peer interaction has already been amply demonstrated. So these preliminary findings are interesting not so much for their own sake but for the questions that they open up for investigation. The major question is simply: Who are these 56 percent of the children who were able to profit from their peer experience, and what are they like? Initial answers to the first part of this question will come from an examination of the backgrounds and group compositions experienced by this 56 percent. But more revealing for the second part will be an analysis of the group debates in which these children participated. This analysis, based upon videotapes of the group debates, will focus on aspects of children's social cognitive performances hypothesized to be particularly connected to short- and long-term changes in reasoning. For this analysis, I am measuring children's perspective-taking and communication behavior as observable during the actual peer encounter. This observational social cognitive measurement system focuses on dimensions such as: a subject's means of initiating discussion with others; a subject's means of reacting to the messages of others; a subject's mode of recognizing and resolving a conflict between his or her own viewpoint and those of others; a subject's choice of attentional focus during the peer encounter; and the nature of a subject's social-interaction style. In addition, I have asked children to view the videotapes of their own performances, and to comment about these in a "post-post" interview. From these interviews I am deriving information about children's recollection of their experience, and about children's reflections upon their own social cognitive processes. All of these dimensions, of course, will be related to children's justice reasoning prior to the interaction as well as to subsequent changes in this reasoning among the 56 percent of children who showed such change.

In this study of change (and others like it, for the major issues will not be resolved by one study, however large its magnitude), the hope is to discern connections, parallels, and divergences between the organizational (or knowledge-structure) and the processing aspects of children's social cognition. In this way we shall be better able to ascertain how children establish and profit from their social interactions, and to identify social interactional styles in children that are developmentally related (or that have developmental consequences). Ultimately we shall have a better grasp of the various roles played by social cognition in the everyday behavior and the intellectual development of children.

Summary and conclusions

The study of children's social cognition, a relatively recent area of interest within developmental psychology, has been proceeding along two fronts. The first has relied upon interviews and other laboratory tasks that test children's understanding of social issues, and has begun charting out broad developmental trends in children's social conceptions. The second has relied upon observations of children's social interactions, and from these observations has made inferences concerning children's early use of social cognitive processes (such as perspective-taking and communication skills). The first line of research has sought to describe the qualitative and organizational features of children's social understanding at different ages, whereas the second has attempted to describe how children establish, maintain, and profit from social interaction and communication.

Although both lines of research may be seen simply as reactions away from traditional psychological approaches to the study of cognition, each has a rationale that goes well beyond mere reaction. The study of children's developing social understanding, with specially designed social tasks, fills an important gap in developmental psychology because social understanding cannot be reduced to cognition about the physcial world.

This is because the social world has interactional properties not present in the inanimate world, and also because the cognizing subject exists in a unique relationship with the rest of the social world. These properties, and the nature of this unique subject/social-world relation, can be defined by principles of social interaction. The core difference between social and nonsocial interaction is that the former entails a mutually intentional coordination of actions and thoughts between persons. Social relations are constituted of such intentional interactions. Interactions with similar intentions may be grouped together into one or another relation (for example, interactions intended to maintain leadership and obedience constitute the authority relation). The child's task in constructing a social understanding is to conceptualize the various forms of mutually intentional interactions between the self and others; and the psychologist's task in constructing a model of social cognitive development is to describe how these social conceptions are organized and reorganized during different periods of life. For both the child and the psychologist, these tasks require the adoption of cognitive categories and principles tailored to the unique features of social interaction.

But psychologists interested in the development of social cognition cannot restrict their efforts to laboratory-based studies of long-term trends in children's social understanding. As a complement to such studies, the moment-to-moment processes of social influence, an equally important aspect of social cognition, must be explored through observations of actual social interactions. It is only in this way that we shall be able to include in our developmental model a full description of the mechanisms of change. Furthermore, the two-way relations between children's developmental levels of social understanding and their abilities to establish, process, and benefit from social interactions must be defined. Some observational studies of children's peer-group interactions have already begun moving in this direction. Continued research efforts, focusing on many types of social interaction in relation to various aspects of intellectual development, hopefully will follow the lead of these beginning attempts.

Notes

1 Of course, not all peer interactions serve the friendship relation, nor do all child–adult relations serve the authority relation. For example, parents may be friends with their children; children may act as leaders and followers to one another. However, it is important to note that the essential characteristics of the relations – friendship and authority – remain the same, regardless of the participants.

2 An exception is the work of Soviet psychologists, such as Luria (1976) who have searched for empirical evidence in such phenomena as individuals' cognitive changes that accompany the collectivization of social institutions.

3 This is the notion that even developmental trends that are best described discontinuously – as in stage models – actually occur in children via small day-to-day increments of change. The discontinuous stage descriptions are necessary to capture the qualitative, organizational differences between children's behavior at different periods of life, but the behavior itself changes gradually and unevenly. Short-term, seemingly tentative behavioral acquisitions are therefore the building blocks of major, permanent developmental movements. For fuller discussion of this notion, and some related social cognitive data, see Damon, in press-b, in press-c.

4 This change was not by an entire developmental level, but rather an increased percentage of reasoning above the child's previous modal response level (see Damon, in press c, for the significance of this change measure in studies of children's social-cognitive development).

References

Asher, S. The development of referential communication skills. In G. Whitehurst (Ed.), *Child language.* NewYork: Academic Press, 1978.

Baldwin, J.M. *Thought and things.* London: Swann Sonnenschein, 1906.

Baldwin, C. P., & Baldwin, A. L. Children's judgments of kindness. *Child Development,* 1970, *41,* 29–47.

Berndt, T. J. The effect of reciprocity norms on moral judgment and causal attribution. *Child Development,* 1977, *48,* 1322–30.

Bigelow, B. Children's friendship expectations: A cognitive-developmental study. *Child Development,* 1977, *48,* 246–53.

Botvin, G. J., and Murray, F. B. The efficacy of peer modeling and social conflict in the acquistion of conservation. *Child Development,* 1975, *46,* 796–9.

Brainerd, C. J. Feedback, rule knowledge, and conversation learning. *Child Development,* 1977, *48,* 404–11.

Bretherton, I., and Bates, E. The emergence of intentional communication. *New Directions for Child Development,* 1979, *4,* 81–100.

Broughton, J. Development of concepts of self, mind, reality, and knowledge. *New Directions for Child Development,* 1978, *1,* 75–101.

Bruner, J. S. The organization of early skilled action. *Child Development,* 1973, *44,* 1–11.

Chandler, M. J. Social cognition: A selective review of current research. In W. F. Overton (Ed.), *Knowledge and development.* New York: Plenum Press, 1977.

Connell, R. W. *The child's construction of politics.* Melbourne, Australia: Melbourne University Press, 1971.

Damon, W. Early conceptions of positive justice as related to the development of logical operations. *Child Development,* 1975, *46,* 301–12.

The social world of the child. San Francisco: Jossey-Bass, 1977.

Why study social-cognitive development? *Human Development,* in press-a.

The nature of social cognitive change in the developing child. In W. Overton and C. Reese (Eds.), *Knowledge and development* (Vol. IV), in press-b.

Patterns of change in children's social reasoning: A two-year longitudinal study. *Child Development,* in press-c.

Doise, W., Mugny, G., and Perret-Clermont, A. N. Social interaction and the development of cognitive operations. *European Journal of Social Psychology,* 1975, *5,* 367–83.

Social interaction and cognitive development: Further evidence. *European Journal of Social Psychology,* 1976, *6,* 245–7.

Doise, W., and Mugny, G. Individual and collective conflicts of centrations in cognitive development. *European Journal of Social Psychology,* 1979, in press.

El Konen, D. B. Toward the problem of stages in the mental development of the child. *Soviet Psychology,* 1972, *10,* 225–51.

Flavell, J. H. *Cognitive development.* Englewood Cliffs: Prentice-Hall, 1977.

Furth, H. Children's societal understanding and the process of equilibration. *New Directions for Child Development,* 1978, *1,* 101–23.

Gerson, R., and Damon, W. Moral understanding and children's conduct. *New Directions in Child Development,* 1978, *2,* 41–60.

Gottman, J.The development of friendship. In A. Pick (Ed.), *Minnesota symposium on child psychology,* in press.

Hubley, P., and Trevarthen, C. Sharing a task in infancy. *New Directions for Child Development,* 1979, *4,* 57–80.

Inhelder, B., Garcia, R., and Vonéche, J. *Epistómologie génétique et equilibration.* Neuchatel, 1976.

Keller, A., Ford, L., and Meacham, J. Dimensions of self-concept in preschool children. *Developmental Psychology,* 1978, *145,* 483–9.

Kuhn, D. Mechanisms of change in the development of cognitive structures. *Child Development,* 1972, *43,* 833–44.

Lewis, M., and Brooks, J. Infants' social perception: A constructionist view. In L. Cohen & P. Salapatek (Eds.), *Infant perception: From sensation to cognition* (Vol. II) New York: Academic Press, 1975.

Lewis, M., and Feiring, C. The child's social world. In R. M. Lerner & G. D. Spanier (Eds.), *Child influences on marital and family interaction: A life-span perspective.* New York: Academic Press, 1978.

Lewis, M., and Brooks-Gunn, J. Toward a theory of social cognition: The development of self. *New Directions for Child Development,* 1979, *4,* 92–114.

Livesley, W. J., and Bromely, D. B. *Person perception in childhood and adolescence.* London: Wiley, 1973.

Macmurray, J. *The self as agent.* London: Faber and Faber, 1957.

Persons in relation. London: Faber and Faber, 1961.

Mead, G. H. *Mind, self, and society.* Chicago: University of Chicago Press, 1934.

Montemayor, R., and Eisen, M. Development of self-conceptions from childhood to adolescence. *Developmental Psychology,* 1977, *13,* 314–19.

Mueller, E., and Lucas, T. A developmental analysis of peer interaction among toddlers. In M. Lewis & L. A. Rosenblum (Eds.), *Friendship and peer relations.* New York: Wiley, 1975.

Mueller, E., and Brenner, J. The origins of social skill and interaction among play-group toddlers. *Child Development,* 1977, *48,* 854–61.

Mugny, G., and Doise, W. Socio-cognitive conflict and structuration of individual and collective performances. *European Journal of Social Psychology,* 1976, *8,* 181–92.

Murray, F. Acquisition of conservation through social interaction. *Developmental Psychology,* 1972, *6,* 1–6.

Perret-Clermont, A. N., Mugny, G., and Doise, W. Une approche psychosociologique du développement cognitif. *Archives de Psychologie,* 1976, *44,* 135–44.

Piaget, J. *The moral judgment of the child.* New York: Free Press, 1965, originally published, 1932.

Logic and psychology. New York: Basic Books, 1957.

Comments on Vygotsky's critical remarks. In L. Vygotsky *Thought and language.* Cambridge, Mass., MIT Press, 1962.

Development and learning. In Ripple & Rockastle (Eds.), *Piaget rediscovered.* Ithaca, N.Y.: Cornell University Press, 1964.

Etudes sociologiques. Geneva: Droz, 1966.

Biology and knowledge. Chicago: University of Chicago Press, 1972.

Shatz, M., and Gelman, R. The development of communication skills: Modifications in the speech of young children as a function of listener. *Monographs of the Society for Research in Child Development.* Chicago: University of Chicago Press, 1973.

Silverman, I. W., and Geiringer, E. Dyadic interaction and conservation induction: A test of Piaget's equilibration model. *Child Development,* 1973, *44,* 815–20.

Smedslund, J. Les origens sociales de la centration. In F. Bresson M. de Montmalin (Eds.), *Psychologie et épistemologie génétiques.* Paris: Dunod, 1966.

Sullivan, H. S. *The interpersonal theory of psychiatry.* New York: Norton, 1953.

Trevarthen, C. Conversations with a two-month-old. *New Scientist,* 1974, *62,* 230–5.

Turiel, E. Social regulations and domains of social concepts. *New Directions for Child Development,* 1978, *1,* 45–75.

8   Relations between social cognition, nonsocial cognition, and social behavior: the case of friendship

Thomas J. Berndt

Research on children's understanding of the social world, their social cognition, is a relatively recent phenomenon. With a few important exceptions, nearly all of the theoretical and empirical studies of the development of social cognition have appeared within the past decade (see Damon, 1978; Flavell, 1977; Shantz, 1975). The rapid emergence of social cognition as a major field of study has led to some uncertainty about the relations of the new field to longer-established areas of research. In this chapter I will first describe research on one aspect of social cognition, children's conceptions of friendship. Then I will use friendship conceptions as an example when discussing relations between social cognition and two other research areas. First, parallels can be drawn between social cognitive research and the vast body of research on nonsocial cognition, or the child's thinking about physical events and logical-mathematical concepts. I will suggest that the most important of these parallels concerns the role of experience in cognitive development. Second, children's thinking about the social world must affect their social behavior. Initial attempts to relate social cognition and social behavior were equivocal or disappointing (Kurdek, 1978; Shantz, 1975), but problems in the reliability and validity of the social cognitive measures may be responsible. I will propose a model for exploring the relations of social cognition to behavior that is an adaptation of previous theories of moral development and of social-psychological views about the links between attitudes and behavior.

Conceptions of friendship

Writers and philosophers discussed friendships for thousands of years before friendship captured the attention of developmental psychologists. Friendships were extolled as the most satisfying and significant part of life, as when Aristotle said, "No one would choose a friendless existence on condition of having all the other good things in the world." Aristotle

176

also noted some of the key features of friendship, including the helpfulness and generosity that one friend extends to another, the intimacy and loyalty of friends, and the constancy of friends' affection for one another. Yet until recently, psychological research focused on only two issues. Similarity between friends has been investigated in a large number of studies going back to the 1920s (see Duck, 1973; Hartup, 1970). In addition, the factors contributing to the formation of friendship, of which similarity is one, have been intensively investigated in research on interpersonal attraction (Duck, 1977; Huston, 1974). Many of the early studies of similarity between friends were done with children, but most of the interpersonal attraction research has been done with adults.

Children's social cognitions about friendship have only been examined in the past few years. A fairly large number of studies have been done (Bigelow, 1977; Bigelow & LaGaipa, 1975; Gamer, 1977; Hayes, 1978; Reisman & Shorr, 1978; Selman & Jaquette, 1977; Youniss & Volpe, 1978), and most have used variations on one method. Children have been interviewed individually, and asked rather open-ended questions about their conceptions of friendship. In my own research, typical questions were "How do you know that someone is your best friend?" and "What would make you decide not to be friends with someone anymore?" After a child gave an initial response, standard probe questions were used to elicit additional responses. The questions assess what friends are, what they should do to one another, and what they should not do to one another. I used these questions in two studies, one with working- and middle-class children and the other with middle- and upper-middle-class children. Each study included ninety-six children who were evenly divided between kindergarten, third, and sixth grades. Half of the children were girls and half were boys.

A content analysis of the responses was done, and similar responses were classified into the same category. Categories were added until the total set included all of the responses and appeared to capture the major distinctions among different answers. The final set included eight categories. Responses to each of the two types of friendship questions were coded separately. For each question chldren's responses were coded as present (1) or absent (0) for each category. Then scores for the two questions were summed, so that the range for each category was from 0 to 2. Mean scores for each age in each study are shown in Table 8.1.

The first and simplest category was for responses mentioning the defining features of friendship: You know someone, you like them, and they say they are your friend. In the second study older children referred to the defining features of friendship less often than younger children. The age change was marginally significant in the first study.

Table 8.1. *Mean scores at each grade for categories of friendship conceptions*

Category	Study 1			Study 2		
	Kindergarten	Third	Sixth	Kindergarten	Third	Sixth
Defining features	.97	1.06	.59	.72	.35	.25
Attributes	.16	.06	.34	.19	.17	.25
Play or association	1.31	1.47	1.22	.90	1.08	.97
Prosocial behavior	.38	.88	.91	.22	.44	.81
Aggressive behavior	.56	1.00	1.00	.75	1.06	1.06
Intimacy or trust	.03	.03	.69	.00	.24	.50
Loyal support	.03	.19	.94	.03	.03	.34
Faithfulness	.31	.16	.44	.00	.25	.28

The second category included answers referring to the attributes of the friend, such as "she's a nice girl" or "he bothers other kids." For this and all categories, responses were included in a category if they represented positive instances, reasons why someone was your friend; or negative instances, reasons why you would not be friends with someone. In Study 1, but not Study 2, references to the attributes of the friend were significantly more common at sixth grade than at the younger grades. The change is analogous to the change with age toward more dispositional or traitlike descriptions of other people (Peevers & Secord, 1973).

The third category referred to play or association. It included answers like "he plays with me" and "she calls me all the time." Responses of this type were extremely common, but their frequency did not change significantly with age. The fourth and fifth categories, which referred to the friends' behavior toward one another, were also common. Children expected friends to behave prosocially toward them, by sharing things with them and helping when they needed help. They expected friends *not* to fight with them, call them names, or behave aggressively toward them in other ways (e.g., "put dynamite next to my house and blow it up"). References to friends' behaving prosocially and avoiding aggression increased significantly with age in both studies. It is worth stressing that the positive behavior of the friends toward one another did not become less important as children grew older. Adolescents' friendships have been reported to be more "ideal," and less dependent on one friend's sharing and helping another (Douvan & Adelson, 1966). If there is a decline in emphasis on friends' prosocial behavior during adolescence, it reverses the earlier trend and is not permanent, for college students regard a friend's help as one of the most important aspects of friendship (LaGaipa, 1977).

The sixth category, intimacy or trust, included responses such as "we can talk freely to one another," and "I can tell secrets to her," as well as the simpler "I can trust him." Intimacy and trust have been described by many writers as the essence of friendship. Therefore it is interesting to see that kindergarten children rarely mentioned them as criteria for friendship, and in Study 1 they were just as rare for third graders. In contrast, sixth graders frequently mentioned intimacy, and the age change was highly significant in both studies.

The seventh category included another type of response that has been taken as stereotypical of friendships – loyal support. To distinguish loyal support from other behaviors, we defined it as supporting the friend when other people are present. The most common responses were "he'll stick with me when I'm in a fight," and "she won't talk about me behind my back." Responses mentioning loyal support increased with age in both studies, and like intimacy responses, they were nearly absent at kindergarten and third grade.

The final category might be defined as another aspect of loyalty – faithfulness. It referred to cases where the friend stayed with the child instead of going off with someone else. It is thus the opposite of desertion, and closely related to jealousy. Older children showed significantly more concern with faithfulness than younger children. The difference was significant in Study 2, but only marginally significant in Study 1.

Similar age trends were obtained when specific questions were used, in the second study, to supplement the open-ended questions. For example, when asked about their intimacy with a friend, whether they would tell a best friend if they did something clumsy or foolish, more of the older children said they would tell. When explaining their answer, older children also referred more often to the need for intimacy in a friendship. In other studies a different set of categories has been used for coding responses, or responses have been assigned to a series of stages for friendship conceptions (see Bigelow, 1977; Selman & Jaquette, 1977). However, a close examination of the data from previous studies indicates developmental changes that are reasonably consistent with those reported in this chapter. Moreover, similar responses were found in what is probably the first psychological study of friendship conceptions, published in a very early volume of the *Psychological Review* (Monroe, 1898). When asked what they liked in a "chum," children most often said they liked chums who were "fond of play" and "not quarrelsome." The responses fit the two categories most frequently used in our studies, play or association and aggressive behavior.

Age changes in friendship conceptions can be most dramatically illustrated by examples. What follows is the full set of responses given by a kindergarten child to the question, "How do you know that someone is your best friend?"

I sleep over at his house sometimes [play or association]. When he's playing ball with his friends he'll let me play [prosocial behavior]. When I slept over, he let me get in front of him in 4-squares [a playground game – prosocial behavior]. He likes me [defining features].

A sixth-grader gave the following answer to the same question:

If you can tell each other things that you don't like about each other [intimacy]. If you get in a fight with someone else, they'd stick up for you [loyal support]. If you can tell them your phone number and they don't give you crank calls [aggressive behavior]. If they don't act mean to you when other kids are around [loyal support].

Social cognition and nonsocial cognition

Parallels can be drawn between developmental changes in friendship conceptions and developmental changes previously described for nonsocial cognition. For example, the increase with age in concern for intimacy reflects an understanding that friends can share thoughts and feelings, as well as sharing activities. To an older child, friendship means a joining of personalities, not simply joining together for play. The age change might be considered part of a general shift from an emphasis on the external and superficial characteristics of objects to their deeper characteristics or an underlying reality (see Flavell, 1977). In nonsocial cognition, the change is shown by the child's success at conservation tasks, which depends on an understanding that the attributes of objects are not always changed by changes in their appearance. Similarly, the increase with age in concern for loyal support reflects an understanding that the relationship between two friends may be affected by influences from a larger social network. In the nonsocial realm, consideration of the network of relations in a physical or chemical system is required for many of Piaget's formal-operational tasks. For example, in the task for colored and colorless chemicals (Inhelder & Piaget, 1958), the child must recognize that addition of a specific chemical to a mixture has different effects depending on what other chemicals are already in the mixture.

On the other hand, strong correlations between measures of social and nonsocial cognition are unlikely. Although parallels can be drawn between the two types of tasks at an abstract level, there are great differences in the content of the tasks. Social cognition deals with persons and their thoughts and feelings; nonsocial cognition deals with objects and their physical connections. Moreover, social and nonsocial tasks may differ in the verbal skills they demand, the strain they impose on memory, or other factors, and the differences may lessen the correlations between the two types of tasks. Essentially the same explanation has been given for the low correlations typically found between different tasks within the domain of nonsocial cognition (Flavell, 1970).

However, the case of social cognition is still more complicated. In studying the development of nonsocial cognition, researchers can rely on children's growing up in a physical environment that is essentially identical for all. The effects of rearrangement on the number of objects in a row, or of a beaker's shape on the height that a quantity of water rises in it, are the same whatever a child's language or culture. For many aspects of social cognition, this universality cannot be assumed. Friendship conceptions provide an especially good illustration. The emergence in preadolescence of a concern for intimacy in friendship indicates the stress on intimacy on close relationships that is found among adults in Western societies. In many other societies, intimacy is not valued or even expected in friendships (Paine, 1974). It is reasonable to suppose that where intimacy is not an important aspect of friendships themselves, it is not important in friendship conceptions. Stated more generally, friendship conceptions are greatly determined by the meaning and nature of friendships in a culture.

Of course, the effects of actual friendships on friendship conceptions can be demonstrated even without cross-cultural research. In a number of studies, sex differences have been found in children's friendships. Girls more often confine their friendships to a single other person, whereas boys more often have a group of friends (Eder & Hallinan, 1978; Maccoby & Jacklin, 1974). When with a friend girls show more negative reactions to a newcomer than boys do (Feshbach, 1969; Feshbach & Sones, 1971). Both results suggest that girls' friendships are more exclusive and more intimate than those of boys. Sex differences also appear in friendship conceptions. In our first study girls mentioned intimacy and faithfulness more than boys did. In the second study sex differences were nonsignificant for the open-ended questions, but on the specific question about intimacy girls more often said they would tell a friend if they did something clumsy or foolish. Unfortunately, no study has examined friendship conceptions and characteristics of friendship in the same children. Sex differences in the two do not guarantee significant correlations within each sex. Significant correlations would not appear if the overall environment of the same-sex peer group has a greater impact on friendship conceptions than experiences in specific friendships.

When children's social cognition varies because they live in different social environments, correlations between social and nonsocial tasks will be still further attentuated. The environmental variation in social cognition will obscure whatever abstract similarities exist between the two types of tasks. In short, studying the relations between social and nonsocial cognition by the correlational method seems unlikely to pay off. A more profitable strategy might be to explore the ways in which cognitive change comes about, the process of development of social cognition and nonsocial cognition. One place to start is by investigating the effects of experience. As just noted, sex differences in friendship conceptions indicate the effects of social experience on social cognition. Children's experiences also affect their performance on nonsocial tasks. It makes sense to consider nonsocial cognition first, because the role of experience in that domain has been vigorously debated and extensively researched.

Nonsocial cognitive development

The focus of the debate is Piaget's (e.g., 1970) proposition that experience with objects has a specific and limited impact on cognitive development. Development can be accelerated by placing children in a stimulating environment, but children cannot be directly taught how to solve a Piagetian task. Cognitive change occurs only through the children's recognizing and responding to the conflicts created when they use an incorrect approach to the task. The conflicts upset the children's cognitive equilibrium, and subsequent attempts to resolve the conflicts lead to the discovery of the correct approach and the achievement of a new equilibrium. These descriptions explain the different labels given to the process: self-discovery, cognitive conflict, and equilibration. The crucial element in the process is children's own mental activity in response to conflicts. For Piaget the process is the only source of cognitive development.

In a recent critique Brainerd (1978) argued that Piaget's position is very poorly supported by empirical research. A variety of methods besides self-discovery are effective in improving children's performance on Piagetian tasks. The methods include providing feedback on the child's responses, direct teaching of the rule or rules that lead to correct performance, and having children observe a model who performs correctly. Because the methods include the components of traditional teaching techniques, Brainerd labeled them tutorial methods. Direct comparisons of the two types of interventions are rare, but comparisons across studies suggest that tutorial methods have stronger effects in less time than self-discovery methods. These results are especially damaging to Piaget's theory.

Flavell (1977) has analyzed the abilities children must have to benefit from self-discovery methods, and his analysis helps explain their limited effectiveness (see also Brainerd, 1978). A child must "(1) attend to or notice both of the apparently conflicting elements in the situation; (2) interpret and appreciate them *as* conflicting . . .; (3) respond to the sensed conflict by progressing rather than regressing, e.g., by trying to explain it rather than clinging defensively to his initial belief or refusing to have anything more to do with the problem; [and] (4) come up with a better conceptualization of the situation that can resolve the apparent conflict . . . (1977, p. 242). The success of tutorial methods can be attributed to their eliminating the need for some of these abilities. For example, when the method of rule instruction is used, children need not devise a better conceptualization of the situation on their own; they can simply adopt the rule stated and demonstrated by the experimenter.

Not all training methods can be unambiguously defined as self-discovery or tutorial. In the social-conflict method, children who take different approaches to a task, such as a conserver and a nonconserver, are asked to discuss the task, resolve their conflict, and agree on a single answer. The technique usually leads to a significant improvement in the nonconserver's performance (e.g., Murray, 1972; Silverman & Geiringer, 1973). The method is similar to self-discovery, because it involves the exposure and resolution of conflicts. It is similar to tutorial methods, because the conserver provides the nonconserver with a better conceptualization of the problem.

The role of social conflict in social cognition

Social-conflict methods are doubly social when they involve conflict with a peer over social cognitive issues. I will argue that the experience of social conflict is a frequent and powerful source of change in social cognition, and friendship conceptions in particular. The hypothesis has a long history. Sullivan (1953) suggested that interactions with a friend can reveal to children their own selfishness or conceit, and lead to changes in their views of themselves and other people. Still earlier, Piaget (1932/1965) suggested that interaction with peers aids in the elimination of egocentrism and fosters mutual respect. Kohlberg (1969, 1976) is the most prominent recent advocate of the hypothesis. He asserts that discussion of moral issues with other people is a significant factor in the advance to higher stages of moral reasoning. The three hypotheses are different in detail, but each contains the assumption that interactions with other people expose conflicts between points of view, and attempts to resolve the conflicts lead to progress in social cognition.

The major problem with the hypotheses lies in their undifferentiated and overly optimistic view of social conflicts. Not all conflicts are alike, and not all conflicts lead to cognitive progress. Various possible outcomes of a social conflict can be described by returning to Flavell's analysis of the conflict-resolution process, using a conflict between friends as an example. Suppose a girl violates her friend's confidence by telling other children a secret that is personally embarrassing to the friend. If the friend takes the matter seriously, she will directly and forcefully inform the child that she is upset. The first move in the conflict process is thus taken: The children recognize that they disagreed about the importance of telling the secret to others. The next move, how the children respond to the conflict, is critical. Each of them could "cling defensively to her initial belief," and they might end the friendship in a clash of accusations and counteraccusations. In this case no progress in the children's friendship conceptions would be expected. However, resolution of the conflict and continuation of the friendship does not guarantee social cognitive change. The girls might "refuse to have anything more to do with the problem," agreeing simply to forget about it. Again no change in their friendship conceptions would be anticipated. Progressive change, indicated by an increased appreciation of the importance of intimacy in friendships, would only be expected if the girls discuss the conflict freely and openly until they understand why it occurred and how similar conflicts can be prevented in the future.

These hypotheses can be tested in various ways. Children could be asked to report on how they typically resolve conflicts with their friends, or how they resolved their most recent conflicts. Alternatively, efforts could be made to observe conflicts in natural settings. Both methods have advantages and disadvantages, but because they are basically correlational they cannot provide conclusive evidence that conflicts play a causal role in social cognitive development. For this purpose a more experimental approach is desirable.

For the experiment children might first be pretested on their conceptions of friendship. Then they would be individually interviewed, and asked to describe conflicts that exist in their friendships and problems that have not yet led to overt conflicts. This procedure has already been used in studies with adults (Harvey, Wells, & Alvarez, 1978; Orvis, Kelley, & Butler, 1976). Then each child would be asked to discuss the conflicts with his or her friend. (The experimenter would be absent but the discussion would be taped.) Immediately following the discussion, or in a separate session a few days later, children would again be asked to describe their conceptions of friendship. Possible long-term effects of the intervention could be examined in a delayed posttest that includes other variables: whether the friendship grew stronger, weaker, or ended; and how frequently the children report that they have conflicts with their friend.

In interpreting the results of the experiment, emphasis should be placed on how well they support the hypotheses about the effects of different responses to the conflicts, different techniques for discussing and resolving (or not resolving) them. If the specific hypotheses are confirmed, alternative explanations for the results will be less plausible. However, one additional aspect of the results is of considerable theoretical significance. In the most favorable case, when children fully and openly discuss their conflicts and problems, two outcomes are possible. Both children might show more mature friendship conceptions on the posttest, or one child might merely attain the level already reached by the other. In the latter case, the results might be attributed to conformity or observational learning (see Botvin & Murray, 1975; Brainerd, 1978). However, if even the more advanced child gains significantly from the intervention, these explanations are inadequate. A process more similar to self-discovery must have occurred, but it is the social analogue to self-discovery. Through discussion with one another the children discovered or created more advanced social concepts.

There is some evidence for a process of social discovery. If two children who have a partial understanding of spatial perspective taking discuss a spatial problem together, they both achieve a more complete understanding of it (Mugny & Doise, 1978). However, current evidence on a social-discovery process is meager. More attention should be given to it and to the variety of other processes that may explain the effects of social conflicts. Because these conflicts may arise with tasks for social cognition and for nonsocial cognition, research that directly compares developmental processes in the two domains can be conducted. This approach seems at the present time to be the best strategy for integrating research on social cognition and nonsocial cognition.

Social cognition and social behavior

In considering the effects of social experience on friendship conceptions, a relation between social cognition and social behavior was assumed. However, the nature of the relation was not examined in detail. In this

$$B \sim BI = (A_{beh})w_0 + SNB(Mc)w_1 + PNB(Mc)w_2$$

Symbols: B   = Behavior
       BI   = Behavioral intention, or intention to perform a behavior
       A_{beh} = Attitude toward performing the behavior
       SNB = Social normative beliefs, beliefs about the expectations of reference group members
       Mc   = Motivation to comply with the expectations of reference group members, or with personal normative beliefs
       PNB = Personal normative beliefs, or the person's beliefs about what he or she should do
       $w_{0,1,2,}$ = Empirically determined weights

Figure 8.1. A model of the relation between social cognition and social behavior.

section of the chapter I will present a model for the relation that is adapted from one originally proposed by Ajzen and Fishbein to explain the relation between attitudes and behavior (Ajzen & Fishbein, 1973; Fishbein & Ajzen, 1975). The model is complicated in certain respects, but its basic form is quite simple (See Figure 8.1) Three components, shown on the right side of the equation, are used to predict intentions to perform a behavior. The correlation between behavioral intentions and actual behavior is variable, but it should be strong if the following conditions are met: People can do the act if they wish – that is, there are no external constraints on their behavior; the measure of intentions is as specific as the behavior (Ajzen & Fishbein, 1977); and intentions are measured shortly before the behavior is measured, so that changes in intentions do not reduce the correlation.

The first component on the right side of the equation, attitudes toward performing the behavior, is assumed to be a function of the perceived consequences of the behavior for the individual, multiplied by the evaluation of those consequences. The operation of the component can be illustrated by an example involving two friends, Johnny and Jimmy. If Johnny believes sharing his bike with Jimmy will make Jimmy a better friend, and Johnny wants Jimmy to be a better friend, then Johnny will have a positive attitude toward sharing his bike with Jimmy.

The second component on the right side of the equation also involves a multiplier, social normative beliefs multiplied by motivation to comply. Social normative beliefs are the actor's beliefs that members of his reference group – family, friends, colleagues, and the like – expect him to perform the behavior. Motivation to comply is the person's general willingness to go along with the expectations of reference group members. In our example, if Johnny believes Jimmy expects him to share his bike, and Johnny is generally agreeable to doing what Jimmy expects, then Johnny will be more likely to share his bike with Jimmy.

The third component, personal normative beliefs multiplied by motivation to comply, is not included in the current Ajzen and Fishbein model. However, it was in the original model and was included in some empirical tests of the model. Furthermore, it has important connections to theories in developmental psychology. Personal normative beliefs refer to a person's own beliefs about whether or not he should perform the behavior. Returning to our example, Johnny may feel he should share his bike with his friend Jimmy, and generally be willing to do what he thinks he should do. His personal beliefs should then increase the likelihood that he will share the bike with Jimmy.

Ajzen and Fishbein (1973) assume that the three components constitute an exhaustive set of the factors influencing behavioral intentions. That is, any other variable that affects behavioral intentions must do so indirectly, through its effect on one or more of the components. The assumption seems reasonably accurate for college students. In one study of blood donations (Pomazal & Jaccard, 1976), variables such as donating experience, perceived cost of donating, and feelings of social responsibility to donate contributed very little to the prediction of behavioral intentions after the contribution of the three components was taken into account.

If the assumption is true for children as well, it has significant implications. Age changes in social behavior must then be due to changes in the factors included in the three components, or in the weighting of the three components. For example, numerous laboratory studies show an increase with age in prosocial behaviors such as donating pennies to needy children (Mussen & Eisenberg-Berg, 1977). The increase might reflect changes in perceptions of the personal consequences of donating (e.g., changes in the value of pennies to the children), changes in the child's understanding of social norms or motivation to comply with them (e.g., changes in responses to the experimenter's implicit demands), changes in children's personal norms or motivation to comply with them (e.g., a change in children's opinions about what they should do), or changes in the relative importance of these factors to the decision. Incidentally, data on age changes in personal norms and understanding of social norms can be found in previous research. Two recent examples are Damon's (1977) studies of what children believe is a fair distribution of resources and rewards, and Turiel's (1978) studies of children's reasoning about social conventions.

Age changes in components' weights

Ajzen and Fishbein (1973) also assume that the weights of the three components vary with different behaviors, different actors, and different situations. They did not attempt to formulate systematic hypotheses about the variations. However, a specific hypothesis about changes with age in the weighting of the components can be derived from cognitive-developmental theories of morality. Each component can be linked to one of the three levels (each level combining two adjacent stages) in Kohlberg's (1969) description of moral reasoning. Individuals at the lowest, preconventional level, emphasize what is in their self-interest, and consequently they should give most weight to the component of attitudes toward the behavior. Individuals at the intermediate, conventional level, emphasize conformity to societal standards, and they should give most weight to the component of social norms. Individuals at the highest, postconventional level, emphasize their own moral principles, and they should give most weight to the personal norms component. The changes with age in social cognition, now described in terms of changes in the weighting of components in the model, should lead to predictable changes in behavioral intentions, and hence to predictable changes in behavior.

Changes in the weighting of the three components should affect both behavioral intentions and behavior, because the model implicitly assumes that there is a strong relation between social cognition and behavior at all ages. Some researchers have asserted instead that the correspondence between cognition and behavior increases with age (e.g., Burton, 1963; Henshel, 1971). However, the evidence used in support of the claim is flawed. The social cognitions that were assessed applied only to the personal norm component. A stronger correlation between personal norms and behavior at older ages is actually support for the hypopthesis that the weighting of the personal norm component increases with age. According to the model, if all three components had been measured, they would in combination have predicted social behavior quite accurately at each age.

The hypothesis regarding age changes in components' weights is not simply a restatement of Kohlberg's theory. His theory is primarily applicable to moral development; the model presented here can be applied to all social behaviors. More importantly, the components in the model are not exactly equivalent to the levels in Kohlberg's typology. The correspondence between the two rests on the assumed sources of motivation for behavior – external rewards and punishments, expectations of others, and personal standards. However, a principled moral reasoner in Kohlberg's system does not merely weight personal norms most heavily. He or she is said to hold a particular set of personal norms, ones that express universal ethical principles (Kohlberg, 1976). The alternative model contains a much greater separation between the content of a person's beliefs and the sources of motivation for the person's behavior. Determining what personal norms are accepted by an individual, and how much his or her behavior is influenced by them, are two different operations. One implication of the differentiation is that age changes in the content of a component must be examined when studying age changes in its relative weight. Otherwise the two types of changes may be confused. An earlier example provides a good illustration. The increase with age in children's donations to needy persons might reflect a change in beliefs about what a person should do, rather than an increased influence of personal standards on behavior.

Competing hypotheses regarding age changes

Despite the differences between the two perspectives, the current model can be used as a framework for discussing the various hypotheses in Kohlberg's theory and the many criticisms of it. Because the literature on the theory is enormous, a comprehensive discussion is impossible. I will concentrate on a hypothesis that is central to the theory and that displays both the potential utility and the problems of the alternative model.

Kohlberg (1969) asserts that an individual's moral reasoning forms a "structured whole." The operational definition of this concept is that "individuals should be consistently at a stage unless they are in transition to the next stage (when they are considered in mixed stages). The fact that almost all individuals manifest more than 50 percent of responses at a single stage with the rest at adjacent stages supports this criterion" (1976, p. 47). The strongest version of the corresponding hypothesis in the three-component model is that only one component has a significant weight for any individual. Children at the lowest level should consider only their attitudes toward the act, children at the intermediate level should consider only social norms, and children (and adults) at the highest level should consider only personal norms. The strongest alternative hypothesis is that regardless of their age, individuals consider all three components when deciding how to behave. Age changes reflect merely the relative weighting of the components.

In considering the two hypotheses, the most interesting questions concern young children who display preconventional moral reasoning and emphasize the component for external rewards and punishment. Kohlberg (1969) assumes that preconventional children do not use higher-level reasoning because they cannot understand it. For example, the social-norm component is not meaningful if a child does not realize that other people have expectations for his or her behavior. Inferring that other people expect you to behave in a specific way demands role taking that can be difficult for young children. Studies showing a correlation between children's moral reasoning and their role-taking ability support this viewpoint, although the correlations are not entirely consistent (Kurdek, 1978). On the other hand, even preschool children show accurate role taking when the situation is familiar to them and the task is a simple one (Flavell, 1977; Shantz, 1975). Therefore, researchers must consider two alternative explanations for an apparent failure of social norms to influence young children's behavior: (1) the children did not appreciate that social norms were relevant, that is, that other people held expectations for their behavior; and (2) the children recognized the other people's expectations but ignored them when deciding how to behave.

For the personal-norms component the question of understanding is more ambiguous. The universal ethical principles that define Kohlberg's highest level are complex and difficult for young children to understand (Rest, 1973). However, many principles are far less complex. Aronfreed (1976) describes a seven-year-old who understood the principle that she should not hit her younger brother, but in one situation she refrained from hitting him only because an adult was present. Her problem was not in understanding but in commitment to the principle. In the three-component model commitment is represented by the motivation to comply element. Unfortunately, little attention has been given to this element in the model. Fishbein and Ajzen (1975) confess that it is poorly understood. In other writings it would be viewed as the affective element in behavior (Dienstbier, 1978; Hoffman, 1976). Its significance has probably been underestimated. One could argue that the Fishbein-Ajzen model contains redundant parameters, that the weights (w_1 and w_2) attached to the normative components are unnecessary, and that the developmental hypothesis about changes in weights would be more parsimoniously expressed in terms of changes in children's motivation to comply with social and personal norms.

Still a third explanation could be offered for cases in which only the attitudinal component seems to influence children's behavior. Young children may consider other's expectations, or personal norms, only by translating these into consequences for the self. The translation might go as follows: "Jimmy expects me to share my bike with him, and if I don't he won't be friends with me." Although the children begin by considering what the friend expects, they end by considering compliance with expectations in terms of self-interest. If young children engage in this form of translation, social norms will not affect behavioral intentions *independently* of attitudes toward the behavior. Somewhat older children may differentiate between attitudes toward the behavior and social norms, but confound social norms with personal norms. The translation would go as follows: "Jimmy expects me to share my bike with him, so I should share my bike with him." Again if the translation occurs, personal norms will not have an independent effect on behavioral intentions. Perhaps the full differentiation between the three components is found only in adulthood, and only then do all three components have significant independent effects on behavior.

The idea of translating normative components into the attitudinal component is the basis for the social-learning critique of Kohlberg's theory. This perspective is concisely expressed by Mischel and Mischel (1976): "even the noblest altruism supported by the 'highest' levels of moral reasoning still depends on expected consequences, although the consequences are often temporally distant, are not in the immediate external environment, are not easily identified, and reside in the actor himself rather than in social agents" (pp. 97–8). The statement can be read as a call for definitions of the three levels in Kohlberg's theory, or the three components in the alternative model, that conceptually and operationally distinguish among them.

Current definitions are clearly inadequate. For example, Kohlberg (1976) states that one reason given by Stage 3 (conventional) individuals for behaving morally is "the need to be a good person in your own eyes and those of others" (p. 34). However, the need to see yourself as a good person might be viewed as the reason for behaving consistently with personal norms, and the need to be seen as a good person might be viewed as a desire for social reinforcement. Of course, Kohlberg's descriptions of each stage are complex, and concentrating on a single statement may be unwise. However, the more extensive presentations of the stage typology provoke similar questions. Each stage is described in great detail, but the distinctions between stages are less clearly and less fully discussed. The same bias in theoretical focus is found in Fishbein and Ajzen's (1975) writings. They blur the distinction between the attitude and social-norm components by suggesting that one factor affecting motivation to comply with other people's expectations is the others' ability to reward and punish the person. Yet as a potential consequence of behavior, rewards and punishments by other people belong in the attitudinal component.

These examples indicate that the social-learning critique derives some of its force from the absence of clear separations between the attitudinal and normative components. Devising more adequate definitions of these basic constructs will partially depend on theoretical analysis, but empirical research will also be needed. Three alternative directions for research can be identified. Examples of the three approaches will be drawn from the three-component model, but comparable examples could be presented for Kohlberg's theory.

Directions for future research

First, instead of studying social cognition by obtaining children's verbal responses, experimental manipulations could be devised that attempt to vary social cognitions in predictable ways. Then the effects of the variations on behavior would be examined. This approach was used in a series of experiments that investigated children's generosity toward others when the children were in a negative mood (Cialdini & Kenrick, 1976; Kenrick, Baumann, & Cialdini, 1979). Mood was manipulated by having the children think about unhappy experiences or neutral experiences. The measure of generosity was how many coupons children donated to other children who would not be able to participate in the experiment. Children were told that the prize they received at the end of the study would depend on the number of coupons they kept for themselves.

Preschool children donated less when in a negative mood than in a neutral mood, apparently because they viewed giving away the rewards as self-punishment. Negative mood thus accentuated their concern with self-interest. School-age children donated more in the negative-mood condition if an experimenter was present, but not if the experimenter was absent. The results suggest the children felt that the experimenter expected them to donate coupons. However, the problem of distinguishing between the attitude and social-norm components arises again. Instead of being motivated to comply with the experimenter's expectations, the children may simply have preferred one type of reinforcement over another, social approval over material rewards (cf. Weisz, 1978). The results would more clearly support the developmental hypothesis if the experimenter had stated his expectation that the children would behave generously, informed the children that he would not actually know how much they donated, and left the room (cf. Grusec, 1972). If negative mood still led to increased donating in this condition, the results could be unambiguously attributed to the influence of social norms. At high school and college age, subjects donated more when in a negative mood even if the donation was anonymous. The findings are consistent with the hypothesis that the subjects viewed donating as a personal norm and found it self-gratifying to act in accordance with personal norms (Schwartz, 1977).

The variety of experiments that could be done to test the developmental hypothesis is virtually unlimited. To establish its generality and boundary conditions, different behaviors could be assessed in different contexts. To gain further understanding of the three components and their construct validity, different experimental manipulations of each component could be used to see if they have similar effects. Finally, more than one component can be varied in an experiment. If both attitudes and social norms are manipulated, and age is a third factor in the design, the results would directly show whether the weighting of the two components changed with age.

A second approach is to continue the assessment of social cognition through verbal responses, following the general procedure of Fishbein and Ajzen (1975). Individuals respond to an interview or questionnaire that contains independent measures of the three components and behavioral intentions. Then estimates of the components are used in a multiple regression equation to predict behavior.

The third approach is a modification of the Fishbein-Ajzen procedure. Instead of obtaining measures of the three components from specific questions and fixed-format response scales, subjects would be asked open-ended questions about how they would behave in a particular situation and why. One advantage of the alternative procedure is that it allows a check of the validity of the a priori classification of reasons for behavior into three components. If coders supplied only with a conceptual definition of the three components can reliably assign all individuals' responses to one of the components, claims that the three components form a mutually exclusive and exhaustive set will be strengthened. Instances in which coders have difficulty in reliably distinguishing the components will suggest the need for refinements in their definitions. This method of construct validation was used in recent studies of interpersonal and achievement attributions (Frieze, 1976; Orvis et al., 1976). Another advantage of the alternative procedure is the possibility of directly assessing how people decided what to do. Techniques for obtaining reports on the decision-making process could be adapted from those used to study problem solving in adults (Newell & Simon, 1972).

Combinations of the three approaches are feasible. When social cognitions are assessed through verbal reports, experimental manipulations that are known to affect people's behavior might be described in the stimuli. For example, subjects in different conditions might be given different information about what other people expect them to do. How the information affects what subjects say they would do, and how they say they made their decision, could be examined. Conversely, when actual behavior is of primary interest, people could be asked to report on the reasons for their behavior.

Will the different methods lead to similar results? According to Nisbett and Wilson (1977), the answer is "no" in many cases. They reviewed experiments in cognitive and social psychology, and presented new data of their own, that almost invariably indicated little or no correspondence between the factors that actually influenced people's behavior and the factors people said influenced their behavior. Nisbett and Wilson's explanation for the general lack of correspondence, and occasional reports of high correspondence, can be summarized in two propositions about people's reports on the causes of their own behavior. First, the reports are not based on a conscious awareness of mental processes, for people do not have conscious awareness of these processes. Second, the reports are based on causal theories, ideas about the possible causes of behavior in particular situations. When powerful causes of behavior are not represented in people's causal theories, verbal reports will be inaccurate. When the causal theories are reasonably accurate, the same will be true for verbal reports. Accuracy is especially likely if people are following an explicit rule in their subculture about how to respond to specific stimuli, and if there is continuing feedback concerning how well people are following the rule.

Although Nisbett and Wilson emphasize the inaccuracy of verbal reports, the cases that are most important from the present perspective may fit the conditions for accurate reports. That is, people's causal theories are likely to include the assumption that self-interest, other people's expectations, and personal standards are important influences on behavior. The theories are likely to contain the idea that decisions must be made by balancing the three influences. Furthermore, people are likely to receive clear and often strong feedback from other people about the correctness of their balancing rule. These assumptions may be valid for children as well as adults. Returning briefly to an earlier example, Johnny may want his bicycle for himself, but feel he should share it with Jimmy. Johnny may recognize the two factors in the dilemma, and accurately report how he weighed them.

These assertions are not to be taken as self-evident truths, but as hypotheses to be tested against alternatives. The correspondence between verbal reports and actual causes of behavior may change with age, because of changes in children's theories of social causation. Developmental research on the topic would be extremely intriguing. It would also bridge social-psychological research on the adult intuitive psychologist (Ross, 1977) and developmental research on metacognition, or children's thinking about their own thinking (Brown, 1978; Flavell & Wellman, 1976). Finally, it would expose an important new relation, between actual social-cognitive processes and people's theories of these processes.

Conclusion

The first theme of this chapter was that research on social cognition stands at the intersection of two older research areas, studies of nonsocial cognition and studies of social behavior. These areas can be related to one another in various ways. Some appear to be more promising than others. Although the relation between social and nonsocial cognition has most often been studied by correlating measures of performance on the two types of tasks, this method is of dubious value. Abstract similarities between the abilities required for the two do exist, but the tremendous differences in the content of the tasks are likely to lead to nonsignificant or low correlations between them. Exploration of similarities and differences in the process of development of social and nonsocial cognition appears to be more valuable. Research has shown that experience, and social experience in particular, influences development in both domains. Investigation of the factors responsible for the effects of experience is likely to most rapidly lead to the integration of research on social and nonsocial cognition.

Conceptual analyses of the relation between social cognition and social behavior are rare in developmental psychology. To describe the relation a model was presented that includes aspects of Kohlberg's theory of moral development and Fishbein and Ajzen's (1975) theory of the relation between attitudes and behavior. The model assumes that social behavior is a function of people's relative weighting of three components: (1) attitudes toward a behavior, which depend on an evaluation of its consequences for the actor; (2) social norms and motivation to comply with them, which reflect the influence of other people's expectations; and (3) personal norms and motivation to comply with them, which reflect an actor's commitment to do what he or she believes should be done. A rough equivalence between the three components and the three levels in Kohlberg's typology for moral reasoning was discussed. Although the model is probably inaccurate in detail, it may be a helpful first step in studying the relations between social cognition and behavior.

The second and equally important theme in this chapter concerns the role of hypothesis testing in social-cognitive research. I presented the hypothesis that social conflicts, conflicts with a peer about the proper viewpoint on a situation or the correct approach to a task, can be an important source of developmental change in social and nonsocial cognition. However, conflicts may not produce cognitive progress in all cases. An analysis of the process of recognizing and responding to conflicts indicated that several different outcomes of a conflict are possible. Each outcome can be expected to have a different effect on cognitive change. Moreover, the effects of conflicts can be explained in various ways. Instances in which two children resolve a conflict after full discussion of each child's viewpoint are most interesting. If both children show increases in understanding as a result of their discussion, the effect can be attributed to a process of social discovery that is analogous to the process of self-discovery (or equilibration) in Piagetian theory. Through discussion with one another the children discover more advanced conceptions than either possessed initially.

I also presented the hypothesis that age changes in social behavior can be attributed to changes in social cognition. Specifically, the relative influences on behavior of attitudes toward a behavior, social norms, and personal norms may change with age. Various factors might explain the developmental changes, for example, a change in children's ability to understand that other people have expectations for their behavior. In addition, examples of three types of research that might be done to test the hypothesis were given. The greatest contrast exists between methods that infer social cognition from people's behavior and methods that assess social cognition through people's verbal reports. The extent to which studies using the two methods would show similar results was considered.

The emphasis on generation and testing of hypotheses may seem surprising, because the first section of the chapter reported a purely normative study of children's conceptions of friendship. However, I believe that we now have fairly complete descriptions of several aspects of social cognitive development. Progress in the field may be enhanced if attention is given to hypotheses that attempt to *explain* the development of social cognition.

References

Ajzen, I., & Fishbein, M. Attitudinal and normative variables as predictors of specific behaviors. *Journal of Personality and Social Psychology*, 1973, *27*, 41–57.

Attitude-behavior relations: A theoretical analysis and review of empirical research. *Psychological Bulletin*, 1977, *84*, 888–918.

Aronfreed, J. Moral development from the standpoint of a general psychological theory. In T. Lickona (Ed.), *Moral development and behavior: Theory, research, and social issues.* New York: Holt, Rinehart & Winston, 1976.

Bigelow, B. J. Children's friendship expectations: A cognitive-developmental study. *Child Development,* 1977, *48,* 246–53.

Bigelow, B. J., & LaGaipa, J. J. Children's written descriptions of friendship: A multidimensional analysis. *Developmental Psychology,* 1975, *11,* 857–8.

Botvin, G. J., & Murray, F. B. The efficacy of peer modeling and social conflict in the acquisition of conservation. *Child Development,* 1975, *46,* 796–9.

Brainerd, C. J. Learning research and Piagetian theory. In L. S. Siegel and C. J. Brainerd (Eds.), *Alternatives to Piaget: Critical essays on the theory.* New York: Academic, 1978.

Brown, A. L. Knowing when, where, and how to remember: A problem of metacognition. In R. Glaser (Ed.), *Advances in Instructional Psychology* (Vol. 1). Hillsdale, N.J.: Lawrence Erlbaum Associates, 1978.

Burton, R. V. Generality of honesty reconsidered. *Psychological Review,* 1963, *70,* 481–99.

Cialdini, R. B., & Kenrick, D. T. Altruism as hedonism: A social development perspective on the relationship of negative mood state and helping. *Journal of Personality and Social Psychology,* 1976, *34,* 907–14.

Damon, W. *The social world of the child.* San Francisco: Jossey-Bass, 1977.

(Ed.), *Social Cognition.* San Francisco: Jossey-Bass, 1978.

Dienstbier, R. A. Attribution, socialization, and moral decision making. In J. H. Harvey, W. Ickes, and R. F. Kidd (Eds.), *New directions in attribution research* (Vol. 2) Hillsdale, N.J.: Lawrence Erlbaum Associates, 1978.

Douvan, E., & Adelson, J. *The adolescent experience.* New York: Wiley, 1966.

Duck, S. W. *Personal relationships and personal constructs.* London: Wiley, 1973.

Duck, S. *Theory and practice in interpersonal attraction.* London: Academic, 1977.

Eder, D., & Hallinan, M. T. Sex differences in children's friendships. *American Sociological Review,* 1978, *43,* 237–50.

Feshbach, N. Sex differences in children's modes of aggressive response toward outsiders. *Merrill-Palmer Quarterly,* 1969, *15,* 249–58.

Feshbach, N., & Sones, G. Sex differences in adolescent reactions toward newcomers. *Developmental Psychology,* 1971, *4,* 381–6.

Fishbein, M., & Azjen, I. *Beliefs, attitudes, intentions, and behavior: An introduction to theory and research.* Reading, Mass.: Addison-Wesley, 1975.

Flavell, J. H. Concept development. In P. H. Mussen (Ed.), *Carmichael's manual of child psychology* (Vol. 1, 3rd ed.). New York: Wiley, 1970.

Cognitive development. Englewood Cliffs, N.J.: Prentice-Hall, 1977.

Flavell, J. H., & Wellman, H. M. Metamemory. In R. V. Kail and J. W. Hagen (Eds.), *Memory in cognitive development.* Hillsdale, N.J.: Lawrence Erlbaum Associates, 1976.

Frieze, I. H. Causal attributions and information seeking to explain success and failure. *Journal of Research in Personality,* 1976, *10,* 293–305.

Gamer, E. Children's reports of friendship criteria. Paper presented at the meeting of the Massachusetts Psychological Association, May 1977.

Grusec, J. E. Demand characteristics of the modeling experiment: Altruism as a function of age and aggression. *Journal of Personality and Social Psychology,* 1972, *22,* 139–48.

Hartup, W. W. Peer interaction and social organization. In P. H. Mussen (Ed.), *Carmichael's manual of child psychology* (Vol. 2, 3rd ed.), New York: Wiley, 1970.

Harvey, J. H., Wells, G. L., & Alvarez, M. D. Attribution in the context of conflict and separation in close relationships. In J. H. Harvey, W. Ickes, and R. F. Kidd (Eds.), *New directions in attribution research* (Vol. 2). Hillsdale, N.J.: Lawrence Erlbaum Associates, 1978.

Hayes, D. S. Cognitive bases for liking and disliking among preschool children. *Child Development,* 1978, *49,* 906–9.

Henshel, A. The relationship between values and behavior: A developmental hypothesis. *Child Development*, 1971, *42*, 1997–2007.

Hoffman, M. L. Empathy, role-taking, guilt, and development of altruistic motives. In T. Lickona (Ed.), *Moral development and behavior: Theory, research, and social issues*. New York: Holt, Rinehart & Winston, 1976.

Huston, T. L. *Foundations of interpersonal attraction*. New York: Academic, 1974.

Inhelder, B., & Piaget, J. *The growth of logical thinking from childhood to adolescence*. New York: Basic, 1958.

Kenrick, D. T., Baumann, D. J., & Cialdini, R. B. A step in the socialization of altruism as hedonism: Effects of negative mood on children's generality under public and private conditions. *Journal of Personality and Social Psychology*, 1979, *37*, 747–55.

Kohlberg, L. Stage and sequence: The cognitive-developmental approach to socialization. In D. A. Goslin (Ed.), *Handbook of socialization theory and research*. New York: Rand-McNally, 1969.

Moral stages and moralization: The cognitive-developmental approach. In T. Lickona (Ed.), *Moral development and behavior: Theory, research, and social issues*. New York: Holt, Rinehart & Winston, 1976.

Kurdek, L. A. Perspective taking as the cognitive basis of children's moral development. A review of the literature. *Merrill-Palmer Quarterly*, 1978, *24*, 1–28.

LaGaipa, J. J. Interpersonal attraction and social exchange. In S. Duck (Ed.), *Theory and practice in interpersonal attraction*. London: Academic, 1977.

Maccoby, E. E., & Jacklin, C. N. *The psychology of sex differences*. Stanford: Stanford University Press, 1974.

Mischel, W., & Mischel, H. N. A cognitive social-learning approach to morality and self-regulation. In T. Lickona (Ed.), *Moral development and behavior: Theory, research, and social issues*. New York: Holt, Rinehart & Winston, 1976.

Monroe, W. S. Social consciousness in children. *Psychological Review*, 1898, *5*, 68–70.

Mugny, G., & Doise, W. Socio-cognitive conflict and structure of individual and collective performances. *European Journal of Social Psychology*, 1978, *8*, 181–92.

Murray, F. B. Acquisition of conservation through social interaction. *Developmental Psychology*, 1972, *6*, 1–6.

Mussen, P., & Eisenberg-Berg, N. *Roots of caring, sharing, and helping: The development of prosocial behavior in children*. San Francisco: Freeman, 1977.

Newell, A., & Simon, H. A. *Human problem solving*. Englewood Cliffs, N.J.: Prentice-Hall, 1972.

Nisbett, R. E., & Wilson, T. D. Telling more than we can know: Verbal reports on mental processes. *Psychological Review*, 1977, *84*, 231–59.

Orvis, B. R., Kelly, H. H., & Butler, D. Attributional conflict in young couples. In J. H. Harvey, W. H. Ickes, and R. F. Kidd (Eds.), *New directions in attribution research* (Vol. 1). Hillsdale, N. J.: Lawrence Erlbaum Associates, 1976.

Paine, R. Anthropological approaches to friendships. In E. Leyton (Ed.), *The compact: Selected dimensions of friendship*. Newfoundland: Memorial University of Newfoundland, 1974.

Peevers, B. H., & Secord, P. F. Developmental changes in attribution of descriptive concepts to persons. *Journal of Personality and Social Psychology*, 1973, *27*, 120–8.

Piaget, J. *The moral judgment of the child*. New York: Free Press, 1965 (Originally published, 1932).

Piaget's theory. In P. H. Mussen (Ed.), *Carmichael's manual of child psychology* (Vol 1., 3rd ed.), New York: Wiley, 1970.

Pomazal, R. J., & Jaccard, J. J. An informational approach to altruistic behavior. *Journal of Personality and Social Psychology*, 1976, *33*, 317–26.

Reisman, J. M., & Schorr, S. I. Friendship claims and expectations among children and adults. *Child Development*, 1978, *49*, 913–16.

Rest, J. The hierarchical nature of moral judgment: A study of patterns of comprehension and preference of moral stages. *Journal of Personality*, 1973, *41*, 86–109.

Ross, L. The intuitive psychologist and his shortcomings: Distortions in the attribution process. In L. Berkowitz (Ed.), *Advances in experimental social psychology* (Vol. 10). New York: Academic, 1977.

Selman, R. L., & Jaquette, D. The development of interpersonal awareness (a working draft): A manual constructed by the Harvard-Judge Baker Social Reasoning Project, January 1977.

Schwartz, S. H. Normative influences on altruism. In L. Berkowitz (Ed.), *Advances in experimental social psychology* (Vol. 10). New York: Academic, 1977.

Shantz, C. U. The development of social cognition. In E. M. Hetherington (Ed.), *Review of child development research* (Vol. 5). Chidago: University of Chicago Press, 1975.

Silverman, I. W., & Geiringer, E. Dyadic interaction and conservation induction: A test of Piaget's equilibration model. *Child Development*, 1973, *44*, 815–20.

Sullivan, H. S. *The interpersonal theory of psychiatry*. New York: Norton, 1953.

Turiel, E. The development of concepts of social structure: Social-convention. In J. Glick and K. A. Clarke-Steward (Eds.), *Personality and Social Development* (Vol. 1). New York: Gardner, 1978.

Weisz, J. R. Choosing problem-solving rewards and Halloween prizes: Delay of gratification and preference for symbolic reward as a function of development, motivation, and personal investment. *Developmental Psychology*, 1978, *14*, 66–78.

Youniss, J., & Volpe, J. A relational analysis of children's friendships. In W. Damon (Ed.), *Social cognition*. San Francisco: Jossey-Bass, 1978.

9 Self-referent thought: a developmental analysis of self-efficacy

Albert Bandura

Much psychological research is aimed at explaining how children gain knowledge of their social and physical environment. An equally important but surprisingly little-studied problem is how children come to know themselves, and how their self-percepts affect their psychosocial functioning. Among the different facets of self-knowledge, perhaps none is more central to people's everyday lives than conceptions of their personal efficacy. Such self-percepts affect not only the courses of action people pursue but their thought patterns, and the emotional arousal they experience (Bandura, 1977a, 1981). This chapter explores the nature and sources of self-efficacy and the ways in which efficacy judgments enter into the determination of behavior. I shall first present a conceptual analysis of self-efficacy and then discuss the developmental aspects of this phenomenon.

Conceptual framework

Competence in dealing with one's environment is not a fixed act or simply a matter of knowing what to do. Rather, it involves a generative capability in which component cognitive, social, and motor skills are organized into integrated courses of action in accordance with certain rules or strategies. A capability is only as good as its execution. Performance of a skill requires continuous improvisation and adjustment to ever changing circumstances. Even routinized activities are rarely performed in exactly the same way. Thus the initiation and regulation of transactions with the environment are partly governed by judgments of operative capabilities. Self-efficacy is concerned with judgments about how well one can organize and execute courses of action required to deal with prospective situa-

The preparation of this paper and research by the author reported here was facilitated by Public Health Research Grant M-5162 from the National Institute of Mental Health.

tions that contain many ambiguous, unpredictable, and often stressful, elements.

Diverse effects of perceived self-efficacy

Perceived efficacy can have diverse effects on behavior, thought patterns, and affective arousal. The behavioral effects take several different forms. Self-percepts of efficacy influence choice of activity and environmental settings. People tend to avoid situations they believe exceed their capabilities, but they undertake and perform with assurance activities they judge themselves capable of handling (Bandura, 1977a). Any factor that helps to determine choice behavior can have profound effects on the course of personal development. Active engagement in activities contributes to the growth of competencies. Shunning enriching activities and environments retards development of potentialities and shields negative self-percepts from corrective change.

Self-efficacy also determines how much effort people will expend and how long they will persist in the face of obstacles or aversive experiences. The stronger the perceived self-efficacy, the more vigorous and persistent are the efforts. In the face of difficulties people who entertain serious doubts about their capacities slacken their efforts or give up altogether, whereas those who have a strong sense of efficacy exert greater effort to master the challenges (Bandura, 1977a; Schunk, 1981). Because knowledge and competencies are achieved through sustained effort, any factor that leads people to give up readily has personally limiting consequences.

People's perceptions of their own capabilities also influence their thought processes and emotional reactions during anticipatory and actual transactions with their environment. Those who judge themselves inefficacious in coping with environmental demands tend to engage in frequent self-appraisals of inadequacy and cognize potential difficulties as more formidable than they really are. Such self-referent preoccupation produces disruptive arousal and impairs performance by diverting attention from the task at hand to self-evaluative concerns (Beck, 1976; Meichenbaum, 1977; Sarason, 1975a). By contrast, people who have a strong sense of efficacy deploy their skills well to the demands of the situation and are spurred by obstacles to greater effort.

Function of self-efficacy judgment

In their daily lives people continuously have to make decisions about whether or not to pursue certain courses of action or how long to continue those they have undertaken. As we have noted, such decisions are partly determined by judgments of personal efficacy. Accurate appraisal of one's own capabilities is therefore of considerable value in successful functioning. Misjudgments of personal efficacy in either direction have consequences. People who grossly overestimate their capabilities undertake activities that are clearly beyond their reach. As a result, they get themselves into considerable difficulties and suffer needless failures, if not injuries. Some of the missteps, of course, can produce serious irreversible harm.

People who underestimate their capabilities also bear costs, although these are more likely to take self-limiting rather than aversive forms. Such individuals typically avoid beneficial environments and activities that cultivate personal potentialities. They cut themselves off from potentially rewarding experiences. Moreover, by approaching tasks with strong self-doubts, they dwell on personal deficiencies and generate debilitating distress, which creates internal obstacles to effective performance.

In the case of habitual routines, people develop their self-knowledge through repeated experiences to the point where they no longer need to judge their efficacy on each occasion they perform the activity. They behave in accordance with what they know they can or cannot do without giving the matter much further thought. However, significant changes in task demands or situational circumstances prompt efficacy reappraisals as guides for action under altered conditions.

There are decided benefits to suspending further self-efficacy appraisals in routinized performances that have proven highly successful. If people had to judge their capabilities anew each time they were about to drive their automobiles or to perform other familiar tasks they would spend much of their cognitive life in redundant self-referent thought. There are considerable personal costs, however, when self-judged inefficacy leads to routinized thoughtless avoidance of activities and situations that can enrich one's life. Langer and her associates (Langer, 1979) document the self-debilitating effects that result when people erroneously judge themselves as incompetent without giving much further thought to their capabilities.

Sources of efficacy information

Self-knowledge is gained through information conveyed by either personal or socially mediated experiences. Judgments of one's own efficacy, whether accurate or faulty, are based on four principal sources of information. These include performance accomplishments; vicarious experiences of observing the performances of others; verbal persuasion and allied types of social influences that one possesses certain capabilities; and states of physiological arousal from which people partly judge their capableness and vulnerability.

Performance accomplishments. Enactive attainments provide the most influential source of efficacy information because they are based on authentic mastery experiences (Bandura, Adams, & Beyer, 1977). Successes raise efficacy appraisals; repeated failures lower them, especially if the failures occur early in the course of events and do not reflect lack of effort or adverse external circumstances. After a strong sense of efficacy is developed through repeated success, occasional failures are unlikely to have much effect on judgments of one's capabilities. Indeed, failures that are overcome by determined effort can instill robust percepts of self-efficacy through experience that one can eventually master even the most difficult obstacles.

Vicarious experience. People do not rely on enactive experience as the sole source of information about their capabilities. Efficacy appraisals are partly influenced by vicarious experiences. Seeing similar others perform successfully can raise efficacy expectations in observers that they too possess the capabilities to master comparable activities (Bandura et al., 1977). They persuade themselves that if others can do it, they should be able to achieve at least some improvement in performance. By the same token, observing others perceived to be of similar competence fail despite high effort lowers observers' judgments of their own capabilities (Brown & Inouye, 1978).

There are several conditions under which efficacy appraisals are especially sensitive to vicarious information. Amount of prior experience is one such factor. Perceived efficacy can be readily changed by relevant modeling influences when people have little previous experience on which to base evaluations of their personal competence. Lacking direct knowledge of their own capabilities, they rely more heavily on modeled indicators (Takata & Takata, 1976).

Although vicarious influences are generally weaker than are direct personal experiences, they can produce significant enduring changes through their performance effects. People convinced vicariously of their inefficacy are inclined to behave in ineffectual ways that, in fact, generate confirmatory behavioral evidence of inability. Conversely, modeling influences that enhance perceived efficacy can weaken the impact of direct failure experiences by sustaining performance in the face of repeated failure (Brown & Inouye, 1978). A given mode of influence can thus set in motion processes that augment its effects or diminish the effects of otherwise powerful influences.

Verbal persuasion. In attempts to influence human behavior, verbal persuasion is widely used because of its ease and ready availability. People are led, through suggestion, into believing that they possess certain capabilities and that they can surmount their difficulties. Although social persuasion alone may be limited in its power to create enduring increases in self-efficacy, it can contribute to successful performance if the heightened appraisal is within realistic bounds. To the extent that persuasive boosts in self-efficacy lead people to try hard enough to succeed, such influences promote development of skills and competencies.

It is probably more difficult to produce enduring increases in perceived efficacy by persuasory means than to undermine it. Illusory boosts in efficacy are readily disconfirmed by the results of one's actions. But the people who are persuaded of their inefficacy tend to avoid challenging activities and give up readily in the face of difficulties. By restricting choice behavior and undermining effort, self-disbeliefs readily create their own validation.

Emotional arousal. Stressful and taxing situations generally elicit emotional reactions of varying intensities. Emotional arousal provides another constituent source of efficacy information. People rely partly on their state of physiological arousal in judging their capabilities and vulnerability to stress. Because high arousal usually debilitates performance, individuals are more likely to expect success when they are not beset by aversive arousal than if they are tense and viscerally agitated. Fear reactions generate further fear through anticipatory self-arousal. By conjuring up fear-provoking thoughts about their ineptitude, people can rouse themselves to elevated levels of distress that produce the very dysfunctions they fear.

Cognitive processing of efficacy information

The discussion thus far has centered on the different sources of information – enactive, vicarious, persuasory, and emotive – that people use in judging their capabilities. A distinction must be drawn between information conveyed by environmental events and information processed, weighted, and integrated into efficacy judgments. The impact of different experiences on perceptions of personal efficacy will depend on how they are cognitively appraised. Cognitive processes in efficacy judgment have two separable aspects: The first concerns the types of cues people use as indicators of personal efficacy; the second concerns the inference rules or heuristics they employ for integrating efficacy information from different sources in arriving at their self-efficacy judgments.

Enactive information. Many factors can affect level of performance that have little to do with ability. Efficacy evaluation is therefore an inferential process in which the relative contribution of ability and nonability factors to performance successes and failures must be weighted. The degree to which people are likely to raise their perceived efficacy through performance successes will depend upon, among other factors, the difficulty of the task, the amount of effort they expend, the amount of external aid they receive, the situational circumstances under which they perform, and the temporal pattern of their successes and failures.

Mastery of an easy task is redundant with what one already knows, whereas mastery of a difficult task conveys new efficacy information for raising one's efficacy appraisal. Successes achieved with external aid carry less efficacy value because they are likely to be credited to external factors rather than to personal capabilities. Similarly, faulty performances under adverse situational conditions will have much weaker efficacy implications than those executed under optimal circumstances.

Cognitive appraisals of effort expenditure may further affect the impact of performance accomplishments on judgments of personal efficacy. Success with minimal effort fosters ability ascriptions but analogous attainments gained through heavy labor connote a lesser ability and are thus likely to have weaker impact on perceived self-efficacy. The rate and pattern of attainments furnish additional information for judging personal efficacy. Individuals who experience periodic failures but continue to improve over time are more apt to raise their perceived efficacy than those who succeed but see their performances leveling off compared to their prior rate of improvement. Studies conducted within the attributional framework (Bem, 1972; Weiner, 1974) have examined how some of these variables affect performance. In a social learning analysis, these types of factors serve as conveyors of efficacy information that influence performance largely through their intervening effects on perceptions of self-efficacy, as when people infer their level of efficacy from effort and task-difficulty cues.

Similar inferential processes operate in efficacy appraisal based on performance failures. Deficient performances are unlikely to lower perceived efficacy much, if at all, when failures are discounted on the grounds of insufficient effort, adverse situational conditions, despondent mood, or debilitated physical state. People who hold a low view of themselves are prone to the opposite judgmental bias – crediting their achievements to external factors rather than to their own capabilities (Bandura, Adams, Hardy, & Howells, 1980). Here the problem is one of inaccurate ascription of personal competency to situational factors. In such cases, stable boosts in self-efficacy require mastery experiences on challenging tasks with minimal external aid that verify personal capabilities (Bandura, 1977a).

Perceived efficacy is affected for better or for worse not only by how performance successes and failures are interpreted, but also by biases in the self-monitoring of the performances themselves. In any given endeavor, some performances surpass, other match, and still others fall below one's typical attainments. Such variations allow some leeway in what aspects of one's performance are observed and remembered. People who selectively attend to the more negative aspects of their performances are likely to underestimate their efficacy even though they may process correctly what they remember. In such instances the problems reside in faulty attentional and memorial processes rather than in the inferential judgments made about the causes of one's successes and failures.

Selective self-monitoring can also magnify percepts of self-efficacy if it is the personal successes that are especially noticed and remembered. Research on self-modeling provides suggestive evidence bearing on this enhancement effect (Dowrick, 1977). In these studies children exhibiting gross deficits in psychomotor and social skills are helped, by a variety of aids, to perform at a level that exceeds their usual attainments. The hesitancies, mistakes, and external aids are then selectively deleted from the videotape recordings to show the children performing much more skillfully than they are normally capable of doing. After observing their videotaped successes they display substantial improvement in performance compared to their baseline level or to other activities that are filmed but not self-observed. Seeing oneself perform errorlessly can enhance proficiency in at least two ways: It provides further information on how to perform appropriately, and it strengthens self-beliefs that one can succeed.

Vicarious information. The cognitive processing of vicariously derived information will similarly depend on efficacy indicants conveyed by modeled events. We noted earlier that people judge their capabilities partly through social comparison with the performances of others. Similarity to the model is one factor that increases the personal relevance of modeled performance information for observers' perceptions of their own efficacy. Persons who are similar or slightly higher in ability provide the most informative compar-ative information for gauging one's own capabilities (Festinger, 1954; Suls & Miller, 1977). Neither outperforming those of lesser ability nor being surpassed by the vastly superior convey much information about one's own level of competence. In general, modeled successes by similar others raise, and modeled failures lower, self-appraisals.

In gauging personal efficacy through social comparison, observers may rely on similarity to the model either in past performances or in attributes presumably predictive of the ability in question. The influential role of prior performance similarity on vicarious efficacy appraisal is revealed in a study by Brown and Inouye (1978). Observers who believed themselves to be superior to a failing model maintained high efficacy expectations and did not at all slacken their efforts despite repeated failure. In con-trast, modeled failure had a devastating effect on observers' self-judged efficacy when they perceived themselves of comparable ability to the model. They expressed a very low sense of personal efficacy and gave up quickly when they encountered difficulties on the task. Regardless of treatment condition, the higher the observers' perceived efficacy the longer they persisted on insoluble tasks.

Efficacy appraisals are often based, not on comparative performance experiences, but on similarity to models on personal characteristics as-sumed to be predictive of performance capabilities. People develop pre-conceptions of performance capabilities according to age, sex, educa-tional and socioeconomic level, race, and ethnic designation, even though the performances of individuals within these groups are extremely varied. Such preconceptions usually arise from a combination of cultural stereo-typing and overgeneralization from salient personal experiences.

Attribute similarity generally increases the force of modeling influences even though the personal characteristics may be spurious indicants of performance capabilities (Rosenthal & Bandura, 1978). Indeed, when model attributes irrelevant to the new task are salient and overweighted in predictive value, irrelevant model characteristics (e.g., age or sex) exert greater sway on observers than do more relevant ability cues (Kaz-din, 1974). When the successes of models who possess similar attributes lead others to try things they would otherwise shun, spurious indicants have beneficial social effects. But comparative efficacy appraisals through faulty preconceptions often lead those who are uncertain about their capabilities to judge valuable pursuits to be beyond their reach. In such instances, judging efficacy by social comparison is self-limiting.

Vicariously derived information alters perceived self-efficacy through ways other than social comparison. Competent models can teach observers effective strategies for dealing with challenging or threatening situations. This contribution is especially important when perceived inefficacy reflects behavioral deficits rather than misappraisals of the skills one possesses. In addition, modeling displays convey information about the nature of environmental tasks, the difficulties they present, and the predictability of environmental events. Modeled transactions may reveal the tasks to be more or less difficult, and potential threats more or less manageable than observers originally believed. Adoption of serviceable strategies and altered perceptions of task difficulty will alter perceived efficacy. In therapeutic applications of modeling what phobic thinking renders frightful, instructive modeling makes predictable and personally controllable (Bandura, Adams, & Reese, 1980).

The influence of modeled strategy information can alter the usual efficacy effects of social comparative information. Seeing a superior other fail through means clearly insufficient can boost self-efficacy in observers who believe they have more suitable strategies at their command. Conversely, observing a similar other barely succeed through the most adroit tactics may lead observers to reevaluate the task as much more difficult than they had previously assumed. To shed new light on vicarious self-efficacy appraisals, future research should concern itself with strategy exemplification and task evaluation as well as with comparative ability indicants.

Persuasory information. People do not always believe what they are told concerning their performance capabilities. Skepticism develops from personal experiences that often run counter to what one has been told. Were this always the case, performers would eventually turn a deaf ear to their persuaders. But there are many occasions when individuals are persuaded to try things they avoid, or to persist at tasks they were ready to discontinue, only to discover, much to their surprise, that they were capable of mastering them. Consequently, persuasory judgments have to be weighted in terms of who the persuaders are and their credibility.

People often voice opinions of what others can do without being thoroughly acquainted with the difficulty of the tasks, or with the circumstances under which they will have to be performed. Therefore, even the judgments of otherwise credible persuaders may be discounted on the grounds that they do not fully understand the task demands.

Arousal information. The information conveyed by physiological arousal similarly affects perceived efficacy through judgmental processes. A number of factors, including appraisal of the sources of arousal, the level of activation, the circumstances under which arousal is elicited, and past experiences on how arousal affects one's performances are likely to figure in the cognitive processing of emotional reactivity. Activities are often performed in situations that contain varied evocative stimuli. The multiplicity of stimuli creates ambiguity about what caused the physiological reactions. The efficacy value of the resultant arousal will therefore vary depending on the factors singled out and the meaning given to them.

Self-appraisal of efficacy from arousal cues raises a number of developmental questions that require empirical clarification: How do young children come to view bodily states as emotional conditions? How do they learn to tell what emotion they are experiencing? How do they learn that arousal cues signifying particular emotions are predictive of level of functioning? In the social learning view, development of knowledge concerning bodily states is heavily dependent on social labeling processes. Arousing experiences contain three significant events – affective elicitors, internal arousal, and expressive reactions. The internal arousal itself cannot play a differentiating role in the social labeling because the arousal is unobservable to others and phenomenologically different emotions appear to have a similar physiological state (Frankenhaeuser, 1975; Levin, 1972; Mandler, 1975). Adults must therefore infer the presence of bodily states in young children from their expressive reactions and from environmental elicitors known to produce particular types of emotions. Drawing on these observable events adults describe and differentiate the emotions children are experiencing (e.g., happy, sad, angry, fearful) and identify their causes. Thus, for example, arousal is interpreted as fear in threatening situations, as joy in pleasurable situations, as anger in thwarting situations, and as sorrow when valued objects are irretrievably lost (Hunt, Cole, & Reis, 1958; Schachter, 1964). Through repeated social linkage of elicitors, expressive reactions, and internal arousal, children eventually learn to interpret and to differentiate their affective experiences. Different personal interpretations of internal arousal (e.g., "frightened," "fired up") will have different impacts on perceived self-efficacy.

The self-efficacy implications of arousal derive from past experiences with how labeled arousal affects performance. For people who generally find arousal facilitory rather than debilitating, arousal will have different efficacy value than those for whom arousal usually portends marred performances. The judgmental process is complicated by the fact that it is not arousal per se, but its level, that usually serves as the performance indicator. As a general rule, moderate levels of arousal facilitate performance, whereas high levels disrupt it. This is especially true in complex activities requiring intricate organization of behavior.

What constitutes an optimal level of arousal depends not only on the nature of the task, but on causal inferences concerning the arousal. People vary in their judgmental sets. Those who are inclined to perceive their arousal as stemming from personal inadequacies are more likely to lower their perceived efficacy than those who regard their arousal as a common transitory reaction that even the most competent experience.

Integration of efficacy information

The preceding discussion explored the efficacy implications of single dimensions of information within each of the four modalities. In forming their efficacy judgments people have to deal not only with different configurations of efficacy-relevant information conveyed by a given modality, but to weigh and integrate efficacy information from these diverse sources. There has been little research on how people process multidimensional efficacy information. However, there is every reason to believe that efficacy judgments are governed by some common judgmental processes.

Studies of judgmental processes show that people have difficulty weighting and integrating multidimensional information (Slovic, Fischhoff, & Lichtenstein, 1977; Slovic & Lichtenstein, 1971; Tversky & Kahneman, 1974). As a result, they tend to rely on simple judgmental rules. This often leads them to ignore or to inaccurately weigh relevant information. When subjective descriptions of their judgmental processes are compared with their actual judgments, the findings show that people tend to underestimate their reliance on important cues and overweigh those of lesser value.

Although common cognitive processes probably operate in both efficacy and nonpersonal judgments, forming conceptions of oneself undoubtedly involve some distinct processes as well. The persons are rare who are entirely dispassionate about themselves. Self-referent experiences are more likely than experiences involving other persons or objects to arouse affective reactions. Emotional arousal can distort self-monitoring, retention, and processing of multidimensional efficacy information.

Developmental analysis of self-efficacy

We noted earlier that accurate appraisal of one's own capabilities is highly advantageous and often essential for effective functioning. Those who seriously misjudge what they can do are apt to behave in ways that produce detrimental consequences. Very young children lack knowledge of their own capabilities and the demands and potential hazards of differ-

ent courses of action. They would repeatedly get themselves into dangerous predicaments were it not for the guidance of others. They can climb
high places, wander into rivers or deep pools, and wield sharp knives
before they develop the necessary skills for managing such situations
safely (Sears, Maccoby, & Levin, 1957). Adult watchfulness and guidance
see young children through this early formative period until they gain
sufficient knowledge of what they can do and what skills different situations require. With development of cognitive capacities, self-efficacy
judgment increasingly supplants external guidance.

Beginnings of perceived efficacy

A comprehensive theory must explain the origin of social cognition as
well as its nature, function, and developmental course. Self-referent
thought is initially derived from action and observational learning from
occurrences of environmental events. The experiences arising from children's commerce with their environment provide the initial basis for development of a sense of personal efficacy. Infants behave in certain ways,
and certain things happen. Waving rattles produces predictable sounds,
energetic kicks shake cribs, and cries bring adults. By repeatedly observing covariations between their actions and environmental effects, they
begin to develop a sense of personal agency – a growing realization that
they can make events occur.

Newborns are neither as helpless nor as insensitive to environmental
events as previously thought (Papoušek & Papoušek, 1979). Nevertheless, their immobility and limited means of action upon the physical and
social environment restrict their domain of influence. The initial experiences that contribute to development of a sense of personal agency are
tied to infants' ability to control sensory stimulation from manipulable
objects and the attentive behavior of those around them. Infants who
experience success in controlling environmental events become more attentive to their own behavior and more competent in learning new efficacious responses than are infants for whom the same environmental events
occur regardless of how they behave (Finkelstein & Ramey, 1977; Ramey
& Finkelstein, 1978). Such rudimentary efficacy experiences in producing
environmental effects foster the type of active responsiveness that builds
competence. Conversely, repeated experience of inefficacy in influencing
events impairs ability to perceive causal agency and depresses responsiveness in later situations in which actions do produce results (Seligman &
Garber, 1980).

Growth of self-efficacy

Familial sources of self-efficacy. There are many spheres in which young children must eventually achieve mastery. They have to develop and test their motor capabilities, their social competencies, their linguistic skills, and their cognitive skills for comprehending and managing the many situations they encounter daily. Development of sensorimotor capabilities greatly expands the infants' available environment and the means for acting upon it. These early exploratory and play activities, which occupy much of their waking hours, provide opportunities for enlarging their repertoire of basic skills. While developing their capabilities during this initial period of immaturity, most of the infants' gratifications must be mediated through adults. Neonates have to depend on others to feed them, clothe them, comfort them, entertain them, and to furnish the play materials for their manipulative exploration. Because of this physical dependency, infants quickly learn how to influence the actions of those around them by their social and verbal behavior. These enactive efficacy experiences in the exercise of personal control are central to the early development of social and cognitive competence. Parents who are responsive to their infants' communicative behavior, who provide an enriched physical environment, and who permit freedom of movement for exploratory experiences have infants who are relatively accelerated in their social and cognitive development (Ainsworth & Bell, 1974; Cohen & Beckwith, 1979; Yarrow, Rubenstein, Pedersen, & Jankowski, 1972).

During the first few months of life, infants do not possess the attentional and memorial capabilities to profit much from contingent experiences when the effects of their actions are delayed (Millar, 1972; Watson, 1979). There is some evidence that during the initial months of life the exercise of influence over the physical environment may contribute more to the development of efficacious responsiveness than does influence over the social environment (Gunnar, 1980b). Manipulation of physical objects produces immediate predictable effects, thus facilitating perception of personal agency. After shaking a rattle repeatedly and hearing the resultant sound, infants cannot help but notice that they are capable of producing environmental effects. In contrast, social responses to infants' behavior, which depend upon the availability and vagary of others, are not only more delayed and variable, but they often occur independently of the infants' behavior. That is, others frequently attend to and initiate activities with infants regardless of what they may be doing at the time. A cry may bring others instantly, some time later, or not at all; others often appear in the absence of crying. Causal agency is more difficult to discern in the noisier social contingencies. However, it is not long before the exercise of control over the social environment begins to play an important role in the early development of self-efficacy.

Acquisition of language provides children with symbolic means to reflect on their experiences and thus to begin to gain self-knowledge of what they can and cannot do. Once they come to understand speech, parents and others comment on the children's performance capabilities to provide guidance in foreseen situations in which the parents may not be present. To the extent that the social efficacy appraisals are adopted, they can affect the rate of personal development by influencing whether, and how, children approach new tasks. Thus, for example, overprotective parents, who are oversolicitous and dwell on potential dangers, undermine development of their children's capabilities (Levy, 1943), whereas the more secure are quick to acknowledge and to encourage their children's growing competencies.

The initial efficacy experiences are centered in the family, but as the growing child's social world rapidly expands peers assume an increasingly important role in children's developing self-knowledge of their capabilities. It is in the context of peer interactions that social comparison processes come most strongly into play. At first the closest comparative agemates are the siblings. There is much interesting work to be done on how different family structures affect a child's developing sense of efficacy. Families differ in number of siblings, how far apart in age they are, and in their sex distribution. These structural variables, either singly or in combination, create different references for comparative efficacy appraisal. Do firstborns and only children differ in how they judge their capabilities from children with older brothers and sisters? Does ordinal position exert differential effects on achievement efficacy (Zajonc & Markus, 1975) and on social efficacy? Do comparative efficacy appraisals for siblings close in age differ from those for siblings spaced farther apart in age? Do siblings of the same sex engage in more competitive ability evaluations than those of different sex? And finally, there is the interesting question of how the evaluative habits developed in sibling interactions affect the salience and choice of comparative referents in self-ability evaluations in later periods of life.

Peers and the broadening and validation of self-efficacy. The nature of children's efficacy-testing experiences changes substantially as they move increasingly into the larger community. It is in peer relationships that they both broaden the scope of, and make finer discriminations in, self-knowledge of their interpersonal capabilities. Peers serve several important efficacy functions. Those who are most experienced and competent provide models of efficacious styles of behavior. A vast amount of social learning occurs, for better or for worse, among peers. In addition, age-mates provide the most informative points of reference for comparative efficacy appraisal and verification. Children are therefore especially sensitive to their relative standing among the peers with whom they affiliate on factors that determine prestige and popularity.

The different ways in which peers contribute to self-efficacy development require systematic examination. Peers are neither homogeneous nor selected indiscriminately. Of special research interest are the processes whereby selective peer association promotes self-efficacy in particular directions, leaving other potentialities underdeveloped (Bandura & Walters, 1959; Bullock & Merrill, 1981; Ellis & Lane, 1963; Krauss, 1964). The influence processes are undoubtedly bidirectional – affiliation preferences affect the direction of efficacy development, and self-efficacy, in turn, partly determines choice of peer associates and activities. Considering that peers serve as a major agency for the development and validation of self-efficacy, a related research issue concerns the effects of disrupted or impoverished peer relationships on the acquisition of self-percepts.

School as an agency for cultivating cognitive self-efficacy. During the crucial formative period of children's lives, the school functions as the primary setting for the cultivation and social validation of cognitive efficacy. It is the place where children develop their cognitive competencies and acquire the knowledge and problem-solving skills essential for participating effectively in the society. Here their knowledge and thinking skills are continually tested, evaluated, and socially compared. There are numerous critics who believe that for many children, the school falls considerably short of fulfilling its purposes. Not only does it fail to prepare the youth adequately for the future, but all too often it undermines the very sense of personal efficacy needed for continued self-development.

There are a number of school practices that, for the less talented or ill prepared, tend to convert instructional experiences into education in inefficacy. These include lock-step sequences of instruction that lose many children along the way; ability groupings that further diminish the self-efficacy appraisal of those cast into subordinate ranks; and competitive practices in which many are doomed to failure for the success of a relative few.

Children have to learn to face displeasing realities about themselves. However, consideration must be given to social practices that contribute to those personal realities. A major aim of research in the scholastic domain is to clarify how different types of educational practices and structures affect the development of social and cognitive efficacy. Educational practices should be gauged not only in terms of the skills and knowledge they impart for the present, but also by what they do to children's perceptions of themselves, which affects how they approach the future.

Growth of self-efficacy through transitional experiences of adolescence. Each period of development brings with it new challenges to coping efficacy. As adolescents approach the demands of adulthood, they must learn to assume full responsibility for themselves in almost every dimension of life. This requires mastering many new skills and the ways of the adult society. Learning how to deal with heterosexual relationships and partnerships becomes a matter of considerable importance. The task of choosing what lifework to pursue also looms large during this period. These are only a few of the areas in which new competencies have to be acquired. Research is needed to detail the ways in which perceived self-efficacy influences this transition from childhood to adulthood.

Self-efficacy concerns of adulthood. Young adulthood is a period when people have to learn to cope with a host of new demands arising from lasting partnerships, marital relationships, parenthood, and a career. As in earlier mastery tasks, a firm sense of self-efficacy is an important motivational contributor to the attainment of further competencies and success. Those who enter adulthood poorly equipped with skills and plagued by self-doubts find many aspects of their adult life stressful and depressing.

By the middle years people settle into established routines that stabilize self-percepts of efficacy in the major areas of functioning. However, the stability is a shaky one because life does not remain static. Rapid technological and social changes constantly require adaptations calling for self-appraisals of capabilities. In the occupational domain, the middle-aged find themselves pressured by younger challengers. Situations in which people must compete for promotions, status, and even work itself, force constant self-appraisals of capabilities through social comparison with younger competitors (Suls & Mullen, 1981). For those whose livelihood and self-esteem rest heavily on physical strength, as in athletic careers, declining physical stamina requires redirection of life pursuits.

It is during the middle years that people confront seriously the limits of their capabilities. Most will have gotten as far as they will in their jobs. They see time and opportunities to realize the ambitions that sustained them over the years slipping away. Visions of a monotonous future give rise to midlife strains, especially for people who harbor doubts that what they are doing serves a worthwhile purpose.

Reactions to stressful stocktaking in the middle years take varied forms. Most people scale down their ambitions and try to pursue their vocation as competently as they can. Because even the same pursuit changes somewhat over time, opportunities for self-development remain. Many who find themselves trapped in routinized jobs do them perfunctorily and seek satisfactions through competence in avocational pursuits. Still others restructure their lives to make them more challenging and fulfilling. They change careers, mates, and locales (Chew, 1976). Some simply drop out for a life free of performance demands and responsibilities.

Reappraisals of self-efficacy with advancing age. The self-efficacy problems of the elderly center on reappraisals and misappraisals of their capabilities. Discussions of aging focus heavily on declining capabilities. Advancing age is said to produce losses in physical stamina, sensory functions, intellectual facility, memory, and in the ability to process information. Many physical capacities do decrease as people grow older, thus requiring reappraisals of self-efficacy for activities in which the mediating biological functions are significantly affected. Gains in knowledge, skills, and expertise may more than offset some loss in physical capacity, but such evidence does not easily dispel the stereotype of deterioration evoked by vivid images of emaciated seniles.

In cultures that revere youth and negatively stereotype its elderly, age becomes a salient dimension for self-evaluation. Once age assumes high significance, changes in performances over time, stemming largely from social factors, are easily misattributed to biological aging. The widespread belief in intellectual decline is a good case in point. Longitudinal studies reveal no universal or general decline in intellectual abilities, but in cross-sectional comparisons of different age groups the young surpass the old (Baltes & Labouvie, 1973; Schaie, 1974). The major share of age differences in intelligence is due to differences in experiences across generations rather than to biological aging. To paraphrase Schaie, cultures age as do people. It is not so much that the old have declined in intelligence but that the young have had the benefit of richer experiences that enable them to function at a higher level.

Misappraisals of performance declines in terms of biological aging undoubtedly occur in other areas of functioning as well. Decreases in sexuality with age that result from stress or boredom may be misattributed mainly to loss of sexual capabilities. Perceived sexual inefficacy diminishes sexual activity. Even declines in physical stamina may partly reflect decriments in self-percepts of efficacy. In laboratory studies of this mediating mechanism, reductions in perceived physical efficacy, induced vicariously through exposure to superior performances of competitors, lower observers' physical endurance (Weinberg, Gould, & Jackson, 1979; Weinberg, Yukelson, & Jackson, 1980). The more perceived physical efficacy is diminished, the greater is the decline in physical stamina. The incomparable Satchel Paige alluded to the self-limiting effects of age-typing when he queried: "How old would you be if you didn't know how old you was?"

Although most people enjoy good health, illnesses in the later years of life take their toll on both psyche and body. The damage to self-percepts of efficacy is no small matter as, for example, in recovery from a heart attack. The heart heals rapidly. But the psychological recovery is slow because patients fear that they lack the physical efficacy to resume their normal activities. The recovery problems stem more from perceived physical inefficacy than from physical debility. The rehabilitation task is to restore a sense of physical efficacy so that victims of a heart attack can lead full, productive lives (Ewart, Taylor, & DeBusk, 1980).

As in earlier periods of development, the major sources of efficacy information provide the elderly with the basis for reappraising their personal efficacy. They evaluate their performance attainments and compare them to their level of functioning at earlier periods of their life (Suls & Mullen, 1981). They read their bodily aches and pains as signs of growing wear and tear. The accomplishments of comparative others provide a further gauge of self-efficacy. The differential age trends in intellectual ability revealed by longitudinal and cross-sectional analysis suggest that the elderly who weigh self-comparison over time more heavily than social comparison with younger cohorts are less likely to view themselves as declining in capabilities. In exploiting the needs, physical changes, and common ailments associated with aging, the television industry stereotypes the elderly either as idle simpletons or as leading impoverished hypochondriacal lives plagued by bowel irregularities, slack dentures, arthritis, tired blood, and age spots. Infirm stereotypes shape cultural expectations and evaluative reactions of inefficacy toward the elderly.

A declining sense of self-efficacy is apt to set in motion self-perpetuating processes that result in declining cognitive and behavioral functioning. People who are insecure about their efficacy not only curtail their range of activities but undermine their efforts in those they undertake. The result is a progressive loss of interest and skill. It is in societies that emphasize the potential for self-development throughout the lifespan rather than psychophysical decline with aging that the elderly are most likely to lead productive, self-fulfilling lives.

Interrelatedness of efficacy influences

The preceding discussion centered mainly on how the major social systems contribute to the growth of self-efficacy for developmental tasks that become crucial at different periods of life. These diverse efficacy influences, of course, operate in an interrelated fashion. This is perhaps best illustrated in the emergence of sex differences in achievement efficacy. Although the findings vary across tasks and age levels, the evidence generally shows that girls view themselves as less efficacious than boys at intellectual activities that are stereotypically linked with males (M. Bandura, 1978; Parsons, Ruble, Hodges, & Small, 1976). These differences stem from a combination of developmental influences, each of which fosters underestimation of the capabilities of girls. The first concerns the pervasive cultural modeling of sex-role stereotypes. Whether it be the television medium, children's play materials and instructional literature, or the social examples around them, children see women cast predominantly in nonachieving roles (Jacklin & Mischel, 1973; McArthur & Eisen, 1976; Sternglanz & Serbin, 1974; Weitzman, Eifler, Hokada, & Ross, 1972). Girls who adopt the stereotypic conception will harbor self-doubts about their own proficiency on achievement tasks. Even by early preschool years children already subscribe to the sexual stereotype of differential intellectual capabilities (Crandall, 1978). To the extent that children's own stereotyping leads them to behave in ways more conducive to intellectual success in boys than in girls, they create further social validation for the preconceptions.

We have previously noted that self-appraisals are influenced by evaluative reactions of others. There is some evidence that parents and teachers have different achievement expectations and vary their attributional explanations for successes and failures depending on the sex of the child. They tend to expect less of girls, to center criticism on the intellectual aspects of their academic work, and to judge their failures more in ability than in motivational terms (Dweck, Davidson, Nelson, & Enna, 1978; Parsons et al., 1976). The cumulative effect of these diverse influences is to create a sense of inefficacy that can only hinder self-development of intellectual capabilities.

Development of self-appraisal skills

With development through exploratory experiences, tuition, and social comparison children gradually improve their self-appraisal skills. This enables them to make efficacy judgments on their own to guide their actions in whatever situations may arise. How children learn to use diverse sources of efficacy information in developing a stable and accurate sense of personal efficacy is a matter of considerable interest.

Accurate appraisal of one's capabilities depends on a number of constituent skills that develop through direct and socially mediated experience. While engaging in activities children must attend simultaneously to multiple sources of efficacy information conveyed by the nature of the task, situational circumstances, characteristics of the performances, and conditional outcomes. Because the activities are performed on repeated occasions, children must be able to transcend particular instances and to integrate efficacy information from performance samples extended over time. This places heavy demands on ability to monitor ongoing events, to evaluate the causes of fluctuations in performances and outcomes, and to represent and retain efficacy information derived from many prior experiences under varying circumstances.

Current research on metacognitive development is exploring how children gain knowledge about cognitive phenomena, such as thoughts about themselves as cognizers, about task goals and strategies for achieving them (Brown, 1978; Flavell, 1978, 1979). Gaining self-knowledge of capabilities as a doer, as well as a thinker, greatly expands the number of different constituent skills that must be appraised. Personal efficacy entails versatile improvisation of multiple cognitive and manual skills in daily transactions with the environment. Activities vary substantially in the demands they make on cognitive and memory skills, motor facility, strength, endurance, and stress tolerance. In addition to gaining self-knowledge, a growing child has much to learn about the difficulty of environmental tasks, the abilities they require, and the types of problems likely to arise in executing different courses of action. Incongruities between self-efficacy and action may stem from misperceptions of task demands as well as from faulty self-knowledge. With wider experience children gain better understanding of themselves and their everyday environment, which enables them to judge their efficacy in particular areas of functioning more realistically.

Because of their limited cognitive skills and experience, young children lack knowledge of their cognitive and behavioral capabilities. They have difficulty in attending simultaneously to multiple efficacy cues, in distinguishing between important and minor indicants, and in processing sequential efficacy information. As a result, their self-appraisals are apt to be heavily dependent on immediate, salient outcomes and hence relatively unstable.

As children become more proficient with age in the constituent skills, reliance on immediate outcomes of performance declines in importance in judging what they can do. These changes are accompanied by developmental increases in children's use of diverse, less salient, and sequential efficacy information (Parsons, Moses, & Yulish-Muszynski, 1977; Parsons & Ruble, 1977). With experience they come to understand how expenditure of effort can compensate for ability (Kun, 1977). Through more extensive utilization of efficacy information across tasks, time, and situations, older children judge their capabilities and limitations more accurately. With increasing development children begin to use inference rules or heuristics in processing efficacy information, as for example, inferring capability from amount of effort expended.

We saw earlier that people judge their capabilities partly through social comparison with the performances of others. Gauging personal efficacy through social comparative information involves greater complexities than self-appraisals based on direct experience. Comparative appraisals of efficacy require not only evaluation of one's own performances, but also knowledge of how others do, cognizance of nonability determinants of their performances, and some understanding that it is similar others who provide the most informative social criterion for comparison. With development, children become increasingly discriminating in their use of comparative efficacy information. Developmental analyses by Morris and Nemcek (1979) show that effective use of social comparative information lags behind perception of ability rankings. Except for the very young (e.g., three-year-olds), who do not discern differences in ability, with increasing age children are progressively more accurate in appraising their own abilities and those of their peers. However, it is not until about age six that they realize that it is the performances of similar others who are slightly better that are most informative for comparative purposes.

It remains a problem of future research to clarify how young children come to know what type of social comparative information is most useful for efficacy evaluation. Such knowledge is probably gained in several ways. One highly plausible process operates through comparative success and failure experiences. Children repeatedly observe their own behavior attainments and the performances of others. We know from the work of Morris and Nemcek that, at least in some areas of functioning, children begin to discern differences in ability at a very early age. Given that they can discriminate ability rankings, they would soon learn that neither the successes of the vastly superior, nor the failures of inept peers, tell them much about how well they are likely to perform the new activity. Rather, it is the attainments of similar others that are most predictive of the children's own operative capabilities. Acting on appropriate comparative self-appraisal thus maximizes the likelihood of success. Attribute similarity would gain informative value for comparative appraisal of ability through the same process. To the extent that children with similar characteristics achieve comparable performance levels, they would more likely use the performances of similar rather than dissimilar others to judge their own efficacy.

Children do not rely solely on the behavioral consequences of comparative efficacy inferences in learning to select similar others for self-ability evaluation. They undoubtedly receive direct tuition from time to time on the appropriateness of various social comparisons. Because of their limited experiences, young children are quick to try what they see others doing even though it is well beyond their reach. Faulty performances can undermine their developing sense of efficacy or, if the activities are potentially dangerous, result in injury. To minimize such consequences, parents explain to their children which comparative referents are appropriate and which are unrealistic for gauging their capabilities.

Measuring efficacy judgments as a function of age can shed some light on developmental trends in children's use of efficacy information in self-appraisals. However, such research does not clarify how proficiency in self-appraisal develops. Understanding of the determinants and processes of efficacy evaluation can be advanced by experimentation designed to create efficacy-appraisal skills where they are lacking. Cognitive modeling provides one effective means for increasing children's understanding of the efficacy value of relevant sources of information.

In cognitive modeling (Debus, 1976; Meichenbaum & Asarnow, 1979), models verbalize aloud their thought processes as they engage in problem-solving and judgmental activities. The covert thought component is thus given overt representation. This mode of tuition has several desirable features that contribute to its effectiveness in producing generalized, durable improvements in cognitive skills. Nonverbal modeling gains and holds attention, which is especially critical with young children. In addition, it provides a meaningful ongoing context within which to imbed verbalized thoughts on how to judge personal efficacy. The judgmental strategies can be reiterated in variant forms as often as needed to impart the cognitive skill without taxing observers' interest simply by using di-

verse exemplars. In applying this procedure to the development of efficacy judgment, while performing different tasks models would identify
efficacy-relevant cues and verbalize rules for interpreting and integrating
the efficacy information. Functional rules for judging social comparative
information can be modeled in a similar fashion.

Research aimed at improving efficacy-appraisal skills offers therapeutic
benefits as well as knowledge about developmental processes. Many children are severely handicapped by perceived inefficacy stemming from
frequent misattributions of performance difficulties to personal limitations and from inappropriate social comparisons. They have much to gain
from changing judgmental orientations that lead them to underestimate
their capabilities.

Microanalytic efficacy methodology

A good theory is obviously of central importance, but effective methods
are also a significant factor in scientific progress. Advancement in a field
therefore requires development of appropriate methodologies that make
the phenomena of interest accessible to study. Some of the processes
relevant to self-efficacy have been examined from other theoretical perspectives in terms of either expectancies for success or causal perceptions
of success and failure. Although both approaches have shed some light on
ability inferences, the methodologies have certain limitations. In the
prototypical expectancy research, children perform a task over a series of
trials and at periodic intervals they are asked to state their likelihood of
success on a subsequent trial. The children do not know specifically what
they will have to do. In fact, ambiguous tasks are often selected so that
success and failure can be varied independently of children's actual performances. Given vagueness of prospective tasks and unrelatedness of
actual performance to success feedback, children's judgments are more
likely to reflect extrapolative outcome guesses from prior feedback than
appraisals of their capabilities. Consequently, such expectancies usually
fluctuate widely with transitory variations in success rates.

In some investigations of performance causal inferences, children are
told how a hypothetical person performed and are given information on a
selected set of possible determinants, such as the difficulty of the task and
the amount of effort expended. They are then asked to rate the causes of
the behavior in terms of a few preselected categories. In another common
approach to the study of causal inference, children actually perform tasks,
after which they are asked to judge the causes of their successes or
failures in terms of a few preselected factors.

These types of methodologies impose some constraints on what one can learn about how children come to judge their capabilities and how their self-referent thought affects their performance. In judging their everyday experiences, children are faced with a welter of information, some of which is highly relevant, some of which is of secondary importance, and much of which is extraneous or redundant. The selection of what is relevant from the array of causal possibilities involves processes that may be as complex as those that operate in forming the self-ability judgments. Forcing children to fit their thinking into the investigators' few preselected categories is likely to yield an incomplete, if not distorted, picture of subjects' evaluations of their capabilities. Moreover, self-appraisals that occur prior to performance must be distinguished from retrospective conjectures about the causes of past behavior. It is probes of antecedent self-appraisals that are best suited for elucidating the relationship between self-referent thought and action.

In testing propositions about the origins and functions of self-efficacy we have employed a microanalytic methodology (Bandura, 1977a). Individuals are presented with efficacy scales representing tasks varying in difficulty, complexity, or threat value. They designate the tasks they judge they can do and their degree of certainty. Efficacy judgments vary on several dimensions that have important performance implications. They differ in *level*. Thus, when tasks are ordered by level of difficulty, the self-judged efficacy of different individuals may be limited to the simpler tasks, extend to moderately difficult ones, or include some of the most challenging and taxing performances. Efficacy judgments also vary in *strength*. Weak self-percepts of efficacy are easily negated by disconfirming experiences, whereas people who have a strong sense of personal mastery will persevere in their coping efforts in the face of dissuading experiences. In addition, self-percepts of efficacy differ in *generality* – they may encompass varied domains or only a few. An adequate efficacy analysis therefore requires detailed assessment of the level, strength, and generality of self-efficacy commensurate with the precision with which behavioral processes are measured. The relationship between self-referent thought and action is most clearly revealed by microanalysis of the congruence between efficacy judgment and performance at the level of individual tasks.

Extension of the microanalytic methodology to children is illustrated in recent studies designed to enhance self-efficacy in cognitive skills (Bandura & Schunk, 1981; Schunk, 1981). In the experiment conducted by Schunk (1981), young children who were demoralized by repeated failure at mathematical tasks were assigned to one of three conditions. Children in a cognitive-modeling treatment first observed individually an adult model solve arithmetic problems and verbalize aloud the cognitive operations she was using to arrive at correct solutions. The children then received guided practice in applying what they had learned with corrective modeling of any constituent operations they failed to grasp. In corrective modeling, which provides the most informative feedback for skill acquisition (Vasta, 1976), troublesome aspects are identified and skilled ways of performing them are exemplified. Children in a didactic treatment condition received verbal instruction in the arithmetic principles from the same adult and the same amount of practice in applying the knowledge they had gained but without the benefit of intensive modeling of cognitive operations. A third group of children participated in the assessment procedures but received no intervening treatment.

Attribution retraining programs in the area of achievement behavior often concentrate on changing children's causal ascriptions of failure to lack of effort (Dweck, 1975). To test whether effort attributions made in the context of competency development affect self-efficacy and achievement performance, causal attributions were also varied. For half the children in each of the two treatments the adult periodically ascribed the children's successes to sustained effort and their failures to insufficient effort. The remaining children received the competency training without causal attributions for their performances.

Both prior to, and after, completing the treatment program all children were first tested for their perceived efficacy and then for their arithmetic attainments. In measuring their arithmetic efficacy, the children were shown at very brief exposures – sufficient to portray the nature of the tasks but much too short even to attempt any solutions – sets of arithmetic problems of varying levels of difficulty. For each sample, children judged their capability to solve that type of problem and the strength of their perceived efficacy. Because the posttreatment tasks tapped new applications of the cognitive skill, children had to rely on generalizable perceptions of their own capabilities in making their judgments. The performance measure consisted of multiple sets of arithmetic problems, many of which required the children to apply the arithmetic principles to new problems that were more complex than any they had encountered before.

Both the didactic and cognitive-modeling treatments enhanced self-efficacy and arithmetic skill, with the cognitive modeling treatment producing the greater gains. In the context of competency development, effort attributions had no significant effect either on perceived efficacy or on arithmetic performance. These findings are consistent with evidence reported by Chapin and Dyck (1976) that the effects of effort ascriptions depend on the performance context in which they occur. When children learn they can succeed despite repeated failure, they show high persistence regardless of whether or not their successes and failures were attributed to how much effort they exerted. When children's competencies are expanded through skill development, children persist on the basis of their self-judged efficacy rather than on effort attributions from others. Microanalysis of the relationship beween efficacy judgments and performance revealed that the stronger the children's perceived efficacy for a given level of task the longer they persisted and the more likely they were to perform successfully.

Related views of personal efficacy

Self-referent processes have been the subject of considerable interest in other approaches to human behavior. The theoretical perspectives differ, however, in how they view the nature and origins of self-percepts and the intervening processes by which they affect behavior.

Self-concept

Self-influences have traditionally been conceptualized in terms of the self-concept (Rogers, 1959; Wylie, 1974). The self-concept is a composite view of oneself that is formed through direct experience and adopted evaluations of significant others. In these approaches self-concepts are measured by having people rate in one way or another descriptive statements that they consider apply to themselves. The principal thesis that self-concepts determine psychological functioning is then tested by correlating self-concepts or disparities between actual–ideal selves with various indexes of adjustment, attitudes, and behavior.

Examining self-processes in terms of the self-concept contributes to understanding how people develop attitudes toward themselves and how their self-attitudes affect their outlook on life. There are several features of self theories of this type, however, that detract from their power to explain and to predict how people are likely to behave in particular situations. For the most part, self theories are concerned with global self-images. A global self-conception does not do justice to the complexity of efficacy self-percepts, which vary across different activities, different levels of the same activity, and different situational circumstances. A composite self-image may yield some modest correlations, but it is not equal to the task of predicting with any degree of accuracy intraindividual variability in performance. Self theories have had difficulty explaining how the same self-concept can give rise to diverse actions.

Effectance motivation

In seeking a motivational explanation of exploratory and manipulative behavior, White (1959, 1960) postulated an "effectance motive," which is conceptualized as an intrinsic drive for transactions with the environment. The effectance motive presumably develops through cumulative acquisition of knowledge and skills in dealing with the environment. In these conceptual papers, White argues eloquently for a competence model of child development. The theory deals at some length with nonorganic motivators of behavior, but there are a number of points on which the theory requires clarification. The process by which an effectance motive emerges from effective transactions with the environment is not spelled out. In this formulation, successful action builds effectance motivation. But there is no place in the theory for the effects of failure experiences, which are by no means insignificant (Harter, 1978). It is difficult to verify the existence of an effectance motive because the motive is inferred from the exploratory behavior it supposedly causes. Without an independent measure of motive strength one cannot tell whether people explore and manipulate things because of a competence motive to do so, or for any number of other reasons.

The theory of effectance motivation has not been formulated in sufficient detail to permit extensive theoretical comparisons. Nevertheless, there are several issues on which social learning and effectance formulations clearly differ. In the social learning view, choice behavior, effort expenditure, and affective arousal are governed in part by percepts of self-efficacy rather than by a drive condition. Because efficacy judgments are defined and measured independently of performance, they provide a basis for predicting the occurrence, generality, and persistence of coping behavior, whereas an omnibus motive does not. People will approach, explore, and try to deal with situations within their self-perceived capabilities but, unless externally coerced, they will avoid transactions with potentially aversive aspects of their environment they perceive as exceeding their coping capabilities.

The alternative views also differ on the origins of personal efficacy. Within the framework of effectance theory, the effectance drive develops gradually through prolonged transactions with one's surroundings. This theory thus focuses almost exclusively on the effects produced by one's own actions. In social learning theory, self-efficacy results from diverse sources of information conveyed vicariously and through social evaluation as well as through direct experience. These differences in theoretical approach have significant implications for how one goes about studying the role of perceived self-efficacy in motivational and behavioral processes.

Judgments of personal efficacy do not operate as dispositional determinants independently of contextual factors. Some situations require greater skill and more arduous performances, or carry higher risk of negative consequences than do others. Judgments will vary accordingly. Thus, for example, the level and strength of perceived efficacy in public speaking will differ depending on the subject matter, the format of the presentation, and the types of audiences to be addressed. Therefore, analyses of how self-percepts affect actions rely on microanalytic procedures rather than on global measures of personality traits or motives of effectance. From the social learning perspective, it is no more informative to speak of self-efficacy in global terms than to speak of nonspecific social behavior. In the microanalysis both the efficacy judgments and the corresponding activities are measured in terms of explicit types of performances rather than on the basis of global indexes.

In effectance theory, producing effects on the environment arouses feelings of pleasure and efficacy. Although this may often be the case, as we have already seen, competent performance does not necessarily enhance perceived efficacy. It depends on how the determinants of the performances are cognitively appraised and how they measure up against internal standards. Nor does the exercise of personal mastery necessarily bring pleasure. When competencies are used for harmful purposes, performers may feel self-efficacious in their triumphs but remain displeased with themselves. A theory of effectance must therefore consider the important role played by personal standards and cognitive appraisal in the affective and self-evaluative reactions to one's own performances. The manner in which internal standards and self-percepts of efficacy operate as interrelated mechanisms of personal agency has been addressed elsewhere and will not be reviewed here (Bandura, 1981).

Effectance motivation presumably comes into play only under certain limited conditions (White, 1959), a point that is often overlooked in overextensions of the theory to wide realms of behavior. The effectance motive is believed to be aroused when the organism is otherwise unoccupied or is only weakly stimulated by organic drives. In the words of White (1960), effectance promotes "spare-time behavior." In the social learning view, efficacy judgments enter into the regulation of all types of performances, except for habitual patterns that have become routinized.

Self-efficacy: an integrative construct

The discussion thus far has addressed mainly questions about the origins of self-efficacy and its relationship to action. People's perceptions of their efficacy influence their thought patterns and emotional arousal as well as their behavior. Indeed, self-efficacy is a broadly integrative construct that encompasses a wide range of psychological phenomena (Bandura, 1981). It is to some of these phenomena of special developmental interest that we turn next.

Self-efficacy conception of fear arousal

Children's perceptions of their own capabilities affect their emotional reactions as well as their behavior. This is especially true of fear reactions to unfamiliar or potentially aversive events. From the social learning perspective, it is mainly perceived inefficacy in coping with potentially aversive events that makes them fearsome. To the extent that one can prevent, terminate, or lessen the severity of painful occurrences there is little reason to fear them. Hence, experiences that increase coping efficacy can diminsh fear arousal and increase commerce with what was previously avoided (Bandura, 1977a).

A sense of controllability can be achieved either behaviorally or cognitively (Averill, 1973; Miller, 1979). In behavioral control, individuals take actions that forestall or modify aversive events. In cognitive control, people believe they can manage environmental threats should they arise. These two forms of controllability are distinguished because the relationship between actual and perceived coping efficacy is far from perfect. Indeed, there are many competent people who are plagued by a sense of inefficacy and many less competent ones who remain unperturbed because they are assured of their coping capabilities.

Behavioral control. The effects of behavioral control on fear reduction and stress responses have been documented with both children and adults. Studies conducted with infants demonstrate that a frightening mechanical object is transformed into a pleasant one when infants can personally activate the very events that frightened them (Gunnar-vonGnechten, 1978). However, in the initial months of life, when infants have difficulty perceiving causal agency, control does not reduce distress. The exercise of behavioral control over possible threats eliminates or decreases autonomic reactions to aversive events in adults as well (Miller, 1979).

To the extent that control over events makes them predictable it reduces uncertainty. It might therefore be argued that it is predictability rather than controllability that is stress reducing. However, the evidence indicates that behavioral control decreases arousal over and above any benefits derived from the ability to predict the occurrence of stressors. If anything, having foreknowledge of when aversive events will occur without being able to do anything about them increases anticipatory stress reactions (Gunnar, 1980a; Miller & Grant, 1979). But because predictability signals safety as well as danger (Seligman & Binik, 1977), it can have opposite effects at different points in time, raising anticipatory arousal just prior to stressful events while reducing arousal during safe interim periods.

Being able to manage what one fears can diminish arousal because the capability is used to reduce or to prevent the occurrence of threatening events. But there is more to the process of fear reduction by behavioral control than simply curtailing unpleasant environmental stimulation. Previously frightening events may continue to occur often, but they become nonthreatening when they are activated personally (Gunnar, 1980a). Here it is the personal agency of causality that reduces fear. And in situations in which the opportunity to wield control exists but is unexercised, it is the self-knowledge of coping efficacy rather than its application that reduces fear arousal (Glass, Reim, & Singer, 1971).

Cognitive control. A painful event has two arousal components to it – the discomfort produced by the physically aversive stimuli and the thought-produced arousal. It is the thought component – the arousal generated by repetitive perturbing ideation – that accounts for much of human distress. Anticipatory cognition that does not exceed realistic bounds has functional value in that it motivates development of competencies and plans for dealing with foreseeable threats. But to those who doubt their coping efficacy, the anxious anticipation becomes a preoccupation that often far exceeds the objective hazards. People who are plagued by an exaggerated sense of coping inefficacy not only magnify the severity of possible threats but worry about perils that rarely, if ever, happen. As a result, they experience a high level of cognitively generated distress.

The way in which self-referent thoughts arouse anxiety and debilitate performance has been examined extensively in the area of achievement anxiety. As Sarason (1975b, 1978) and Wine (1971) have shown, in evaluative situations, people who are prone to anxiety over achievement impair their performances by excessive preoccupation with their personal deficiencies. In contrast, the low anxious are spurred by evaluative pressures to higher performances by mobilizing their efforts and concentrating on the requirements of the task. The arousing and performance-debilitating effects of negative self-referent thought have been well documented by Meichenbaum (1977) and Beck (1976) in other areas of functioning.

Because stress-inducing thought plays a paramount role in human arousal, perceived personal control can reduce the level of arousal before, during, and after a trying experience. In laboratory tests, people who believe that they can exercise some influence over the occurrence of aversive events display less autonomic arousal and impairment in performance than those who do not believe they have personal control, even though both groups are subjected to the same aversive stimulation (Miller, 1979). In these situations it is the perception, rather than the actuality, of control that is stress reducing. Mere belief in coping efficacy similarly increases ability to withstand pain (Neufeld & Thomas, 1977).

Self-efficacy as a mediating mechanism. That perceived self-efficacy may be a cognitive mechanism by which controllability reduces fear receives support in research designed to enhance coping efficacy in severe phobics (Bandura et al., 1980). In these studies, after completing various forms of treatment, phobics designate the strength of their perceived efficacy in performing different tasks varying in threat value. During later behavioral tests, they report the intensity of fear arousal they experience in anticipation of performing each task, and again while they are performing the activity. People experience high anticipatory and performance fear on tasks in which they perceive themselves to be inefficacious, but as the strength of their self-judged efficacy increases, their fear arousal declines. At high strengths of self-efficacy, threatening tasks are performed with virtually no apprehensiveness. Fear arousal on the same task varies inversely as a function of differential levels of self-efficacy (Bandura, Adams, & Reese, 1980).

The efficacy formulation provides a unified conceptual framework not only for studying the determinants and processes of fear arousal, but also for devising effective treatments and explaining their mode of operation. Results of a series of studies confirm that treatments relying on enactive, vicarious, or cognitive mastery experiences increase the level, strength, and generality of self-efficacy in coping with threats (Bandura & Adams, 1977; Bandura et al., 1977; Bandura et al., 1980). The greater the perceived efficacy at the completion of treatment, the lower is the fear arousal and the higher are the performance accomplishments. In microanalyses of degree of congruence between self-efficacy judgment and performance, self-efficacy is an accurate predictor of performance on threatening tasks regardless of whether coping efficacy is enhanced by enactive, vicarious, emotive, or cognitive means. Consistent with self-efficacy theory, enactive mastery serves as the most powerful vehicle of change. The most generalized durable changes are achieved by participant mastery methods using performance aids initially to establish successful functioning, then removing the external supports to authenticate personal efficacy, then providing self-directed mastery to strengthen and generalize self-percepts of coping efficacy.

Cultivation of intrinsic interest through self-efficacy development

Most of the things that people enjoy doing for their own sake originally had little or no interest for them. Young children do not come innately interested in singing operatic arias, playing tubas, deriving mathematical formulas, writing sonnets, or propelling heavy shot-put balls through the air. But with appropriate learning experiences almost any activity, however silly it may appear to many observers, can become imbued with consuming significance.

The process by which children develop interest in activities in which they initially lack skill, interest, and self-efficacy is an issue of considerable developmental significance. Proponents of behavioral approaches have sought to promote such changes through the use of positive incentives. Some writers (Deci, 1975; Lepper & Greene, 1978) have questioned the wisdom of such an approach on the grounds that rewarding people for engaging in an activity is more likely to reduce than to increase subsequent interest in it. Extrinsic incentives are presumed to decrease interest by shifting causal attributions for performance from internal motivators to external rewards.

Extensive research on this issue reveals that extrinsic incentives can increase interest in activities, reduce interest, or have no effect (Bandura, 1977b; Kruglanski, 1975; Ross, 1976). These variable results have prompted efforts to specify the limiting conditions under which rewards might undermine interest. Lepper and Greene (1978) postulate four necessary conditions for the occurrence of reductive effects: The relationship between task performance and reward must be clearly noticeable; there should be sufficient initial interest in the activity to permit room for attributional shifts; tests for the effects of reward should be conducted under conditions free of social surveillance, demands, or expectation of continued reward; and finally, there should be no performance improvements that could provide sources of satisfaction. However, evidence that even under these limiting conditions extrinsic incentives can sometimes enhance interest leaves the issue still unsettled (Arnold, 1976; Davidson & Bucher, 1978).

In evaluating the role of rewards in the development of interest it is important to distinguish between whether incentives are used to regulate performance or to promote competencies. Conceptual analyses of intrinsic interest assign competence a mediating role (Deci, 1975; Lepper &

Greene, 1978), but there is little experimentation on this issue. In most of the studies in this area rewards are given merely for performing over and again an activity that is already of interest. Moreover, to minimize the possibility of performance improvements, children are rewarded for engaging in the activity regardless of how well they perform. The controversy over the effects of performance-irrelevant reward on high interest has led to a neglect of the developmentally important question of whether incentives made conditional upon progressive mastery of activities that would otherwise be avoided cultivate interest and self-percepts of efficacy.

Competence-contingent incentives. There are several ways in which contingent incentives can contribute to the growth of interest and self-efficacy. Positive incentives foster performance accomplishments. The resulting acquisition of knowledge and skills heightens interest and perceived efficacy. Success in attaining desired outcomes through challenging performances additionally verifies existing competencies. This is because people usually do not perform optimally although they possess the constituent skills. It is under incentives that lead them to try hard that they find out what they are able to do. By mobilizing high effort, incentives help to substantiate talents even though no new skills are acquired in the process.

Rewards also assume efficacy informative value when performance appraisals rely more heavily on subjective social criteria than on factual aspects of the performances themselves. To complicate further the competence validation process, most activities involve diverse facets so their perceived adequateness may vary widely depending on how the different factors are subjectively weighted. Because of these ambiguities, level of reward imparts social information on the quality of performance. In this process, competent performances are perceived as the reason for the rewards rather than the rewards being viewed as the cause of competent performances (Karniol & Ross, 1977). Studies of how the experience of causal efficacy affects children's interest show that personal causation of rewarding events heightens interest in the instrumental activity (Kun, Garfield, & Sipowicz, 1979; Nuttin, 1973).

Results of several studies lend validity to the view that positive incentives can enhance interest when they either promote or authenticate personal efficacy. Both children and adults increase or maintain their interest in activities when rewarded for performance attainments, whereas their interest declines when rewarded for undertaking activities irrespective of quality of performance (Boggiano & Ruble, 1979; Ross, 1976). The larger the reward for performances signifying competence, the greater is the increase in interest in the activity (Enzle & Ross, 1978). But even incentives for undertaking a task rather than for performance mastery can enhance interest if engagement in the activity provides information about personal competence (Arnold, 1976). When material reward for each task completion is accompanied by self-verbalization of competence, children sustain high interest in the activity (Sagotsky & Lewis, 1978). Results of these different lines of research lend support to the view that the effects of incentives on interest and continued performance of an activity without extrinsic reward are partly mediated by perceived efficacy.

Proximal self-motivation. Contingent incentives are not necessarily the best vehicles for enlisting the type of sustained involvement in activities that builds interest and self-efficacy where they are lacking. In social learning theory, an important cognitively based source of motivation operates through the intervening processes of goal setting and self-evaluative reactions (Bandura, 1977b, 1978). This form of self-motivation requires internal standards against which to evaluate performance. By making self-satisfaction conditional on matching selected standards, people give direction to their behavior and create self-inducements to persist in their efforts until their performances match self-prescribed goals. Sustained involvement in activities is best achieved through proximal subgoals that lead to larger future ones.

Adopting proximal subgoals for one's own behavior can have at least three major psychological effects. As already alluded to, they have *motivational effects.* Proximal subgoals provide immediate incentives and guides for performance, whereas distal goals are too far removed in time to effectively mobilize effort or to direct what one does in the here and now.

Proximal goals can also serve as an important vehicle in the *development of self-percepts of efficacy.* Without standards against which to measure their performances, people have little basis for judging how they are doing or for gauging their capabilities. Subgoal attainments provide indicants of mastery for enhancing self-efficacy. By contrast, distal goals are too far removed in time to provide sufficiently clear markers of progess along the way to ensure a growing sense of self-efficacy.

Proximal subgoals can also contribute to *enhancement of interest* in activities in at least two ways. (1) When people aim for and master desired levels of performance, they experience a sense of satisfaction (Locke, Cartledge, & Knerr, 1970). The satisfactions derived from subgoal attainments can build intrinsic interest. When performances are gauged against lofty distal goals, the large negative disparities between standards and attainments are likely to attenuate the level of self-satisfaction experienced along the way. In addition, a sense of personal efficacy in mastering challenges is apt to generate greater interest in the activity than is self-perceived inefficacy in producing competent performances. (2) To the extent that proximal subgoals promote and authenticate a sense of causal agency, they can heighten interest through their effects on perception of personal causation.

In testing the effects of proximal self-influence (Bandura & Schunk, 1981), children who exhibited gross deficits and disinterest in mathematical tasks pursued a program of self-directed learning under conditions involving either proximal subgoals, distal goals, or without any reference to goals. Under proximal subgoals children progressed rapidly in self-directed learning, achieved substantial mastery of mathematical operations, and developed a sense of personal efficacy and intrinsic interest in arithmetic activities that initially held little attraction for them. Distal goals had no demonstrable effects. In addition to its other benefits, goal proximity fostered veridical self-knowledge of capabilities as reflected in high congruence between judgments of mathematical self-efficacy and subsequent mathematical performance. Perceived self-efficacy was positively related to accuracy of mathematical performance and to intrinsic interest in arithmetic activities.

Summary

This chapter analyzes human development in terms of changes in self-efficacy, which plays an influential role in most aspects of human functioning throughout the lifespan. Self-percepts of efficacy affect the courses of action people pursue, their thought patterns, and the emotional arousal they experience. Among the various issues addressed, those of special interest concern the nature of self-efficacy, its developmental determinants, and the mechanisms through which it exerts its diverse effects. Self-efficacy theory affords another perspective from which to study problems of human thought, affect, and action and their interrelatedness. The task ahead is to explore in greater detail how self-knowledge of efficacy is acquired and how it, in turn, shapes the course of personal development.

References

Ainsworth, M. D. S., & Bell, S. M. Mother-infant interaction and the development of competence. In K. Connolly & J. Bruner (Eds.), *The growth of competence.* London: Academic Press, 1974.

Arnold, H. J. Effects of performance feedback and extrinsic reward upon high intrinsic motivation. *Organizational Behavior and Human Performance,* 1976, *17,* 275–88.

Averill, J. Personal control over aversive stimuli and its relationship to stress. *Psychological Bulletin,* 1973, *80,* 286–303.

Baltes, P. B., & Labouvie, G. V. Adult development of intellectual performance: Description, explanation, and modification. In C. Eisdorfer & M. P. Lawton (Eds.), *The psychology of adult development and aging.* Washington, D.C.: American Psychological Association, 1973.

Bandura, A. Self-efficacy: Toward a unifying theory of behavioral change. *Psychological Review,* 1977, *84,* 191–215. (a)

Social learning theory. Englewood Cliffs, N.J.: Prentice-Hall, 1977. (b)

The self system in reciprocal determinism. *American Psychologist,* 1978, *33,* 344–58.

The self and mechanisms of agency. In J. Suls (Ed.), *Social psychological perspectives on the self.* Hillsdale, N.J.: Erlbaum, 1981, in press.

Bandura, A., & Adams, N. E. Analysis of self-efficacy theory of behavioral change. *Cognitive Therapy and Research,* 1977, *1,* 287–308.

Bandura, A., Adams, N. E., & Beyer, J. Cognitive processes mediating behavioral change. *Journal of Personality and Social Psychology,* 1977, *35,* 125–39.

Bandura, A., Adams, N. E., Hardy, A. B., & Howells, G. N. Tests of the generality of self-efficacy theory. *Cognitive Therapy and Research,* 1980, *4,* 39–66.

Bandura, A., Adams, N. E., & Reese, L. *Microanalysis of action and fear arousal as a function of differential levels of self-efficacy.* Unpublished manuscript, Stanford University, 1980.

Bandura, A., & Schunk, D. H. Cultivating competence, self-efficacy, and intrinsic interest through proximal self-motivation. *Journal of Personality and Social Psychology,* 1981, in press.

Bandura, A., & Walters, R. H. *Adolescent aggression.* New York: Ronald Press, 1959.

Bandura, M. M. *Sex differences in predictions of success, confidence level, and performance on a math and verbal task following failure feedback.* Masters thesis, Pennsylvania State University, 1978.

Beck, A. T. *Cognitive therapy and the emotional disorders.* New York: International Universities Press, 1976.

Bem, D. J. Self-perception theory. In L. Berkowitz (Ed.), *Advances in experimental social psychology* (Vol. 6). New York: Academic Press, 1972.

Boggiano, A. K., & Ruble, D. N. Competence and the overjustification effect: A developmental study. *Journal of Personality and Social Psychology,* 1979, *37,* 1462–8.

Brown, A. L. Knowing when, where, and how to remember: A problem of metacognition. In R. Glaser (Ed.), *Advances in instructional psychology.* Hillsdale, N.J.: Erlbaum, 1978.

Brown, I., Jr., & Inouye, D. K. Learned helplessness through modeling: The role of perceived similarity in competence. *Journal of Personality and Social Psychology,* 1978, *36,* 900–8.

Bullock, D., & Merrill, L. The impact of personal preference on consistency through time: The case of childhood aggression. *Child Development,* 1980, *51,* 808–14.

Chapin, M., & Dyck, D. G. Persistence in children's reading behavior as a function of N length and attribution retraining. *Journal of Abnormal Psychology,* 1976, *85,* 511–15.

Chew, P. *The inner world of the middle-aged man.* New York: Macmillan, 1976.

Cohen, S. E., & Beckwith, L. Preterm infant interaction with the caregiver in the first year of life and competence at age two. *Child Development,* 1979, *50,* 767–76.

Crandall, V. C. Expecting sex differences and sex differences in expectancies: A developmental analysis. In *Role of belief systems in the production of sex differences.* Symposium presented at the meeting of the American Psychological Association, Toronto, August 1978.

Davidson, P., & Bucher, B. Intrinsic interest and extrinsic reward: The effects of a continuing token program on continuing nonconstrained preference. *Behavior Therapy*, 1978, *9*, 222–34.

Debus, R. L. *Observational learning of reflective strategies by impulsive children.* Paper presented at the 21st International Congress of Psychology, Paris, July 1976.

Deci, E. L. *Intrinsic motivation.* New York: Plenum Press, 1975.

Dowrick, P. W. *Videotape replay as observational learning from oneself.* Unpublished manuscript, University of Auckland, 1977.

Dweck, C. The role of expectations and attributions in the alleviation of learned helplessness. *Journal of Personality and Social Psychology*, 1975, *31*, 674–85.

Dweck, C. S., Davidson, W., Nelson, S., & Enna, B. Sex differences in learned helplessness: II. The contingencies of evaluative feedback in the classroom and III. An experimental analysis. *Developmental Psychology*, 1978, *14*, 268–76.

Ellis, R. A., & Lane, W. C. Structural supports for upward mobility. *American Sociological Review*, 1963, *28*, 743–56.

Enzle, M. E., & Ross, J. M. Increasing and decreasing intrinsic interest with contingent rewards: A test of cognitive evaluation theory. *Journal of Experimental Social Psychology*, 1978, *14*, 588–97.

Ewart, C. K., Taylor, C. B., & DeBusk, R. F. *Increasing self-efficacy after heart attack: Effects of treadmill exercise.* Paper presented at the meeting of the American Psychological Association, Montreal, 1980.

Festinger, L. A theory of social comparison processes. *Human Relations*, 1954, *7*, 117–40.

Finkelstein, N. W., & Ramey, C. T. Learning to control the environment in infancy. *Child Development*, 1977, *48*, 806–19.

Flavell, J. H. Metacognitive development. In J. M. Scandura & C. J. Brainerd (Eds.), *Structural/process theories of complex human behavior.* Alphen a. d. Rijn, The Netherlands: Sijthoff and Noordhoff, 1978.

Metacognition and cognitive monitoring: A new area of cognitive-developmental inquiry. *American Psychologist*, 1979, *34*, 906–11.

Frankenhaeuser, M. Experimental approaches to the study of catecholamines and emotion. In L. Levi (Ed.), *Emotions: Their parameters and measurement.* New York: Raven Press, 1975.

Glass, D. C., Reim, B., & Singer, J. Behavioral consequences of adaptation to controllable and uncontrollable noise. *Journal of Experimental Social Psychology*, 1971, *7*, 244–57.

Gunnar, M. R. Control, warning signals, and distress in infancy. *Developmental Psychology*, 1980, *16*, 281–9. (a)

Contingent stimulation: A review of its role in early development. In S. Levine & H. Ursin (Eds.), *Coping and health.* New York: Plenum Press, 1980. (b)

Gunnar-vonGnechten, M. R. Changing a frightening toy into a pleasant toy by allowing the infant to control its actions. *Developmental Psychology*, 1978, *14*, 147–52.

Harter, S. Effectance motivation reconsidered: Toward a developmental model. *Human Development*, 1978, *21*, 34–64.

Hunt, J. McV., Cole, M. W., & Reis, E. E. S. Situational cues distinguishing anger, fear, and sorrow. *American Journal of Psychology*, 1958, *71*, 136–51.

Jacklin, C. N., & Mischel, H. M. As the twig is bent – Sex role stereotyping in early readers. *The School Psychology Digest*, 1973, *2*, 30–8.

Karniol, R., & Ross, M. The effect of performance-relevant and performance-irrelevant rewards on children's intrinsic motivation. *Child Development*, 1977, *48*, 482–7.

Kazdin, A. E. Covert modeling, model similarity, and reduction of avoidance behavior. *Behavior Therapy*, 1974, *5*, 325–40.

Krauss, I. Sources of educational aspirations among working-class youth. *American Sociological Review*, 1964, *29*, 867–79.

Kruglanski, A. W. The endogenous-exogenous partition in attribution theory. *Psychological Review*, 1975, *82*, 387–406.

Kun, A. Development of the magnitude-covariation and compensation schemata in ability and effort attributions of performance. *Child Development*, 1977, *48*, 862–73.

Kun, A., Garfield, T., & Sipowicz, C. *Causality pleasure: An experimental study of mastery motivation*. Paper presented at the meeting of the Society for Research in Child Development, San Francisco, March 1979.

Langer, E. J. The illusion of incompetence. In L. C. Permuter & R. A. Monty (Eds.), *Choice and perceived control*. Hillsdale, N.J.: Erlbaum, 1979.

Lepper, M. R., & Greene, D. Overjustification research and beyond: Toward a means–end analysis of intrinsic and extrinsic motivation. In M. R. Lepper & D. Greene (Eds.), *The hidden costs of reward: New perspectives on the psychology of human motivation*. Hillsdale, N.J.: Erlbaum, 1978.

Levi, L. (Ed.) Stress and distress in response to psychosocial stimuli. *Acta Medica Scandinavica*, 1972, *191*, Supplement No. 528.

Levy, D. M. *Maternal overprotection*. New York: Columbia University Press, 1943.

Locke, E. A., Cartledge, N., & Knerr, C. S. Studies of the relationship between satisfaction, goal-setting, and performance. *Organizational Behavior and Human Performance*, 1970, *5*, 135–58.

Mandler, G. *Mind and emotion*. New York: Wiley, 1975.

McArthur, L. Z., & Eisen, S. V. Achievements of male and female storybook characters as determinants of achievement behavior by boys and girls. *Journal of Personality and Social Psychology*, 1976, *33*, 467–73.

Meichenbaum, D. *Cognitive-behavior modification: An integrative approach*. New York: Plenum Press, 1977.

Meichenbaum, D., & Asarnow, J. Cognitive-behavior modification and metacognitive development: Implications for the classroom. In P. C. Kendall & S. D. Hollon (Eds.), *Cognitive-behavioral interventions: Theory, research, and procedures*. New York: Academic Press, 1979.

Millar, W. S. A study of operant conditioning under delayed reinforcement in early infancy. *Monographs of the Society for Research in Child Development*, 1972, *37*(2, Serial No. 147).

Miller, S. M. Controllability and human stress: Method, evidence, and theory. *Behavior Research and Therapy*, 1979, *17*, 287–304.

Miller, S. M., & Grant, R. P. *Predictability and human stress: Evidence, theory, and conceptual clarification*. Unpublished manuscript, University of Pennsylvania, 1979.

Morris, W. N., & Nemcek, D. *The development of social comparison motivation among preschoolers: Evidence of a step-wise progression*. Unpublished manuscript, Dartmouth College, 1979.

Neufeld, R. W. J., & Thomas, P. Effects of perceived efficacy of a prophylactic controlling mechanism on self-control under pain stimulation. *Canadian Journal of Behavioural Science*, 1977, *9*, 224–32.

Nuttin, J. R. Pleasure and reward in human motivation and learning. In D. E. Berlyne & K. B. Madsen (Eds.), *Pleasure, reward, preference*. New York: Academic Press, 1973.

Papoušek, H., & Papoušek, M. Early ontogeny of human social interaction: Its biological roots and social dimensions. In M. vonCranach, K. Foppa, W. Lepenies, & D. Ploog (Eds.), *Human ethology: Claims and limits of a new discipline*. Cambridge: Cambridge University Press, 1979.

Parsons, J. E., Moses, L., & Yulish-Muszynski, S. The development of attributions, expectancies, and persistence. In *Success and failure attributions and student behavior in the classroom*. Symposium presented at the meeting of the American Psychological Association, San Francisco, 1977.

Parsons, J. E., & Ruble, D. N. The development of achievement-related expectancies. *Child Development*, 1977, *48*, 1075–9.

Parsons, J. E., Ruble, D. N., Hodges, K. L., & Small, A. W. Cognitive-developmental factors in emerging sex differences in achievement-related expectancies. *The Journal of Social Issues*, 1976, *32*, 47–62.

Ramey, C. T., & Finkelstein, N. W. Contingent stimulation and infant competence. *Journal of Pediatric Psychology*, 1978, *3*, 89–96.

Rogers, C. R. A theory of therapy, personality, and interpersonal relationships, as developed in the client-centered framework. In S. Koch (Ed.), *Psychology: A study of a science. (Vol. 3). Formulations of the person and the social context.* New York: McGraw-Hill, 1959.

Rosenthal, T. L, & Bandura, A. Psychological modeling: Theory and practice. In S. L. Garfield & A. E. Bergin (Eds)., *Handbook of psychotherapy and behavior change: An empirical analysis* (2nd ed.). New York: Wiley, 1978.

Ross, M. The self perception of intrinsic motivation. In J. H. Harvey, W. J. Ickes, & R. F. Kidd (Eds.), *New directions in attribution research.* Hillsdale, N.J.: Erlbaum, 1976.

Sagotsky, G., & Lewis, A. *Extrinsic reward, positive verbalizations, and subsequent intrinsic interest.* Paper presented at the meeting of the American Psychological Association, Toronto, 1978.

Sarason, I. G. Anxiety and self-preoccupation. In I. G. Sarason & C. D. Spielberger (Eds.), *Stress and anxiety* (Vol. 2). Washington, D.C.: Hemisphere, 1975. (a)

  Test anxiety and the self-disclosing coping model. *Journal of Consulting and Clinical Psychology*, 1975, *43*, 148–53. (b)

  The test anxiety scale: Concept and research. In C. D. Spielberger & I. G. Sarason (Eds.), *Stress and anxiety* (Vol. 5). Washington, D.C.: Hemisphere, 1978.

Schachter, S. The interaction of cognitive and physiological determinants of emotional state. In L. Berkowitz (Ed.), *Advances in experimental social psychology* (Vol. 1). New York: Academic Press, 1964.

Schaie, K. W. Translations in gerontology – from lab to life: Intellectual functioning. *American Psychologist*, 1974, *29*, 802–7.

Schunk, D. H. Modeling and attributional effects on children's achievement: A self-efficacy analysis. *Journal of Educational Psychology*, 1981, in press.

Sears, R. R., Maccoby, E. E., & Levin, H. *Patterns of child rearing.* Evanston, Ill.: Row, Peterson, 1957.

Seligman, M. E. P., & Binik, Y. M. The safety signal hypothesis. In H. Davis & H. Hurwitz (Eds.), *Pavlovian-operant interaction.* Hillsdale, N.J.: Erlbaum, 1977.

Seligman, M. E. P., & Garber, J. (Eds.), *Human helplessness: Theory and research.* New York: Academic Press, 1980.

Slovic, P., Fischhoff, B., & Lichtenstein, S. Behavioral decision theory. In M. R. Rosenzweig & L. W. Porter (Eds.), *Annual review of psychology* (Vol. 28). Palo Alto, Calif.: Annual Reviews, 1977.

Slovic, P., & Lichtenstein, S. Comparison of Bayesian and regression approaches to the study of information processing in judgment. *Organizational Behavior and Human Performance*, 1971, *6*, 649–744.

Sternglanz, S. H., & Serbin, L. A. Sex role stereotyping in children's television programs. *Developmental Psychology*, 1974, *10*, 710–15.

Suls, J., & Mullen, B. From the cradle to the grave: Comparison and self-evaluation across the life-span. In J. Suls (Ed.), *Social psychological perspectives on the self*. Hillsdale, N.J.: Erlbaum, 1981, in press.

Suls, J. M., & Miller, R. L. (Eds.). *Social comparison processes: Theoretical and empirical perspectives*. Washington, D.C.: Hemisphere, 1977.

Takata, C., & Takata, T. The influence of models on the evaluation of ability: Two functions of social comparison processes. *The Japanese Journal of Psychology*, 1976, *47*, 74–84.

Tversky, A., & Kahneman, D. Judgment under uncertainty: Heuristics and biases. *Science*, 1974, *185*, 1124–31.

Vasta, R. Feedback and fidelity: Effects of contingent consequences on accuracy of imitation. *Journal of Experimental Child Psychology*, 1976, *21*, 98–108.

Watson, J. S. Perception of contingency as a determinant of social responsiveness. In E. B. Thoman (Ed.), *Origins of the infant's social responsiveness*. (Vol. 1) New York: Halsted Press, 1979.

Weinberg, R., Gould, D., & Jackson, A. Expectations and performance: An empirical test of Bandura's self-efficacy theory. *Journal of Sport Psychology*, 1979, *1*, 320–31.

Weinberg, R. S., Yukelson, D., & Jackson, A. Effect of public and private efficacy expectations on competitive performance. *Journal of Sport Psychology*, 1980, in press.

Weiner, B. *Achievement motivation and attribution theory*. Morristown, N.J.: General Learning Press, 1974.

Weitzman, L. J., Eifler, D., Hokada, E., & Ross, C. Sex-role socialization in picture books for preschool children. *American Journal of Sociology*, 1972, *77*, 1125–50.

White, R. W. Motivation reconsidered: The concept of competence. *Psychological Review*, 1959, *66*, 297–333.

Competence and the psychosexual stages of development. In M. R. Jones (Ed.), *Nebraska Symposium on Motivation, 1960*. Lincoln: University of Nebraska Press, 1960.

Wine, J. Test anxiety and direction of attention. *Psychological Bulletin*, 1971, *76*, 92–104.

Wylie, R. C. *The self-concept: A review of methodological considerations and measuring instruments* (rev. ed.). Lincoln: University of Nebraska Press, 1974.

Yarrow, L. J., Rubenstein, J. L., Pedersen, F. A., & Jankowski, J. J. Dimensions of early stimulation and their differential effects on infant development. *Merrill-Palmer Quarterly*, 1972, *18*, 205–18.

Zajonc, R. B., & Markus, G. B. Birth order and intellectual development. *Psychological Review*, 1975, *82*, 74–88.

10   Metacognition and the rules of delay

Walter Mischel

The nature, extent, and origin of people's knowledge about psychological processes has been one of the most enduring questions in psychology; the answer has profound implications for one's view of the human being. At different times in the history of the field, dramatically different conclusions have been reached about the degree to which people possess such psychological knowledge. In its extreme form, radical behaviorism suggested an image of human organisms responding automatically to stimuli and remained mute about people's possible knowledge of the psychological principles or rules that govern their own behavior. And in spite of the "cognitive revolution" of the last decade, which allocates an extensive role to cognition in human conduct (e.g., Bandura, 1977; Mischel, 1973), the status of people as intuitive psychologists remains highly controversial (e.g., compare Mischel, 1977 and Nisbett & Wilson, 1977; see Nisbett & Ross, 1980).

The child as intuitive psychologist

As part of a larger research program on cognitive social learning person variables (Mischel, 1973, 1979), we have been exploring the development of various facets of the child's cognitive competencies. We view children as potentially sophisticated (albeit fallible) intuitive psychologists who come to know and use psychological principles for understanding social behavior, for regulating their own conduct, and for achieving increasing mastery and control over their environments. In one direction, to study the development of children's cognitive competencies we have begun to explore their growing understanding of psychological principles that un-

The research reported in this chapter is also presented in Mischel, 1980, in press a, and in press b, and was supported in part by Grant MH06830 from the National Institute of Mental Health and by Grant HD MH09814 from the National Institute of Child Health and Human Development.

240

derlie social behavior. Having often bantered at parties about how our grandmothers knew most of the things we psychologists work so busily to discover empirically, we decided to actually explore the potential wisdom of young children (our grandmothers were no longer available). We wanted to see which insights, if any, from the fundamental principles of our field would become known to youngsters early in the course of development. For this goal, we devised objective tests with highly specific multiple-choice questions that asked fourth grade and sixth grade children to predict the probable outcome of classical experiments in psychology (Mischel & Mischel, 1979b).[1] These were described in detail, but with the jargon removed and phrased in age-appropriate ways. For example, research on the effect of intermittent reinforcement on extinction was described by introducing pictures of a white pigeon and a gray pigeon in their Skinnerian worlds. We then carefully described (and illustrated) each pecking at a bar, with pieces of food dropping into a cup continuously for each of many bar presses for one pigeon, opposed to reward delivery on an intermittent schedule for the other pigeon.

After the cessation of food for bar pressing was described, the child had to indicate which sentence below says best what each pigeon will do when food never drops into the cup anymore:

1. The gray pigeon (who had gotten food some of the time it pressed the bar) will completely stop pressing the bar sooner than the white pigeon.
2. The gray pigeon (who had gotten food some of the time it pressed the bar) and the white pigeon (who had gotten food every time it pressed the bar) will both completely stop pressing the bar at the same time.
3. The white pigeon (who had gotten food every time it pressed the bar) will completely stop pressing the bar sooner than the gray pigeon.

The experiments we sampled ranged from Skinner's investigations of reinforcement schedules to Asch's study on conformity, from Bandura's research on modeling to Pavlov's demonstration of classical conditioning. A complete list of the principles and experiments, the sources from which they were drawn, and the predictions made by children at each grade level appear in Table 10.1.

Even the ten-year-olds proved to know an impressive amount about the basic principles of social behavior. For example, they knew at $p < .001$ that children who have seen an adult playing aggressively will subsequently play more aggressively; that live modeling with guided participation is more effective in reducing snake phobic behavior than covert desensitization or modeling alone; that frightened baby monkeys prefer to cling to a soft surrogate mother rather than a wire one that provides milk; and that not attending to either immediate or delayed rewards

Table 10.1. *Summary of children's predictions of psychological principles*

Experiment or principle	Prediction					
	Grade	χ^2	df	Right	Wrong	NS
Group pressure can distort visual judgment (Asch, 1956).	4	25.28	1		$< .001$	
	6	.082	1			X
Not attending to the rewards facilitates delay (Mischel, Ebbesen, & Zeiss, 1972).	4	38.42	3	$< .001$		
	6	30.59	3	$< .001$		
The same water temperature feels cooler on a hot day than on a cool day (based on principle of effect of context, Helson, 1964).	4	12.80	2	$< .002$		
	6	54.03	2	$< .001$		
Classical conditioning: After repeated pairing of light and food, dog will salivate to food alone (Pavlov, 1927).	4	2.14	1			X
	6	4.0	1		$< .05$	
Children who have seen an adult behave aggressively will subsequently behave more aggressively than a control group (Bandura, Ross, & Ross, 1961).	4	21.16	3	$< .001$		
	6	78.26	3	$< .001$		
Modeling with guided participation is more powerful than covert desensitization or modeling alone in the treatment of phobic behavior (Bandura, Blanchard, & Ritter, 1969).	4	59.26	3	$< .001$		
	6	103.08	3	$< .001$		
The absence of object permanence at age 3 months (Piaget, 1954).	4	16.96	2	$< .001$		
	6	4.2	2			X
The attainment of object permanence by age 1½ years (Piaget, 1954).	4	2.53	2			X
	6	12.87	2	$< .002$		
Narrative stories are an aid to memory for lists of words (Bower & Clark, 1969).	4	10.04	2	$< .007$		
	6	48.38	2	$< .001$		

Finding					
Frightened, infant monkeys prefer soft surrogate mothers to wire ones that produce milk (Harlow & Zimmerman, 1959).	4	21.54	2	< .001	
	6	23.35	2	< .001	
Memory performance is better when measured by recognition vs. recall (Achilles, 1920).	4	44.15	2	< .001	
	6	70.71	2	< .001	
Inhibition of bystander intervention					X
(a) Two person groups are less likely than an individual alone to offer help to an injured woman (Latané & Rodin, 1969).	4	4.23	2	< .001	
(b) Two person groups are less likely than an individual alone to report a fire (Latané & Darley, 1968).	6	15.87	2	< .001	
Extinction of a response is more rapid following continuous vs. intermittent reinforcement (Ferster & Skinner, 1957).	4	12.72	2	.002	
The absence of conservation of quantity of liquid at age 4 years (Piaget, 1965).	4	44.89	4	< .001	
The attainment of conservation of quantity of liquid by age 10 years (Piaget, 1965).	4	114.89	4	< .001	
Physical appearance is more important in determining future dating behavior than opinions, intelligence, or school grades (Walster, Aronson, Abrahams, & Rothman, 1966).	6	51.17	3	< .001	
Attitude change is greater after a $1 reward for forced compliance than after a $20 reward (Festinger & Carlsmith, 1959).	6	34.02	2	< .001	

facilitates delay. Fourth graders did not know that a bystander will be more likely to help when alone than when in a group; they did know this widely cited nonobvious insight of social psychology by the time they were in grade six.

Before premature conclusions are reached, we must emphasize that the children's psychological knowledge was not limitless. The youngsters for example, did not know Pavlov's discovery about classical conditioning (although they did know that intermittent reinforcement makes Skinner's pigeons peck longer after the food stops). And they were wrong about conformity in the Asch situation; the importance of physical attractiveness in future dating behavior; and the effects of cognitive dissonance. The fact that by grade six we obtained correlations as high as .93 (in a small sample, $N = 10$) with intelligence test scores, encourages us to believe that spontaneous knowledge of psychological principles about social behavior may indeed be a significant feature of personal and cognitive competence that merits more systematic study.

In a more focused way we have been investigating children's understanding of psychological principles for self-regulation, using a two-pronged strategy. We try first to identify the objective conditions that make self-regulation (and particularly delay of gratification and resistance to temptation) either difficult or easy (e.g., Mischel, 1974; Mischel & Moore, 1980; Mischel & Patterson, 1976; Moore, Mischel, & Zeiss, 1976). Second, we are studying the child's own developing understanding of effective strategies for self-regulation.

Until recently there were few clear-cut empirical findings against which one could evaluate the relative efficacy of different strategies for self-control. This lack may help explain why children's developing awareness of self-control strategies has been neglected. Evidence about the conditions that help or hurt delay of gratification in children (e.g., Mischel, 1974; Miller & Karniol, 1976a, 1976b; Toner & Smith, 1977) now offers a basis for appraising the child's developing understanding against objective standards and that is exactly what we have been trying to do.

The aspect of delay of gratification that seems to have especially interesting theoretical implications is the role of reward-relevant ideation. Given the crucial importance of the concept of reinforcement in psychology, it is surprising how little has been learned until recently about the way in which mental representations of rewards and outcomes affect the individual's pursuit of them. Our recent research has focused especially on the problem of reward representation in situations in which people attempt to delay immediate smaller gratification for the sake of more desirable but deferred goals. Our intent has been to better understand how the mental representation of the relevant rewards in a contingency might influence voluntary delay for those outcomes. In this chapter I will summarize first our work on the "objective" rules of effective reward representation and then our research on children's knowledge of those rules.

The origins of delay

Freud's (1911) analysis of the transition from primary to secondary process provides one of the few theoretical discussions of how delay of gratification may be bridged. The psychoanalytic formulation suggests that ideation arises initially when there is a block or delay in the process of direct gratification discharge (Rapaport, 1967). During such externally imposed delay, Freud suggested, the child constructs a "hallucinatory wish-fulfilling image" of the need-satisfying object. As a result of frequent association of tension reduction with goal objects, and the development of greater ego organization, the imposed delay of satisfying objects gradually results in the substitution of hallucinatory satisfactions and other thought processes that convert "free cathexes" into "bound cathexes" (e.g., Freud, 1911; Singer, 1955). Unfortunately, however, the exact process remains unclear, although there has been much psychoanalytic theorizing about the function of the mental representation of blocked gratifications in the development of delaying capacity.

From a very different theoretical direction it also seemed plausible that "time-binding" (the capacity to bridge delay of gratification) might depend on self-instructional processes through which the individual increases the salience of the delayed consequences of his behavior. From that viewpoint, any factors (situational or within the individual) that make delayed consequences more vivid should facilitate impulse control. Such a view, although focusing on the self-instructional components of attention to delayed outcomes, also implies covert self-reinforcement processes through which the individual may reinforce his own delay behavior by vividly aniticipating some of the rewarding consequences that his waiting will produce. Finally, one could also expect that young children would easily forget the deferred outcomes for which they are waiting, and therefore stop waiting unless they are reminded of the relevant contingencies and rewards during the delay period.

In light of these arguments, conditions that help the individual to attend mentally to the delayed reward for which he is waiting should help him to continue to delay. Thus any cues that make the delayed gratifications more salient, vivid, or immediate (for example, by letting the person look at them, by picturing them in imagination, or by thinking of the object for which he is waiting) should enhance waiting behavior. These anticipations also seem consistent with findings from previous research on choice of immediate smaller versus delayed but larger rewards (Mahrer, 1956; Mischel & Metzner, 1962; Mischel & Staub, 1965; Mischel, 1966). These earlier investigations indicated that an important determinant of preference for delayed rewards is the person's expectation ("trust") that he will really get the delayed (but more valuable) outcome. When the child can always see the relevant rewards fewer doubts might arise about their ultimate availability than when the rewards are hidden from view. Therefore conditions in which the delayed gratification is visible may increase the individual's willingness to wait by increasing his expectancy that the delayed outcome will really still be there at the conclusion of the delay.

These considerations led us to predict initially that voluntary delay behavior would be enhanced when the individual converts the delayed object into more concrete form by making it psychologically more immediate, as by providing himself with representations or physical cues about it. To test that notion, the most direct way to increase the salience of the deferred outcomes and to focus attention on them would be to have them physically present in front of the subject so that he could attend to them vividly and easily. To explore how attention to delayed and immediate outcomes influences waiting behavior for them, we varied the availability of those outcomes for attention during the delay period.

Effects of attention to outcomes on waiting behavior

For this purpose we needed a paradigm in which very young children would be willing to stay in an experimental room, waiting by themselves for at least a short time without becoming excessively upset (Mischel & Ebbesen, 1970). As a first step (after the usual play periods for rapport building) each child was taught a "game" in which he could immediately summon the experimenter by a simple signal. This procedure was practiced until the child obviously understood that he could immediately end his waiting period alone in the room by signaling for the experimenter. The experimenter always returned immediately from outside the door when the child signaled. The child was then introduced to the relevant contingency. Specifically, he was shown two objects (e.g., snack food treats) one of which he clearly preferred (as determined by pretesting), but to get the preferred object he had to wait for it until the experimenter returned "by himself." However, the child was free throughout this delay period to signal anytime for the experimenter to return; if he signaled he could have the less preferred object at once but would forego the more desirable one later.

In order to systematically manipulate the degree to which children could attend to the rewards while they were waiting, the reward objects were available to the child's view in all combinations, creating four conditions with respect to the object available for attention. The children in one condition waited with both the immediate (less preferred) and the delayed (more preferred) rewards facing them in the experimental room so that they could attend to both outcomes. In a second group, neither reward was available for the child's attention, both rewards having been removed from his sight. In the remaining two groups either the delayed reward only or the immediate reward only was left facing the child and available for attention while he waited. The length of time before each child voluntarily terminated the waiting period was the dependent measure.

Our initial theorizing about delay behavior led us to predict results that were the opposite of what we found. We had expected that attention to the delayed rewards in the choice situation while waiting would facilitate delay behavior. We found, instead, that attention to the rewards significantly and dramatically decreased delay of gratification. The children waited longest when *no* rewards faced them during the delay period; they waited significantly less long when they faced the delayed reward, or the immediate reward, or both rewards, as Figure 10.1 indicates (with no significant differences between the reward conditions but a trend for shortest delay when facing both rewards).

To explore what caused these unexpected results, we tried to see just what the children were doing while they were waiting. Therefore we observed them closely by means of a one-way mirror throughout the delay period as they sat waiting for their preferred outcomes in what had proved to be the most difficult situation, that is, with both the immediate and delayed outcomes facing them. These observations were helped by "Mr. Talk Box," a device that consisted of a tape recorder and a microphone that announced its name to the youngsters and cheerfully said, "Hi, I have big ears and I love it when children fill them with all the things they think and feel, no matter what." Thereafter, Mr. Talk Box adopted a Rogerian nondirective attitude and acceptingly "uhemed" and "ahad" to whatever the child said to him. In fact, many children seemed to quickly treat Mr. Talk Box as an extension of their psyche and engaged in elaborate, animated discussions with themselves.

Observations of the children during the delay period itself gradually

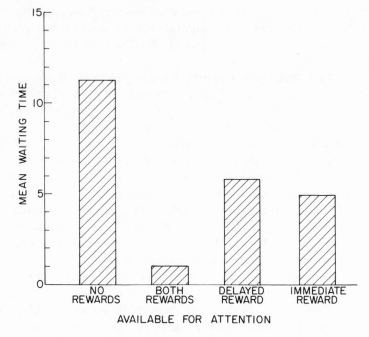

Figure 10.1. Mean minutes of voluntary waiting time for the delayed reward in each attention condition (from Mischel & Ebbesen, 1970).

gave us some clues about the mechanisms through which they seemed to mediate and facilitate their own goal-directed waiting. The most effective delay strategies employed by some children were remarkably simple. These youngsters seemed able to wait for the preferred reward for long periods apparently by converting the aversive waiting situation into a more pleasant nonwaiting one. They managed this by elaborate self-distraction techniques through which they spent their time psychologically doing almost anything other than waiting. Instead of focusing their attention prolongedly on the rewards they avoided them. Some of the children covered their eyes with their hands, rested their heads on their arms, and discovered other similar techniques for averting their gaze from the rewards. Many children also seemed to try to reduce the frustration of delay of reward by generating their own diversions: They talked quietly to themselves, sang ("This is such a pretty day, hurray"), created games with their hands and feet, and when all other distractions seemed exhausted even tried to go to sleep during the waiting time – as one child successfully did, falling into a deep slumber in front of the signal bell. These tactics, of course, are familiar to anyone who has ever been trapped in a boring lecture.

Our observations of the children seem consistent with theorizing that emphasizes the aversiveness of frustration and delayed rewards. If the subject is experiencing conflict and frustration about wanting to end the delay but not wanting to lose the preferred, delayed outcome, then cues that enhance attention to the elements in the conflict (i.e., the two sets of rewards) should increase the aversiveness of waiting. More specifically, when the child attends to the immediate reward his motivation for it increases and he becomes tempted to take it but is frustrated because he knows that taking it now prevents his getting the preferred reward later. When the subject attends to the preferred but delayed outcome he becomes increasingly frustrated because he wants it more now but cannot have it yet. When attention is focused on both objects, both of these sources of frustration occur and further delay becomes most aversive; hence the child acts to end the waiting period quickly (as indeed happened). This reasoning would suggest that conditions that decrease attention to the rewards in the choice contingency and that distract the person (through internal or overt activity) from the conflict and the frustrating delay would make it less aversive to continue goal-directed waiting and thus permit longer delay of gratification. That is, just as cognitive avoidance may help one to cope with anxiety so may it help to deal with such other aversive events as the frustration of waiting for a desired but delayed outcome and the continuous conflict of whether or not to end the waiting period.

The role of cognitive distraction

The foregoing theorizing suggests that delay of gratification and frustration tolerance should be facilitated by conditions that help the individual to transform the aversive waiting period into a more pleasant nonwaiting situation. Such a transformation could be achieved by converting attention and thoughts away from the frustrating components of delay of gratification. Thus voluntary delay of reward should be enhanced by any overt or covert activities that serve as distractors from the rewards and thus ease the aversiveness of the situation. By means of such distraction the person should convert the frustrating delay-of-reward situation into a less aversive one. Activities, cognitions, and fantasy that could distract the individual from the reward objects therefore should increase the length of time that he would delay gratification for the sake of getting the preferred outcome.

But how can one influence what the child is going to think about? After many poor starts we discovered that even at ages three and four our

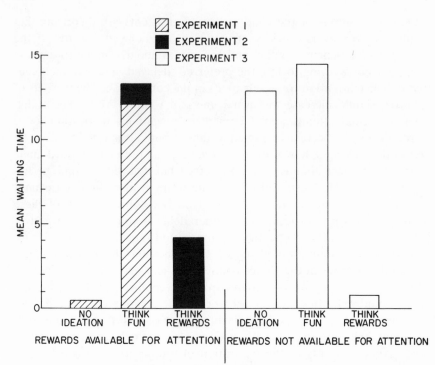

Figure 10.2. Mean minutes of voluntary waiting time for treatment conditions in Experiments 1, 2, and 3, comparing different ideation instructions with controls (from Mischel, Ebbesen, & Zeiss, 1972).

subjects could give us elaborate, dramatic examples of the many events that made them feel happy, like finding frogs, or singing, or swinging on a swing with mommy pushing. In turn, we instructed them to think about these fun things while they sat waiting alone for their preferred outcomes. In some of these studies the immediate and delayed rewards were physically not available for direct attention during the waiting period. We manipulated the children's attention to the absent rewards cognitively by different types of instructions given before the start of the delay period. The results showed that cognitions directed toward the rewards substantially reduced, rather than increased, the amount of time that the children were able to wait. Thus attentional and cognitive mechanisms that enhance the salience of the rewards greatly decreased the length of voluntary delay time. In contrast, overt or covert distractions from the rewards (e.g., by prior instructions to think about fun things) facilitated delay of gratification (Mischel, Ebbesen, & Zeiss, 1972), as Figure 10.2 illustrates.

The overall results undermine theories that predict that mental attention to the reward objects will enhance voluntary delay by facilitating "time binding" and tension discharge (through cathexes of the image of the object). The data also undermine any "salience" theories that would suggest that making the outcomes salient by imagery, cognitions, and self-instructions about the consequences of delay behavior should increase voluntary delay. The findings unequivocally contradict theoretical expectations that images and cognitions relevant to the gratifications sustain delay behavior. Instead, either looking at the rewards or thinking about them in their absence decreases voluntary delay of gratification. Effective delay thus seems to depend on suppressive and avoidance mechanisms to reduce frustration during the delay period; it does not appear to be mediated by consummatory fantasies about the rewards.

These results suggest that the person can delay most effectively for a chosen deferred gratification if during the delay period he shifts his attention from the relevant gratifications and occupies himself internally with cognitive distractions. Situational or self-induced conditions that shift attention from the reward objects appear to facilitate voluntary waiting times appreciably. In order to bridge the delay effectively, it is as if the child must make an internal notation of what he is waiting for, perhaps remind himself of it periodically, but spend the remaining time attending to other less frustrating internal and external stimuli, thereby transforming the noxious into the easy and taking the thinking and the worrying out of waiting and "will power."

As early as 1890, William James noted a relationship between attention and self-control and contended that attentional processes are the crux of the self-control phenomena usually subsumed under the label "will" (or, since James's time, under the concept "ego strength"). As James (1890) put it: "Attention with effort is all that any case of volition implies. The essential achievement of will is to attend to a difficult object . . ." (p. 549). Starting with the work of Hartshorne and May (1928) some correlations have been obtained between indexes of moral behavior and measures of attention or resistance to distraction on mental tests (e.g., Grim, Kohlberg & White, 1968). Such correlations have led to the suggestion that a person's ability to resist temptation may be facilitated by how well he attends to a task. "Yielding to temptation" (e.g., cheating) in most experimental paradigms hinges on the subject's becoming distracted from the main task to which he is supposed to be attending. In such paradigms a subject's ability to focus attention *on* the task and to resist distraction automatically may make it easier for him to resist such temptations as cheating, as Grim et al. (1968) have noted.

Our findings, however, reveal a quite different relation between attention and self-control: *Not* attending to the goal was what facilitated self-control most dramatically. But it should be recognized that the mental transformations and distractions that occur during delay do not erase or undo the role of the reward contingencies in the waiting situation. This was evident from data that showed that there was little persistence in "thinking fun" or playing with a toy when there was no reward contingent upon waiting. The distracting activity itself, although pleasant and distracting enough to maintain the waiting for a contingent reward, did not in itself keep the children in the room for more than a minute when the contingency was removed. Additional evidence that the contingency was available mentally throughout the waiting period is that the children easily reproduced, verbally or by appropriate action, the contingencies at the end of the waiting period. Children who had been busily distracting themselves for the full fifteen minutes, playing with a toy or singing songs, immediately and spontaneously ate the appropriate food reward when the experimenter returned. Obviously then, the transformation of the aversive waiting into a pleasant play period does not efface the task-oriented purpose of the behavior and presumably the two processes somehow coexist. Subjects were guided by their goals, even when seemingly absorbed in distractions designed to obscure these goals. Just how the contingency was operating is an interesting point for speculation. The contingency may have been available but never reproduced mentally until the end of waiting; even more likely, subjects may have reminded themselves of the contingency periodically throughout the waiting period. As mentioned previously, verbalizations of the contingency often occurred when subjects momentarily left their distracting play and seemed about to terminate the waiting period. It is as if the subject periodically reminds himself of the goal for which he is waiting, distracts himself from it to make delay less frustrating, and then repeats the process.

Although the present studies provided reliable findings based on several replications and diverse convergent data, we obviously cannot generalize from them the role of cognition in forms of self-control other than the delay of gratification paradigm. Thus, for example, it might be adaptive to ideate about desired or needed but currently unavailable goal objects, but only in situations in which the subjects' actions can be potentially instrumental in producing the desired outcome. When attainment of a positive outcome is contingent on the person's own problem-solving behavior, it might help the person to think about the goal object while seeking means for achieving or reaching it in reality. In the present delay of gratification paradigm, in contrast, attainment of the preferred goal required only passive waiting; beyond delaying there was absolutely noth-

ing the subject could do to influence the occurrence of the desired outcome. Moreover, even his delay behavior (while a necessary condition for
attainment of the preferred outcome) could in no way affect the time at
which gratification ultimately would occur.

Thus the conclusion that aversive stimuli are avoided cognitively may
be restricted to paradigms in which the person believes that thinking
about the aversive stimulus cannot change the contingencies in the situation. In contrast, when the aversive stimulus (such as an electric shock)
can be avoided, subjects may tend to become vigilant, correctly perceiving the stimulus more quickly than do controls (e.g., Dulany, 1957;
Rosen, 1954). That is, when people can potentially control painful events
perhaps they think about them more and become vigilantly alert to them.
To the extent that the delay-of-gratification situation produces an aversive frustration effect, people are likely to delay better if they avoid
ideating about the rewards, but perhaps only if their own behavior during
delay cannot affect the time at which the frustration will be terminated.
Whether people react to potentially frustrating or painful stimuli by
"blunting" and trying to avoid them cognitively or by "monitoring" and
becoming vigilantly alert to them thus may depend in part on what they
can do to control them (e.g., Miller, 1979; in press).

The findings up to this point suggest that the capacity to sustain self-
imposed delay of reinforcement depends on the degree to which the
individual avoids (or transforms) cues about the frustration of the delay
situation; cues that remind him of what he expects and wants but is
prevented (interrupted, blocked, delayed) from getting. This hypothesis
would apply equally to the externally imposed delays or interruptions that
characterize "frustration" (Mandler, 1964) and to the self-imposed delay
behavior that marks "self-control." To increase subjective frustration a
person then would have to focus cognitively on the goal objects (e.g., by
engaging covertly in anticipatory goal responses); to decrease frustration
he would have to suppress the goal objects by avoiding them cognitively.
In the delay paradigm, "frustration tolerance" would depend on the subject's ability to suppress his attention to the blocked rewards while remaining in the frustrating situation until the goal is attained. More recent
studies by other investigators have confirmed repeatedly that effective
self-imposed delay of gratification in preschool children partly hinges on
the degree to which the individual can avoid attending to the rewards
(outcomes) in the delay contingency (e.g., Miller & Karniol, 1976a,
1976b; Schack & Massari, 1973; Toner, Lewis, & Gribble, 1979; Toner &
Smith, 1977). These studies consistently indicate that attention and ideation directed at the goal objects in the self-imposed delay of gratification

paradigm make it extremely difficult for young children to sustain goal-directed waiting.[2]

The role of symbolically presented rewards

In view of the complex cognitive activity that seems to mediate delay behavior it becomes important to consider and control more precisely the covert activities in the subject during the waiting period. The most relevant condition for further study is the one in which the subject is attending cognitively to the reward objects although the rewards are physically absent. In his formulation of delay of gratification, Freud (1911) suggested that delay capacity begins when the child develops images (mental representations) of the delayed reward in the absence of the object itself. According to that view, the hungry infant may gain some satisfaction by forming a "hallucinatory" image of the mother's breast when she is physically unavailable. Whereas we tried to manipulate attention to the actual rewards by varying their presence or absence in the child's visual field, how could one manipulate the availability of an *image* of the relevant objects when they were absent physically? A study by Mischel and Moore (1973) tried to approximate this condition at least crudely by *symbolic* presentations of the absent objects during the delay period. For this purpose subjects were exposed to slide-presented images of the absent reward objects while waiting for them. The design compared the effect on delay behavior of exposure to such images of the "relevant" objects (i.e., the rewarding outcomes for which the subject was waiting) with exposure to images of similar objects that were irrelevant to the delay contingency.

In this study preschool children first had to choose between two rewards. Then they were allowed to wait for their choice or to signal at any time to obtain the less preferred outcome immediately, just as in the Mischel et al. (1972) study. Two different pairs of reward choices were employed; half the subjects chose between two marshmallows and a pretzel and half between two pennies and a token. During the delay period, experimental subjects were exposed to realistic color slide-presented images on a screen that faced them. In one condition the images were slides of the rewards that the subjects had chosen ("relevant imagery"); in another condition the slides depicted the objects that the subject had not seen before ("irrelevant imagery"). For example, if a subject had been given a choice between two marshmallows and a pretzel, each "relevant imagery" slide would depict those reward objects, whereas each "irrelevant imagery" slide would show the other objects (two pennies and a token) to which he had not been exposed previously (i.e., the "irrelevant" rewards with respect to the contingency). Subjects in a third condition were exposed to a blank slide (no picture but illuminated screen). A "no-slide" control group constituted the fourth condition.

In all conditions the slides with *relevant* imagery produced the longest delay times, with the contents of slide-presented images yielding a highly significant main effect ($p < .001$). Thus the effects of relevant slide-presented rewards proved to be the opposite of those found for exposure to the real rewards. Attention to the real rewards makes it much harder for preschool children to delay for them, whereas slide-presented symbolic presentations of those rewards were found to facilitate waiting time. Moreover, these opposite effects occurred reliably within the same basic subject population and experimental paradigm at the same preschool. Why?

In a recent experiment we (Mischel & Moore, 1980) tried to resolve this discrepancy and to illuminate why symbolic reward presentations enhance self-imposed delay whereas attention to the actual outcomes impedes it. We reasoned that the highly significant effects found for the mode of presentation of the reward stimuli (real versus slide presented) occurred because they led children to ideate about the rewards in different ways. Extrapolating from Berlyne's (1960) and Estes's (1972) distinctions, a stimulus may have a motivational (consummatory, arousal) function and an informational (cue) function. The actual reward stimuli (i.e., the real objects) are apt to have a more powerful motivational effect than do their symbolic representations (i.e., slide images). In contrast, symbolic representations of the objects (e.g., through slide pictures) would have a more abstract cue function. Viewing the actual goal objects increases the child's motivation for them, whereas a picture of the rewards serves to remind him of them but with less affective arousal. The motivational arousal generated by attention to the rewards themselves is frustrating because it increases the subject's desire to make the blocked consummatory responses appropriate to the outcome (e.g., eat it, play with it). This arousal function of the real stimulus increases the frustration effect (because the person cannot let himself make the consummatory response), thereby making delay more difficult and shorter (Mischel et al., 1972). In contrast, the cue (informative) function of the symbolic reward stimulus may guide and sustain the person's goal-directed delay behavior. It may do that by reminding the subject of the contingency in the delay situation (a reminder of what the person will get if he delays) without being so real and arousing as to be frustrating.

Thus, exposure to the real reward stimuli themselves may lead the preschool child to become excessively aroused in the self-imposed delay of gratification paradigm. Such arousal is frustrating because it makes the child ready to perform the terminal response in a situation in which he or she cannot do so, and hence leads to shorter delay. But exposure to the symbolic representations of the objects in the form of pictures (as on the slides) may retain their cue function without generating excessive arousal; one cannot consume a picture.

To test our conceptualization more systematically, we (Mischel & Moore, 1980) attempted to vary the child's consummatory ideation by manipulating (through instructions) their attention to the arousing qualities of the reward objects. Simultaneously, we varied the slide-presented stimulus content facing the subject during the delay period. In this fashion it should be possible to isolate the role of consummatory ideation and of symbolic presentations of the rewards in delay of gratification.

We hypothesized that the crucial variable would be the nature of the child's ideation about the rewards and not their physical representation during the delay period. Specifically, we attempted to replicate the major Mischel and Moore (1973) finding that exposure to slides of the rewards in the delay contingency leads to significantly longer delay than does exposure to slides of comparable rewards that are irrelevant to the delay contingency. Second, we predicted that this enhancing effect of the slide-presented rewards can be completely wiped out and even reversed when subjects are instructed (before the delay period) to ideate about the consummatory qualities of the relevant rewards while waiting for them (Mischel & Moore, 1980).

In a self-imposed delay-of-gratification paradigm, (e.g., Mischel et al., 1972), preschool children waited for preferred but delayed rewards. (Details of the design are in Mischel and Moore, 1980). We systematically varied the contents of slide-presented images of the rewards and instructions about ideation during the delay. The findings unequivocally supported the hypotheses. First, the data replicated the original finding that exposure to slides of the relevant rewards leads to significantly longer self-imposed delay than does exposure to slides of the comparable rewards that are irrelevant to the delay contingency (Mischel & Moore, 1973). But more important, the study also showed that the delay-enhancing effects of the relevant slides can be completely wiped out when subjects are instructed (before the delay interval) to ideate about the consummatory qualities of the relevant rewards (e.g., the taste and texture of food objects) while waiting for them. Presumably the delay-enhancing effects of exposure to the symbolic presentation of the rewards in the waiting contingency hinge on their helping the child to ideate about them but in a nonconsummatory fashion. In contrast, consummatory ideation about the relevant rewards, whether induced by instructions as in this study, or by exposure to the actual rewards (Mischel & Ebbesen, 1970; Mischel et al., 1972), prevents effective delay of gratification.

Specifically, the child's consummatory ideation (induced by instructions before the delay period) about the rewards, and not the content of the slide-presented image facing him during the waiting period, was found to be the crucial determinant of voluntary delay of gratification. Instructions to focus on the consummatory qualities of the rewards in the delay contingency consistently produced the shortest delay times. When instructed to ideate about the consummatory qualities of the objects in the waiting contingency ("relevant rewards") the children delayed gratification significantly less long than when they were given the same instructions focused on comparable rewards irrelevant to the delay contingency. Moreover, the debilitating effect of consummatory ideation regarding the rewards in the contingency occurred regardless of the physical stimulus facing the subject during the delay period (see Figure 10.3).

Cognitive operations to transform the stimulus

Thus the effects of attention to the rewards upon delay behavior probably depend on *how* the subject attends to them rather than simply on whether or not he does. In that case, if attention is focused at the nonconsummatory (more abstract, informative) cue properties of the reward stimuli, delay behavior should be facilitated. In contrast, attention to the motivational or arousing qualities of the rewards should increase the frustration of delay and interfere with effective self-control. If Freud's (1911) conceptualization of the positive role of the "hallucinatory image" of the blocked gratification in the development of delay of gratification refers to the motivational properties of the image, he was probably incorrect. But if his formulation referred to the nonconsummatory, more abstract cue properties of the image it may still prove to be of value.

To test these theoretical possibilities, some of our studies have explored how the impact of attention to the rewards in the delay paradigm can be modified by the specific *cognitive transformations* that the subject performs with regard to them. In these studies, just before the start of the delay period, children are given brief instructions designed to encourage them to ideate in different ways during the actual delay time. For example, one study compared the effects of instructions to ideate about the motivational (consummatory) qualities of the "relevant" rewards with comparable instructions to ideate about their nonmotivational (nonconsummatory) qualities and associations (Mischel & Baker, 1975). The same two types of instructions also were used for the "irrelevant" re-

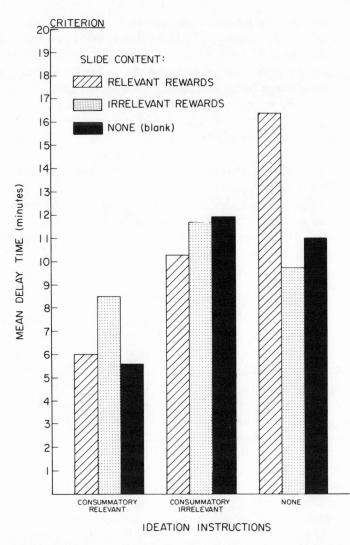

Figure 10.3. Effects of ideation and slide content on delay time (from Mischel and Moore, 1979).

wards. "Relevant" and "irrelevant" were operationalized as in the Mischel and Moore studies. All children had to wait while facing the relevant rewards in the contingency.

We found that through instructions the child can cognitively transform the reward objects that face him during the delay period in ways that either permit or prevent effective delay of gratification. If the child has been instructed to focus cognitively on the consummatory qualities of the

Table 10.2. *Mean delay time in each ideation instruction condition*

	Content of ideation	
Rewards in ideation	Consummatory	Nonconsummatory
Relevant[a]	5.60	13.51
Irrelevant[a]	16.82	4.46

Note: Maximum possible delay time is twenty minutes. All subjects facing the rewards. Data are in minutes.
[a]To contingency in the waiting situation.
Source: Mischel & Baker, 1975.

relevant reward objects (such as the pretzel's crunchy, salty taste or the chewy, sweet, soft taste of the marshmallows) it becomes difficult for him to wait. Conversely, if he cognitively transforms the stimulus to focus on nonconsummatory qualities (by thinking about the pretzel sticks, for example, as long, thin brown logs, or by thinking about the marshmallows as white, puffy clouds or as round, white moons) he can wait for long time periods (Mischel & Baker, 1975). The main results are shown in Table 10.2.

Note that transformations of the reward objects that focus on their nonconsummatory qualities provide more than mere cognitive distraction. The Mischel and Baker study compared, in this regard, the effects of instructions that focus on nonconsummatory qualities of the relevant reward objects (i.e., those for which the subject is actually waiting) with the same instructions for irrelevant rewards. When the children had been instructed to ideate about nonconsummatory qualities of the relevant rewards their mean delay time was more than thirteen minutes (twenty minutes was the maximum possible). In contrast, when subjects had been given the same instructions with regard to the irrelevant rewards (i.e., comparable but not in the delay contingency) their average delay time was less than five minutes. Thus attention to the nonconsummatory qualities and associations of the actual reward objects in the delay contingency substantially enhances the ability to wait for them, and does so more effectively than when the same ideation instructions focus on comparable objects irrelevant to the delay contingency.

One might argue that the relatively low delay time obtained when instructions dealt with ideation for the "irrelevant" rewards reflects that young children simply have trouble thinking about reward objects that are not present. Note, however, that the longest mean delay time (almost seventeen minutes) occurred when subjects were instructed to ideate about those same objects but with regard to their consummatory qualities (see Table 10.2). This finding is also provocative theoretically. It suggests that consummatory ideation about a potentially available object makes it difficult to delay gratification, whereas similar consummatory ideation about an outcome that is simply unattainable in the situation (i.e., the "irrelevant" rewards), rather than being aversive, is highly pleasurable and may serve to sustain prolonged delay behavior. That is, consummatory ideation about reward objects that are not expected and not available in the delay contingency (the irrelevant rewards) may serve as an interesting effective distractor, hence facilitating waiting. In contrast, similar ideation about the relevant but blocked rewards heightens the frustration of wanting what one expects but cannot yet have and, by making the delay more aversive, reduces the length of time that one continues to wait.

Further support for the powerful role of cognitive transformations in delay behavior comes from studies showing that through instructions the children can easily transform the real objects (present in front of them) into an abstract version (a "color picture in your head"), or they can transform the picture of the objects (presented on a slide projected on a screen in front of them) into the "real" objects by imagining that they are actually there on a plate in front of them, with predictable opposite effects on their delay time. Specifically, Moore, Mischel, and Zeiss (1976) exposed preschool subjects either to a slide-presented image of the rewards, or to the actual rewards. In each of these conditions half the children were instructed before the start of the delay period to imagine a "picture" of the reward objects during the delay period. For example:

. . . Close your eyes. In your head try to see the picture of the _____ (immediate and delayed rewards). Make a color picture of (them); put a frame around them. You can see the picture of them. Now open your eyes and do the same thing. (more practice . . . From now on you can see a picture that shows _____ (immediate and delayed rewards) here in front of you. The _____ aren't real; they're just a picture . . . When I'm gone remember to see the picture in front of you.

Conversely, half the children in each of the conditions were instructed before the delay period (with similar techniques) to imagine the *real* rewards actually present in front of them while waiting. Details of the instructions were adapted to make them plausible in each condition and a maximum delay time of twenty minutes was possible. The results indicated that the crucial determinant of delay behavior was the subject's cognitive representation, regardless of what was actually in front of the

Table 10.3. *Mean delay time as a function of cognitive transformations*

Objectively facing subject	Cognitive representation of rewards as:	
	Pictures	Real
Picture of rewards	17.75	5.95
Real rewards	17.70	7.91

Note: Maximum possible delay time is twenty minutes. Data are in minutes.
Source: Moore, Mischel, & Zeiss, 1976.

child. When imagining the rewards as a picture, the mean delay time was almost eighteen minutes, regardless of whether the real rewards or a picture of them actually faced the child. But when representing the rewards cognitively as if they were real, subjects' delay time was significantly and substantially lower, regardless of whether the slide or the actual set of rewards was objectively in front of them (see Table 10.3).

Our overall findings on cognitive stimulus transformations clearly reveal that how children represent the rewards cognitively (not what is physically in front of them) determines how long they delay gratification. Regardless of the stimulus in their visual field, if they imagine the real objects as present they cannot wait very long for them. But if they imagine pictures (abstract representations) of the objects they can wait for long time periods (and even longer than when they are distracting themselves with abstract representations of objects that are comparable but not relevant to the rewards for which they are waiting). By means of instructions (given before the child begins to wait) about what to imagine during the delay period, it is possible to completely alter (in fact, to reverse) the effects of the physically present reward stimuli in the situation, and to cognitively control delay behavior with substantial precision. Although arousal-generating cognitions about the real objects in the contingency significantly impede delay, cognitions about their nonconsummatory (nonmotivational) qualities or about their abstract representations enhance delay.

Thus *how* the subject ideates about the outcomes (rather than whether or not he does) appears to be crucial. In the delay paradigm, cognitive representations of the rewards (goals, outcomes) that emphasize their motivational (consummatory, arousal) qualities, we suggest, prevent effective delay by generating excessive frustration, at least in young children. The more the subject focuses on the arousing qualities of the blocked goals, the more intense and aversive the choice conflict and the delay become, and the sooner he terminates the situation. Conversely, cognitive representation of the same objects that focuses on their nonconsummatory (more abstract, less arousing) qualities appears to facilitate the maintenance of goal-directed behavior. In future research it will be important to explore the exact mechanisms that underlie this facilitation. It seems likely that abstract cognitive representations of the rewards permit the subject to remind himself of the contingency, and to engage in self-reinforcement for further delay, without becoming debilitatingly aroused and frustrated; the specific processes he uses require further study. Such work should continue to clarify not only the mechanisms in delay of gratification but also how the mental representation of goal objects ("rewards") motivates and guides complex waiting and working. The present studies have demonstrated that the specific ways in which rewards are represented cognitively, rather than their physical presence or absence, determine the impact of those rewards on the subject's ability to control his behavior in pursuit of them. Future efforts should provide an increasingly comprehensive analysis of the cognitive mechanisms that permit human beings to achieve such self-control.

The child's knowledge of the delay rules

The results summarized in earlier sections provide evidence about conditions that may facilitate waiting for deferred outcomes. But remarkably little is known about the child's own understanding and strategies for coping with various types of delay. (For example, does the preschool child know that consummatory ideation about the rewards will make self-imposed delay more difficult?) Thus until recently we knew a considerable amount about delay-enhancing stimulus conditions but almost nothing about children's awareness of effective attentional strategies during delay of gratification. To begin to fill this gap, in one recent set of studies we began to explore young children's verbal preferences and actual use of different attentional strategies for sustaining delay of gratification (Mischel, Mischel, & Hood, 1978; Mischel, Mischel, & Hood, 1978; Mischel & Mischel, 1979a; Yates & Mischel, 1979). Our results ultimately should help clarify the degree to which young children know and utilize delay-facilitating attentional strategies when faced with situations requiring them to wait for deferred outcomes and should illuminate the development and implications of such strategies.

To begin to investigate children's preferred attentional strategies for delaying gratification, we (Yates & Mischel, 1979) modified the delay paradigm developed by Mischel et al. (1972). Instead of placing fixed stimuli in front of the child for the entire delay, we designed equipment that allowed the subject to self-regulate the presentation of stimuli throughout the delay period. Each child had available for self-presentation one of the two types of stimuli that facilitate self-imposed delay (SID)[3] and one of the two types of stimuli that hinder it. Different groups of children had available for viewing one of the four possible pairings of the two SID-facilitating and two SID-hindering stimuli. We recorded the amount of time that the children actually viewed the different types of stimuli during either a self-imposed delay of gratification (SID) or during an externally imposed delay (EID) of equal duration, and also assessed their preferences verbally after completion of the delay.

The results of this series of four experiments led to several conclusions concerning the nature and consequences of young children's preferred attentional strategies during delay of gratification. To summarize briefly, Experiment 1 showed that during both self-imposed delay (SID) and externally imposed delay (EID), preschool children prefer to view real stimuli rather than symbolic (pictorial) representations of stimuli, regardless of their relevance to the rewards in the delay contingency. No differences in preference patterns were found in SID versus EID. The same pattern of preferences was replicated in Experiment 2, which also found no significant effects of age within the three age categories sampled (ages 3 to 4.25 years, 4.50 to 5.75 years, and 6.00 to 7.00 years).

Experiment 3 allowed us to distinguish clearly between children's attentional preferences during delay when they are oriented to attend to the stimuli that they want to view (wish strategy) as opposed to those stimuli that they believe would help them wait most (efficacy strategy). The results revealed that when following a wish strategy children attended significantly more to the real rewards than to their more abstract (pictorial) representations, further replicating the findings of Experiments 1 and 2. But when following an efficacy strategy the children did not show any systematic preference for viewing relevant real as opposed to relevant symbolic stimuli: Presumably they simply did not know which of these two types of stimuli would help more and chose quite randomly.

The data from the older children (grades one, two, and three) obtained in Experiment 4 were dramatically different and suggest a change in delay strategies in the course of development, beginning around age seven years. Specifically, when waiting for food, these older children systematically preferred viewing reward irrelevant stimuli and were aware that this strategy would help them delay gratification best. This was true in externally imposed as well as in self-imposed delay situations. The fact that the older children preferred to view the irrelevant stimuli during externally imposed food delay as well as during self-imposed delay raises serious questions about whether the attentional strategies that facilitate EID as opposed to SID are really different and suggests that Miller and Karniol's conclusions about the facilitating effects of attention to the rewards during EID (but not SID) may be premature. Given the potential theoretical importance of the EID–SID distinction, further work to closely assess its empirical status seems crucial.

The Yates and Mischel (1979) finding that the younger children spontaneously prefer to view the real stimuli during delay of gratification seems to be congruent with Freud's (1911) classical theory of wish-fulfilling ideation during delay: When the desired object is blocked, the frustrated child tries to self-present it, to "have it." But our previous research suggests that in so doing, the young child is making self-imposed delay not less but more difficult for himself! That happens because reward-relevant ideation increases his desire and hence enhances the frustration of the delay (e.g., Mischel, 1974), especially if this ideation is consummatory rather than more abstract (Mischel & Baker, 1975; Moore et al., 1976). The youngster is then trapped in a delay-defeating cycle, attending to the consummatory qualities of what he really wants and becoming increasingly frustratively aroused, thereby making it even harder to wait successfully. Thus the young child's preference for attending to the real rewards rather than to more symbolic representations of them helps to explain why it is so difficult for him to tolerate voluntary delay of gratification. By attending to the real rewards the young child may make such delay especially frustrating and arousing, thereby defeating his own ability to wait for what he wants. These interpretations are supported by the fact that it has been demonstrated repeatedly that attention to the real stimuli increases the frustration of self-imposed delay and reduces the length of voluntary waiting (Mischel, 1974; Schack & Massari, 1973; Toner & Smith, 1977).

The young children's preferences for real stimuli over abstract or symbolic ones in the delay situation, and their inability to discriminate between effective and ineffective delay strategies, probably reflects their cognitive-developmental immaturity. With greater cognitive development, the child comes to recognize and prefer attentional strategies (e.g., focusing on irrelevant rather than relevant rewards) that avoid frustrating arousal (Experiment 4). As children increase their ability to deal with stimuli more abstractly, they also can transform them in delay-facilitating ways (Mischel, 1974; Moore et al., 1976). Specifically, we suggest that the older child can focus more on the abstract rather than consummatory qualities of incentives, thereby avoiding excessive frustration while remaining oriented to, and guided by, preferred but delayed goals. Support for that hypothesis, however, still requires empirical work.

Although Yates and Mischel found that their younger subjects did not systematically prefer effective delay strategies, it would be premature to conclude that such young children are totally unaware of the conditions that facilitate delay. Yates and Mischel confined their investigation to preferences that would require a fairly complex level of knowledge about delay. For example, one group of children was asked to choose between viewing the real object for which they were waiting and a picture of this reward, another group to choose between a picture of the reward for which they were waiting and a picture of another (irrelevant) object. Although young children do not correctly select the best delay strategies from such complex choices, they might be aware of more basic rules for successful delay. Indeed, as Gelman (1978) perceptively noted, the traditional account of the younger child has been couched in terms of the capacities he or she *lacked;* we share, instead, Gelman's focus on exploring what the young child *can* do and are impressed by how much at least some preschool children seem to know about effective ways to delay gratification as revealed in our preliminary work. It will be a challenge to assess whether different measurement conditions might reveal systematic knowledge of effective delay at earlier ages; studies exploring such early knowledge are now in progress.

To illustrate, in one study (Mischel et al., 1978), in a delay of gratification paradigm, children of different ages (preschool and grades three and six) were asked whether it would help them wait if the delayed rewards were exposed or covered during the delay period. They were then instructed to suppose that the rewards would be exposed and were asked what they could *think* about to help them to wait. After the children's spontaneous ideas were elicited, pairs of alternative ways of ideating about the rewards were presented with the instruction to choose the one from each pair that would most help the child to wait for the rewards (Table 10.4). One choice was between the consummatory ("hot") properties of the delayed rewards and their abstract, nonconsummatory ("cool") properties. A second choice was between "hot" ideation about the rewards and task-contingency ideation. The sequence in which the choice pairs, and the items in each pair, were presented was random. Following each choice the child was asked the reason for choosing as she or he had. To test for possible preferences for "hot" or "cool" ideation apart from the delay of gratification context, one half of the subjects in each group served as their own controls, first making the choice between

Table 10.4. *Ideation alternatives*

Hot: "The marshmallows taste yummy and chewy."
Cool: "The marshmallows are puffy like clouds."
Task-contingency: "I am waiting for the two marshmallows."

Note: Subjects chose between hot versus cool and hot versus task-oriented ideation. (The table shows the alternatives when the delayed rewards were two marshmallows.)
Source: Mischel, Mischel, & Hood, 1978.

"hot" and "cool" ideation about the reward objects in a nondelay situation and later choosing in the delay context. This control allowed us to assess whether any age-related changes in hot–cool ideational preferences reflected the child's changing knowledge of delay rules or merely reflected developmental changes in preferences for hot–cool ideation regardless of its value for effective delay.

The growth of self-control competencies

We (Mischel & Mischel, 1979a) have been finding that children's spontaneous delay strategies show a clear developmental progression in knowledge of effective delay rules. A few preschoolers suggest a self-distraction strategy or even rehearsal of the task contingency. Most children below the age of five years however, do not seem to generate clear or viable strategies for effective delay; instead they tend to make waiting more difficult for themselves by focusing on what they want but cannot have. By the age of five to six years they know that covering the rewards will help them wait for them while looking at them or thinking about them will make it difficult. By third grade children spontaneously generate and reasonably justify a number of potentially viable strategies and unequivocally understand the basic principles of resistance to temptation: For example, avoid looking at the rewards because: "If I'm looking at them all the time, it will make me hungry . . . and I'd want to ring the bell." Often they focus on the task and contingency, reminding themselves of the task requirement and outcomes associated with each choice ("If you wait you get _____; if you don't, you only get _____"). They also often indicate the value of distraction from the rewards or of negative ideation designed to make them less tempting ("Think about gum stuck all over them"). A small minority still suggest that positive ideation about the rewards ("The marshmallow looks good and fluffy") will help, and one wonders if these are the very youngsters for whom delay is likely to be most difficult. Most third graders clearly know that task-contingency ideation helps delay more than hot reward ideation but they still do not know that cool reward ideation is better than hot reward ideation. By the time they reach sixth grade, the children's spontaneous strategies (just like their formal preferences), show considerable sophistication. At this age most of these youngsters seem to clearly recognize the advantage of delay of cool rather than hot ideation about the rewards. The basic delay rules have been firmly mastered.

Perhaps, most important, we are finding the same meaningful developmental sequence in children's growing knowledge of effective self-control rules when we explore the everyday self-control situations they deal with in their lives (waiting for birthdays, cookies, Christmas, the family ski trip) as we find when we examine their delay knowledge in our experimental situations.

A comprehensive, coherent account of the genesis of knowledge about delay of gratification seems to be emerging. In the course of development children show increasing awareness of effective delay rules and come to generate the strategies necessary for effectively reducing frustration and temptation. They progress from a systematic preference for seeing and thinking about the real blocked rewards and hence the worst delay strategy (Yates & Mischel, 1979), to randomness, to a clear avoidance of attention to the rewards and particularly of consummatory hot reward ideation. Systematically they come to prefer distraction from the temptation, self-instructions about the task contingency, and cool ideation about the rewards themselves. These developmental shifts seem to reflect a growing recognition by the child of the principle that the more cognitively available and "hot" a temptation the more one will want it and the more difficult it will be to resist. Armed with this insight the child can generate a diverse array of strategies for effectively managing otherwise formidable tasks, and for overcoming "stimulus control" with self-control.

Some further questions

Our research so far is providing some answers to the question: At what points in development do children begin to know and understand (or misunderstand) basic rules for delay of gratification (and other behavioral principles)? It leaves unanswered a host of related questions that may deserve further research. It would be interesting to explore not only "who knows what rules when?" but also how such knowledge is linked to other aspects of the child's developing understanding and self-awareness as well as to his or her actual self-control performance under various in vivo temptation conditions.

It will be important to analyze further not only the development of the growth of the child's knowledge, understanding, and cognitive competencies but also the timetable and mechanisms for their effective application to relevant self-control tasks as well as the conditions that might impede or enhance the developmental progression. Although knowledge of self-control rules is only one component of the growth of effective self-control, it appears to follow a predictable developmental sequence of potential theoretical and practical importance. In the future we will want to understand more fully the links between cognitive competence and self-regulatory behavior. We will want to trace not only when do children know and understand what rules, but also what determines the cognitive availability, the accessibility of those rules when they are needed, and their activation to guide behavior.

A cognitive social learning analysis distinguishes between cognitive competencies – the capacities to understand and generate or construct particular actions – and the actual enactment (performance) of those actions (Mischel, 1973). Whereas construction competencies hinge on the growth of the child's knowledge and understanding of how the world works (i.e., its "rules"), performance itself in any given situation depends on such person variables as the individual's relevant expectations, values, and self-regulatory system (e.g., moment-to-moment self-monitoring) as they apply to that particular situation. To allow accurate prediction of behavior, according to this view, we need to estimate both the individual's competencies for generating the relevant performance and the other person variables that will influence its enactment. We are now designing studies with preschool children that attempt such predictions in the domain of delay of gratification, using both indexes of the children's knowledge and understanding of delay rules and of other performance-relevant person variables. Questions that seem worth exploring in this venture include the degree to which young children show generalized knowledge of the rules of self-regulation (e.g., for delay of reward and for resistance to temptation), the coherence and stability of such knowledge, its correlates and antecedents, and the specific links between cognitive competencies and successful self-control.

Notes

1 A form for use with preschoolers and primary grade school children has been developed and piloted with a small number of subjects. The attempt to question young children about psychological principles seems feasible and promising, but our efforts in this direction are still only preliminary.

2 Although the present interpretation seems reasonable, close observation of the children's behavior while they engaged in voluntary delay indicates that it may be both incomplete and too simple. Sheer suppression or distraction from the frustration of the situation seems to be one important determinant of frustration tolerance but it is unlikely to be the only one. Observation of the children's actions and verbalizations while waiting suggested that those who waited effectively were also engaged in complex self-instructions and internal activities (Mischel et al., 1972).

During earlier studies it was noted, for example, that while the child was waiting for the delayed outcome he would often repeat the contingency aloud to himself (alone in the empty room): "If I wait I get . . ." (naming the more preferred object), ". . . but if I ring the bell I get . . ." (naming the less preferred). To maintain his delay behavior effectively, it appeared as if he made an internal notation of what he was waiting for (possibly reminding himself of it by repeating the contingency from time to time), and also reminding himself of the alternative consequences of continuing to delay or of terminating the delay. Intermittently, when not so occupied, he would spend his time distracting himself from the frustration of the delay situation (e.g., by singing to himself), thus transforming the noxious delay into a more pleasant activity. Often it seemed as if the subject also supported his own delay behavior by covert self-reinforcement for waiting. Thus many children performed diverse covert self-congratulatory reactions as they continued to sustain their goal-directed waiting, and created special subjective contingencies of their own. For example, "If I just wait a little more I'll get it for sure – yes, he'll come back soon now – I'm sure he will, he must."

3 In an important series of related subsequent studies, Miller and Karniol (1976a, 1976b, 1979), have distinguished between self-imposed delay (SID) of the sort studied in the paradigm of Mischel and his associates, and externally imposed delay (EID) in which the subject cannot voluntarily terminate the delay in favor of an alternative immediate but less preferred reward. Miller and Karniol believe that the findings of Mischel and associates apply to SID but not to EID. They argue that when individuals have no choice but to endure the delay it is adaptive to focus on the rewards and they have provided some empirical support for their view. Miller and Karniol's conclusions should still be seen as tentative, but their work does underline the need to distinguish between the two types of delay and therefore we have been examining both the SID and EID paradigms separately to determine whether different rules apply.

References

Bandura, A. *Social learning theory*. Englewood Cliffs, N.J.: Prentice-Hall, 1977.

Berlyne, D. E. *Conflict, arousal, and curiosity*. New York: McGraw-Hill, 1960.

Dulany, D. E., Jr. Avoidance learning of perceptual defense and vigilance. *Journal of Abnormal and Social Psychology*, 1957, *55*, 333–8.

Estes, W. K. Reinforcement in human behavior. *American Scientist*, 1972, *60*, 723–9.

Freud, S. Formulations regarding the two principles in mental functioning. In *Collected papers* (Vol. 4). New York: Basic Books, 1959. (Originally published in 1911.)

Gelman, R. Cognitive development. In M. R. Rosenzweig & L. R. Porter (Eds.), *Annual review of psychology* (Vol. 29). Palo Alto, CA: Annual Reviews, 1978.

Grim, P. F., Kohlberg, L., & White, S. H. Some relationships between conscience and attentional processes. *Journal of Personality and Social Psychology*, 1968, *8*, 239–52.

Hartshorne, H., & May, M. A. *Studies in deceit*. New York: MacMillan, 1928.

James, W. *The principles of psychology* (Vol. 1). New York: Holt, 1890.

Mahrer, A. R. The role of expectancy in delayed reinforcement. *Journal of Experimental Psychology*, 1956, *52*, 101–5.

Mandler, G. The interruption of behavior. In D. Levine (Ed.), *Nebraska symposium on motivation*. Lincoln: University of Nebraska Press, 1964.

Miller, D. T., & Karniol, R. Coping strategies and attentional mechanisms in self-imposed and externally imposed delay situations. *Journal of Personality and Social Psychology*, 1976, *34*, 310–16. (a)

The role of rewards in externally and self-imposed delay of gratification. *Journal of Personality and Social Psychology*, 1976, *33*, 594–600. (b)

The process of reward re-evaluation in delay of gratification situations. Paper presented at the meeting of the Society for Research in Child Development. San Francisco, March 18, 1979.

Miller, S. M. Controllability and human stress: Method, evidence and theory. *Behavior Research and Therapy*, 1979, *17*, 287–304.

When is a little information a dangerous thing? Coping with stressful events by monitoring versus blunting. In S. Levine & H. Ursin (Eds.), *Coping and health: Proceedings of a NATO conference*. New York: Plenum Press, in press.

Mischel, H. N., Mischel, W., & Hood, S. Q. *The development of knowledge about self-control.* Unpublished manuscript, Stanford University, 1978.

Mischel, W. Theory and research on the antecedents of self-imposed delay of reward. In B. A. Maher (Ed.), *Progress in experimental personality research* (Vol. 3). New York: Academic Press, 1966.

Toward a cognitive social learning reconceptualization of personality. *Psychological Review*, 1973, *80*, 252–83.

Processes in delay of gratification. In L. Berkowitz (Ed.), *Advances in experimental social psychology* (Vol. 7). New York: Academic Press, 1974.

The interaction of person and situation. In D. Magnusson & N. S. Endler (Eds.), *Personality at the crossroads: Current issues in interactional psychology*. Hillsdale, N.J.: Erlbaum, 1977.

On the interface of cognition and personality: Beyond the person-situation debate. *American Psychologist*, 1979, *34*, 740–54.

Ideation in the development of delay capacity. In L. S. Liben (Ed.), Piaget and the foundation of knowledge. Hillsdale, N.J.: Lawrence Erlbaum, 1980.

Objective and subjective rules for delay of gratification. In D. Lens (Ed.), *Cognition in human motivation and learning*. Hillsdale, N.J.: Erlbaum, in press. (a)

The growth of insight into self-control principles. In S. Yussen (Ed.), *The development of reflection*. New York: Academic Press, in press. (b)

Mischel, W., & Baker, N. Cognitive appraisals and transformations in delay behavior. *Journal of Personality and Social Psychology*, 1975, *31*, 254–61.

Mischel, W., & Ebbesen, E. B. Attention in delay of gratification. *Journal of Personality and Social Psychology*, 1970, *16*, 329–37.

Mischel, W., Ebbesen, E. B., & Zeiss, A. R. Cognitive and attentional mechanisms in delay of gratification. *Journal of Personality and Social Psychology*, 1972, *21*, 204–18.

Mischel, W., & Metzner, R. Preference for delayed reward as a function of age, intelligence, and length of delay interval. *Journal of Abnormal and Social Psychology*, 1962, *64*, 425–31.

Mischel, W., & Mischel, H. N. *The development of children's knowledge of self-control.* Paper presented at the meeting of the Society for Research in Child Development. San Francisco, March 18, 1979. (a)

Children's knowledge of psychological principles. Unpublished manuscript, Stanford University, 1979. (b)

Mischel, W., Mischel, H. N., & Hood, S. Q. *The development of knowledge of effective ideation to delay gratification.* Unpublished manuscript, Stanford University, 1978.

Mischel, W., & Moore, B. Effects of attention to symbolically-presented rewards on self-control. *Journal of Personality and Social Psychology,* 1973, *28,* 172–9.

The role of ideation in voluntary delay for symbolically presented rewards. *Cognitive Therapy and Research,* 1980, *4,* 211–21.

Mischel, W., & Patterson, C. J. Substantive and structural elements of effective plans for self-control. *Journal of Personality and Social Psychology,* 1976, *34,* 942–50.

Mischel, W., & Staub, E. Effects of expectancy on working and waiting for larger rewards. *Journal of Personality and Social Psychology,* 1965, *2,* 625–33.

Moore, B., Mischel, W., & Zeiss, A. Comparative effects of the reward stimulus and its cognitive representation in voluntary delay. *Journal of Personality and Social Psychology,* 1976, *34,* 419–24.

Nisbett, R. E., & Ross, L. D. *Human inference: Strategies and shortcomings of social judgment.* Century Psychology Series. Englewood Cliffs, N.J.: Prentice-Hall, Inc., 1980.

Nisbett, R. E., & Wilson, T. D. Telling more than we can know: Verbal reports on mental processes. *Psychological Review,* 1977, *84,* 231–59.

Rapaport, D. On the psychoanalytic theory of thinking. In M. M. Gill (Ed.), *The collected papers of David Rapaport.* New York: Basic Books, 1967.

Rosen, A. C. Change in perceptual threshold as a protective function of the organism. *Journal of Personality,* 1954, *23,* 182–95.

Schack, M. L., & Massari, D. J. Effects of temporal aids on delay of gratification. *Developmental Psychology,* 1973, *8,* 168–71.

Singer, J. L. Delayed gratification and ego development. Implications for clinical and experimental research. *Journal of Consulting Psychology,* 1955, *23,* 428–31.

Toner, I. J., Lewis, B. C., & Gribble, C. M. Evaluative verbalization and delay maintenance behavior in children. *Journal of Experimental Child Psychology,* 1979, *28,* 205–10.

Toner, I. J., & Smith, R. A. Age and overt verbalization in delay-maintenance behavior in children. *Journal of Experimental Child Psychology,* 1977, *24,* 123–8.

Yates, B. T., & Mischel, W. Young children's preferred attentional strategies for delaying gratification. *Journal of Personality and Social Psychology,* 1979, *37,* 286–300.

11 Monitoring social cognitive enterprises: something else that may develop in the area of social cognition

John H. Flavell

The purpose of this chapter is to suggest some new objects of developmental study. These suggestions result from the application to social cognition of previous ideas concerning the nature and development of nonsocial cognition. I refer here to ideas about the role of metacognition (roughly, knowledge and cognition about cognition) in the management of memory, comprehension, and other kinds of tasks (e.g., Brown, 1978; Flavell, 1978a, 1978b, 1979, in press; Flavell & Wellman, 1977; Markman, in press). Most of the suggestions presented in this chapter had their origins in a recent paper on cognitive monitoring (Flavell, in press).

What are "social cognitive enterprises" and what does it mean to "monitor" them? With Damon (1977), I would prefer to define such enterprises broadly rather than narrowly (Flavell, 1977). Thus, I take them to include all intellectual endeavors in which the aim is to think or learn about social or psychological processes in the self, individual others, or human groups of all sizes and kinds (including social organizations, nations, and "people in general"). Thus, what is thought about during a social cognitive enterprise could be a perception, feeling, motive, ability, intention, purpose, interest, attitude, thought, belief, personality structure, or any other such process or property of self or other(s). It could also be the social interactions and relationships that occur among individuals, groups, nations, or other social entities. A social cognitive enterprise can be very brief (e.g., "I sense that my last remark hurt your feelings") or very extended (e.g., "I feel I am still learning new things about the kind of person you are, even after all these years of trying to understand you").

Monitoring a social cognitive enterprise roughly means keeping track of how it is going and taking appropriate measures whenever it needs to go differently. Because this last suggests a regulatory as well as a feedback

The preparation of this paper was supported by National Institute of Child Health and Human Development Grant HDMH 10429.

272

function for the monitoring process, "monitoring" subsumes and includes "regulation" in this chapter. It is proposed that the monitoring of social cognitive enterprises occurs through the actions of and interactions among four classes of phenomena: *metacognitive knowledge, metacognitive experiences, goals* (or tasks), and *actions* (strategies) (Flavell, 1979, in press).

Metacognitive knowledge means all the knowledge and beliefs you have acquired and stored in long-term memory that concern anything pertinent to social cognition. It can be thought of as that segment of your world knowledge that has specifically to do with people as social cognizers and with their diverse social cognitive tasks, goals, actions, and experiences. As with any other form of stored world knowledge, portions of it may be either automatically or intentionally accessed and used when you are engaged in activities (here, social cognitive ones) to which that knowledge pertains. Examples of metacognitive knowledge are the acquired beliefs that you are often a poor judge of character and that one way to find out how another person feels is to ask her.

Metacognitive experiences refer to any conscious cognitive and/or affective experiences or states of awareness that accompany and relate to a social cognitive enterprise. You can experience all manner of feelings, thoughts, attitudes, and judgments about yourself and others as social cognizers and about the social cognitive tasks, goals, and actions you and they undertake. Examples of metacognitive experiences include the sudden awareness that you don't know what your interlocutor is up to, and the judgment, made while reading an article on the subject, that you are finally making some progress in understanding the differing perspectives of the United States and Russia with respect to the arms race. Metacognitive knowledge and experiences are not assumed a priori to be qualitatively different in nature from nonmetacognitive knowledge and experiences; my present assumption is that the differences lie only in the content and function, not in the form or process.[1]

Goals and subgoals (tasks and subtasks) refer to the various objectives that may be pursued during a social cognitive enterprise. For example, you may try to make inferences about your previous encounters with a certain person (subgoal) to help yourself evaluate his credibility as an informant in a present encounter (goal). Actions (strategies) refer to the cognitions or other behaviors that you carry out to attain these goals and subgoals. Examples are asking questions and attending to nonverbal cues in an effort to learn more about what another person is like.

I shall now discuss these classes of phenomena in more detail and show how they might relate to one another in the monitoring of social cognitive enterprises (cf. Flavell, 1979, in press). Particular attention will be given to the nature and functions of metacognitive knowledge and metacognitive experiences, with goals and actions described in the course of discussing these first two.

Metacognitive knowledge

Like other world knowledge, metacognitive knowledge can vary in clarity, explicitness, and complexity or elaborateness. Similarly, it can also be inaccurate, internally inconsistent, or otherwise flawed. Some of it seems more procedural in nature, some of it more propositional or declarative. Most of it can be characterized as knowledge or beliefs about what factors or variables act and interact in what ways to affect the course and outcome of social cognitive enterprises. Three major categories of such factors or variables can be distinguished: *person, task,* and *strategy.*

Person variables

This category includes all the things you could come to know or believe about yourself and other people (groups, etc.) as social cognizers. This knowledge can be further subdivided into acquired beliefs about intraindividual (or intragroup) differences, about interindividual (or intergroup) differences, and about universals of social cognition.

An illustration of the first would be your belief that you are more skillful in picking up people's covert feelings than in unmasking their efforts to mislead or deceive you; that is, you tend to think of yourself as socially sensitive and empathic but a bit on the gullible side. Alternatively, you could harbor the same belief about a friend, about most clinical psychologists, and so forth.

An example of the second would be your belief that your husband is better at sizing up certain types of people than you are, although less skilled at divining the political strategy of the Republican party for the forthcoming election. Earlier-developing instances might be a ten-year-old's recognition that, unlike herself, her four-year-old brother will believe anything anyone tells him, or always has to be told he is irritating people rather than being able to figure it out for himself from their behavior toward him. It is thus assumed that social comparison processes operate in this skill domain as in any other.

Universals of social cognition refer to beliefs and generalizations about universal properties of human beings as social cognitive devices. Most older children and adults have probably accumulated much naive theory of this sort and this theory may have frequent and important influences on their social cognition and behavior. The following are some generalizations that could develop.

You know that there are various levels and kinds of social understanding: You can know different sorts of things about people and you can know them at greater or lesser depth. You know, for example, that how a person appears and acts is not the same as knowing what is going on inside her, or what she is "really like" as a person; a person (group organization) has an interior as well as an exterior.

As in the nonsocial domain, you can fail to understand a social object in two quite different ways: not understand it and misunderstand it. Not understanding is of course more readily diagnosed than misunderstanding, because misunderstandings "feel" just like correct understandings. You also know that it can sometimes be difficult to judge just how well you understand someone. In particular, you may not easily be able to find out if you know a person at the depth or in the manner needed for your present purposes (goal, task) – to hire her, trust her to keep a secret, marry her and so on. Thus, you know that social cognition can fail in various ways as well as succeed. You know that your understanding of any social object can be insufficient, misdirected (e.g., understanding goal-irrelevant things), incorrect, or otherwise inadequate.

You may also recognize that your and other people's social cognition can be biased by ignorance, prejudice, and egocentrism (in the technical, Piagetian sense). As an example of egocentrism, when you are in physical or psychological distress, you are likely to have little mental energy left over for any sort of social cognition, except perhaps concerning yourself and your troubles. Moreover, what social cognition you may engage in is more liable to error and distortion than when you are functioning normally. When your own current state (perspective) is marked by intense affect, either negative or positive, you are likely to misjudge other perspectives – especially, perhaps, your *own* perspective at other times and in other circumstances. For example, it can be hard to really believe that you could be well or happy next week if you feel terribly ill or unhappy today. Conversely, it is hard to imagine yourself feeling depressed when you feel wildly happy; indeed, it may be easier (albeit not easy) to imagine another's depression than your own when you feel this way. Interestingly, then, some of our most difficult perspective-taking problems can be those in which we try to make inferences about *ourselves* under other than present internal and external conditions; that is, taking your *own* perspective can sometimes be harder than taking another's. In sum, your metacognitive knowledge in the person category may include not only the generalization that people's social cognition can be inaccurate as well as accurate but also knowledge of some of the conditions under which it is particulary susceptible to error. When and how we acquire this kind of metacognitive knowledge is an interesting question.

Finally, you are likely to know that much social behavior is not mediated or accompanied by conscious social cognition at all; it is to a greater or lesser extent thoughtless or, to use Langer's (1978) term, "mindless." A familiar example is your knowledge that people can hurt your feelings without even knowing it, much less without doing it on purpose.

Task variables

One subcategory has to do with the information available to you during a social cognitive enterprise. It can be abundant or sparse, consistent or inconsistent, trustworthy or untrustworthy, and so on. The metacognitive knowledge consists of your knowing what such variations in the quantity and quality of the available information about the target person, social relationship, or group imply for how the enterprise should be carried out and how successful its outcome is likely to be. As an example, you may have acquired the metacognitive generalization that the quantity and quality of the obtainable data or evidence about a social object may not always be sufficient for a confident attribution.

Another subcategory has to do with task demands or goals and their implications. You may have developed a fair amount of sensitivity as to which situations do and which situations do not call for any sort of effort at social cognition.[2] For instance, you have learned to turn on your social cognitive sensors when you hear something relevant (e.g., threatening) to your personal relationship with someone you care about, as contrasted with something that neither concerns nor interests you. Thus, there could be a great deal to learn about what circumstances do and do not warrant the spontaneous establishment of a social cognitive task and goal. Once such a task and goal are established, whether self-generated or imposed by others, there is also much you can know about what the task demands are and what they imply. Some tasks and goals call for a lot of accurate social cognition, because there is a great deal that needs to be learned about the social object and there are serious consequences if the learning is inadequate. For instance, you are likely to realize that more and better social cognition is required when trying to decide whether to take Mary on as your business partner than when trying to decide whether to hire Joan as a part-time store clerk. There are undoubtedly childhood counterparts of these sorts of knowledge. More than the younger child, for example, the older child may sense that he had better try to verify the knowledgeability, credibility, and good sense of the peer who tries to talk him into a dangerous or possibly illegal venture, as contrasted with the one who merely tries to talk him into playing a card game.

Strategy variables

There is also a great deal you could have learned about what strategies (means, processes, actions) are likely to achieve what subgoals and goals in what sorts of social cognitive enterprises. Some of the strategies you can use are the same for social objects as for nonsocial objects. Examples are consulting experts, making inferences, testing hypotheses, and noting co-occurrences or other regularities. You can use the "experimental method" in the social as well as the nonsocial domain: Deliberately do or say something to a social object, see what kind of response you get, and draw appropriate conclusions. Other means can only be used in understanding social objects (cf. Gelman & Spelke, this volume), although the division is not precise. For instance, you can ask a social object to tell you about himself. You can also ask yourself how you would feel if you were in his situation and assume that he probably feels much as you would. Also, as will be explained, you can learn strategies for finding out how well you are progressing toward your social cognitive goal as well as strategies for progressing toward it.

Interactions among variables

Most of the metacognitive knowledge described so far implicitly or explicitly concerns interactions among person, task, and strategy variables. You may have come to believe, for instance, that you (and/or a certain strategy) will fare better in this cognitive enterprise than in that, because of the available information or task demands (task variables) involved in this enterprise.

The role of metacognitive knowledge in the monitoring of social cognitive enterprises

Metacognitive knowledge can be retrieved and used to influence what happens in a social cognitive enterprise. In some instances you might deliberately search this knowledge store in hopes of retrieving some needed bit of procedural or propositional information concerning social cognition. For example, when buying a car you may search your memory for something you know you once heard about how to tell when a car salesman is and is not likely to lower his asking price further. Similarly, you may consciously search for some means (strategy) of obtaining some needed information about someone. In most instances, however, the relevant metacognitive knowledge is probably activated automatically by retrieval cues within the social cognitive enterprise. Likewise, metacognitive knowledge can become conscious, whether retrieved via deliberate search or via involuntary activation. Any item of metacognitive knowledge that becomes conscious would be classified as a metacognitive experience in the present model. However, it is also assumed that metacognitive knowledge can be activated and used to influence the enterprise without entering consciousness, just as other sorts of knowledge can. For example, your knowledge that social cognition is error prone can surely influence your social cognitive conduct without ever being consciously articulated as a principle. Some metacognitive knowledge may once have been conscious (e.g., when first acquired) but seldom if ever becomes conscious now. Other metacognitive knowledge may never become conscious.

What sorts of influence can metacognitive knowledge exert? It can lead you to select, establish, evaluate, revise, and terminate social cognitive tasks, goals, and strategies, taking into consideration their relationships with one another and with your own perceived skills and interests in this area. It can lead to innumerable varieties of conscious metacognitive experiences concerning self, tasks, goals, and strategies, and it can help you interpret the significance and behavioral implications of these metacognitive experiences. In sum, it is what you know about this sector of your cognitive life, and it can have all of the effects – conscious and unconscious, intentional and unintentional – that any other body of knowledge can have. Needless to add, it can also sometimes fail to be activated when needed, fail to have any influence if activated, and fail to have a beneficial influence if influential – again, just like any other body of knowledge.

Metacognitive experiences

As stated at the beginning of this chapter, metacognitive experiences include any conscious cognitive and/or affective experiences that concern social cognitive enterprises. These experiences can be brief or lengthy in duration, simple or complex in content. To illustrate, you may experience the fleeting sense, not further attended to, that you didn't quite understand something that just happened in an unimportant social exchange; in contrast, you may endlessly construct and revise elaborate theories about what some significant other thinks of you and why. Experiences of the latter sort are believed to first become common during adolescence (El-kind, 1967). Metacognitive experiences can occur at any point before, after, or during a social cognitive enterprise. As examples of the first two possibilities, you may have the uneasy feeling that a problematic social cognitive enterprise is on the horizon, or that you were not at your best in one that happened last week.

Metacognitive experiences of the person, task (and goals), strategies, and interactions varieties are easy to think of. You suddenly feel unsure about the letter of recommendation you are currently writing because you remember that you often make incorrect predictions about how people are going to turn out (person, or person-task interaction). It occurs to you that you may not yet have enough information about the values and goals of a certain political organization to decide whether you should join it (task). You decide that imagining you are in Bill's situation and thinking accordingly will probably not yield accurate knowledge in Bill's case; he is just too different from you (strategy, or strategy-task interaction). In social cognitive as in other cognitive enterprises (Flavell, in press), many metacognitive experiences have to do with where you are in the enter-prise and what sort of progress you are making. For example, you sense that you are now just beginning to understand John, finally have a pretty good idea why Jean dislikes Janet so much, and haven't a prayer of ever really figuring out why Joe and Edith get along so well. Similarly, you thought you understood your boss's (for a child – teacher's, coach's) opin-ion of your abilities but now no longer feel sure, and you are surprised that you seem to know Elaine so well on such short acquaintance ("I feel like I've known her all my life"). Your metacognitive experiences can also be strongly emotional: You feel utterly frustrated by your inability to figure out A, very relieved when you finally clear up B, proud of your ability to decipher C, and sorry beyond measure that you ever learned D about a close friend.

When are metacognitive experiences most likely to occur? Not surpris-ingly, they are especially likely to occur in situations where you are doing a lot of intentional, conscious social thinking; such situations obviously provide many opportunities for thoughts and feelings about social cogni-tions to arise. Certain situations seem particularly apt to lead you to engage in deliberate, conscious social cognition (cf. Langer, 1978), thereby increasing the probability of having various sorts of metacognitive experiences. Some situations may explicitly demand conscious social cog-nition, such as interviewing or reading material on patients, clients, and job applicants. Other examples are situations in which you have to behave in new and unaccustomed ways, such as in a new school or on your first date. Because you do not have any overlearned habits or "scripts" (Schank & Abelson, 1977) available for these situations, much thought and attention is likely to be paid to behavioral detail and to how you might appear to others. In certain situations (including some of the foregoing) it is very important to you that your social judgment be as accurate as possible, and so you are liable to attempt a lot of careful, thoroughgoing, and heavily monitored social cognition. What you decide to do in these situations has grave consequences for you or others, and that weighty decision must be guided largely by your social cognition. Instances include some already mentioned, such as deciding whether to marry someone or to invite someone to be your business partner. Making a career choice based upon an appraisal of your interests and aptitudes is another example.

Metacognitive experiences about social cognition are also liable to occur whenever your social expectations are not confirmed, your previous social judgments are shown to be in error, your progress in social thinking is for any reason slowed down or blocked – in general, whenever your present or past social cognitions seem to you to have something wrong with them. This sense that something is wrong need not have been immediately preceded by any conscious social cognition, although of course it could have been. For instance, you can suddenly be led to question your previous impression of someone by something she does, even though you had not just previously been thinking about what sort of person she is. Finally, at least the more complex and extended forms of metacognitive experiences (e.g., a sustained evaluation of your social judgment as contrasted with a fleeting sense of noncomprehension) obviously require considerable space in working memory. Consequently, you are likelier to have such experiences when more compelling nonmetacognitive events or experiences are not preempting that space.

Are all metacognitive experiences items of metacognitive knowledge that have become conscious? Some are, but not all. The sudden feeling that you don't understand someone you thought you did ("He suddenly seems like a stranger") is clearly a metacognitive experience but it is not an item of previously acquired metacognitive knowledge that has just entered consciousness. In contrast, a subsequent conscious thought like "Wow, here's one *more* proof of my longstanding belief that you never can *really* be sure you know a person" does sound like a stored metacognitive generalization that has temporarily become conscious. Thus, some metacognitive experiences are not retrieved metacognitive knowledge (although informed or interpreted by the latter, in many instances), just as some metacognitive knowledge rarely or never becomes a conscious metacognitive experience.

Effects of metacognitive experiences on goals, metacognitive knowledge, and actions

Metacognitive experiences can have important effects on social cognitive goals. To illustrate, a friend does something that strikes you as "out of character" and hence puzzling. This experience then leads you to establish the goal of finding the cause. Metacognitive experiences can cause you to alter or abandon goals as well as establish them. If you discover that your data base is just too inadequate to provide a full and detailed appraisal of some person or group, for instance, you may settle for a rough guess or, if that will not do, abandon the whole enterprise as hopeless.

Metacognitive experiences can affect your store of metacognitive knowledge by adding to, deleting from, or revising that store. You can notice and store as metacognitive knowledge relationships among various social cognitive goals, means (actions), metacognitive experiences, and outcomes. For instance, you can observe and retain the fact that this social cognitive goal was harder to achieve than that one, that X proved to be a good strategy for reaching goal Y, that feelings of puzzlement about the motives and intentions of people that matter to you need to be taken seriously and clarifed, that snap judgments about people based upon minimal or superficial evidence are especially prone to error, and the like. Thus, metacognitive experiences are assumed to play a very important role in the development of metacognitive knowledge, as well as in the monitoring and guiding of social cognitive enterprises.

Metacognitive experiences can engender actions that are aimed at either or both of two types of goals (cf. Flavell, in press). On the one hand, these experiences can instigate actions designed to bring you closer to the main goal of your social cognitive enterprise. To illustrate, you feel that you do not yet know as much as you want or need to know about person A, interpersonal relationship B, or group C, and this feeling (metacognitive experience) leads you to try to learn more about A, B, or C by engaging in further social cognition or some other behavior (action). On the other hand, your metacognitive experience may be the judgment that you aren't sure how close you are to your main social cognitive goal, and this judgment leads you to try to find out how close you are by taking some appropriate, feedback-producing action. What you find out by taking that action will be information about your social cognitive progress, how difficult your social cognitive task is, or the like, and the reception and appraisal of this information is of course another metacognitive experience. Notice that the immediate aim of this feedback-producing action is not to *make* progress toward the main goal but rather to *monitor* that progress.

If we think of the mental and behavioral actions taken in these two cases as strategies, the first is a straightforward *cognitive* strategy, one that is initiated for the purpose of moving you closer to your (social) cognitive goal. In contrast, the second is a *metacognitive* strategy, one aimed at providing you with metacognitive experiences that will inform you about your present relation to that goal. Therefore, part of your acquired metacognitive knowledge about strategies consists of knowledge about the nature and use of metacognitive as well as cognitive strategies.

There are a number of imaginable metacognitive strategies in this as in other areas (cf. Flavell, 1979, in press). You can make a quick appraisal of someone to get a preview of how hard it is going to be to learn whatever you think you need to learn about him (much as you might skim through a course text to see how much work you have ahead of you). You can check presently incoming impressions about an organization (school club, neighborhood gang) to see if they are consistent with your previous impressions of it. You can question someone or paraphrase what she has just told you about her feelings to make sure you have understood them correctly. Not all metacognitive experiences are the outcomes of metacognitive strategies deliberately carried out to engender such experiences. They also frequently occur as the unintended and automatic byproducts of establishing a social cognitive goal, of initiating a cognitive strategy, or any of a variety of other events (Markman, in press). Needless to say, they can be used to monitor and guide the social cognitive enterprise equally well whether intentionally or unintentionally generated.

I said at the beginning of this chapter that the monitoring of social cognitive enterprises proceeds via the actions of and interactions among metacognitive knowledge, metacognitive experiences, goals (tasks), and actions (strategies). It should be fairly clear by now what this sort of monitoring can look like, but a final example might still be helpful. Let us begin at the point where some self-imposed or externally imposed social cognitive task and goal gets formed. Your metacognitive knowledge leads to the conscious metacognitive experience that this particular goal will be time consuming and rather difficult to reach, and both metacognitive knowledge and that experience lead in turn to the more or less automatic (nonconscious) selection of the goal-directed action (cognitive strategy) of, say, asking questions. The answers to these questions create additional metacognitive experiences about how the enterprise is going. These experiences, again informed and guided by whatever pertinent metacognitive knowledge you have, instigate the metacognitive strategy of thinking about what you have learned to see if it is internally consistent, fits with other knowledge as it should, and is sufficient to meet goal requirements. This thinking (also a set of metacognitive experiences, of course) turns up shortcomings of one sort or another, with the consequent enactment of additional cognitive and/or metacognitive strategies, and so things proceed until the enterprise is terminated.

Speculations about development

The ideas presented in this chapter suggest some possible developmental acquisitions in this area. I assume that most of these acquisitions would take place toward the middle-childhood and adolescence end of ontogenesis, although it would be interesting to identify and study early childhood instances or precursors of social cognition monitoring.

To begin with the person-variables category of metacognitive knowledge, children may gradually develop differentiated concepts of themselves and others as social cognizers. Attributions like "I think I am (she is) not easily fooled by others" or "I tend to give people the benefit of the doubt" are possible outcomes of development. In the subcategory of universals, early in development the child may distinguish only between succeeding and not succeeding in learning something he wants to know about another person (not understanding vs. understanding). Subsequently, he may realize that what he has learned when he does succeed can be either accurate or inaccurate (misunderstanding vs. understanding). The acquisition of this distinction may in turn provide the developmental foundation for still later achievements. Examples might be the recognition that accuracy of social cognition may be hard to assess, hard to attain, or both, and knowledge of some of the person variables that may decrease accuracy, such as prejudice, intense affect, and mental and physical illness. It is possible, however, that some forms of the latter knowledge may develop fairly early, such as the recognition that one's friend is not thinking straight about people because he is upset, in a bad mood, and so forth.

In the same category, children could also acquire skills and knowledge for assessing when the social behaviors of others are and are not accompanied by social cognitions, and in the case when they are, for assessing the nature of the relations between the cognitions and the behaviors. In the early years, no social cognitions of any sort are imputed to others.

Later, the child may automatically assume that social cognitions of others are always congruent with their social behaviors – for example, that helpful acts must reflect the intent to help and harmful acts the intent to harm. Still later, the child may recognize that both kinds of acts may reflect either no intent or an incongruent one – a helpful act done unintentionally, for purely selfish reasons, or even with the intent of achieving ultimate harm.

In the task-variables category, there is much to learn about how to evaluate the quantitative and qualitative adequacy of the available evidence you have concerning the object of your social cognitive inquiry. As in other areas of cognitive endeavor, the child has to learn how to assess the basis for his judgments and inferences. It is a fair guess that young children do not do much of this evaluation and assessment. I suspect that part of what develops is the ability and disposition to weight different pieces of evidence, relate one to another, and the like. For example: He acts as if he likes me more than the other kids right now (one piece), but I also notice he is trying to talk me into loaning him my new bicycle (another piece, given heavier weight).

In the task-demands subcategory, the child may gradually learn how to regulate what she does in accordance with task demands. She may learn how to adjust her time, effort, strategies, and attempts at quality control to fit the nature, difficulty, and importance of her social cognitive enterprise. For instance, she may try especially hard to obtain full and accurate knowledge about the likes and dislikes of another child with whom she wants to become close friends. She needs to know how to find out what depth and accuracy of understanding is needed to achieve an acceptable level of probability of reaching her goal. The disposition to do this sort of adjusting would seem to presuppose some measure of acquired planfulness, together with the acquired insights (person-variables category) that social cognitive objects can be understood at different depths and with different degrees of accuracy.

There must be a great deal that could develop in the strategy-variables category, both about cognitive strategies for achieving social cognitive goals and about metacognitive strategies for monitoring the pursuit of those goals. How and when do children learn various means of gaining information about others, as well as various metacognitive activities for monitoring the effectiveness of those means and the adequacy of that information? It is probable that they acquire more direct and obvious strategies before more indirect and subtle ones. The former might include simple observaion of social cognitive objects, asking them direct questions about themselves, and asking other people about them. Young children certainly observe others and occasionally ask them questions about their wants and feelings. When do they start asking third parties about them? The latter might include active hypothesis testing, using either observational or "experimental" methods. We may acquire sophisticated strategies for obtaining information when constraints are imposed, such as when the social cognitive object does not want us to know the information we seek and/or when we do not want the object to know we are seeking it. Under such conditions we do not take all voluntarily given information at face value, we try to observe surreptitiously, we attempt to probe without seeming to, we look for subtle, nonverbal clues, we try to be on the lookout for, or even create, situations in which the object drops its guard, and so on. The same or different strategies could be used for metacognitive or monitoring purposes – for example, to double check the obtained information for accuracy. The nature and development of cognitive and metacognitive strategies in this area strikes me as a particularly interesting and promising research topic.

The development of children's understanding of how person, task, and strategy variables may interact to affect the outcome of social cognitive endeavors could also be investigated. Developmental changes in such understanding have recently been demonstrated in the area of memory (Wellman, 1978); similar research efforts could be initiated in the area of social cognition.

Children may also need to learn that it can be useful to make a deliberate, conscious search of one's store of metacognitive knowledge when trying to solve certain social cognitive problems, such as trying to recall how accurate your previous social judgments and predictions had been in situations like the one you currently face. It is doubtful if young children engage in much intentional search of this sort. If this is the case, one thing that may develop in this area is the ability to get the most out of the metacognitive knowledge you have acquired.

Finally, there may be things for children to discover about how to respond to metacognitive experiences. They may have to learn to attend to them and to take them seriously, even the briefer and less salient ones. For example, they need to learn that even momentary feelings of uncertainty in making a social attribution may indicate that the attribution is not as well founded as previously assumed. They may also need to learn how to interpret these experiences and use them as a guide for subsequent action. Thus, another thing that may develop in this area is the ability to get the most out of the metacognitive experiences that come your way.

Finally, the acquisition of monitoring skills is a topic that also has implications for the rearing, education, and welfare of children and adolescents:

In many real life situations, the monitoring problem is not to determine how well you understand what a message means but rather to determine how much you ought to believe it or do what it says to do. I am thinking of the persuasive appeals the young receive from all quarters to smoke, drink, commit aggressive or criminal acts, have casual sex without contraceptives, have or not have the casual babies that often result, quit school, and become unthinking followers of this year's flaky cults, sects, and movements. (Feel free to revise this list in accordance with *your* values and prejudices.) Perhaps it is stretching the meanings of meta-cognition and cognitive monitoring too far to include the critical appraisal of message source, quality of appeal, and probable consequences needed to cope with these inputs sensibly, but I do not think so. It is at least conceivable that the ideas currently brewing in this area could some day be parlayed into a method of teaching children (and adults) to make wise and thoughtful life decisions as well as to comprehend and learn better in formal educational settings (Flavell, 1979, p. 910).

Summary

It is proposed that social cognitive enterprises are monitored (i.e., over-seen, appraised, regulated, guided) through the actions of and interac-tions among metacognitive knowledge, metacognitive experiences, goals (or tasks), and actions (or strategies). Metacognitive knowledge is stored knowledge about people as agents of social cognition, about social cogni-tive tasks, and about strategies for achieving social cognitive goals and monitoring the pursuit of those goals. Metacognitive experiences are con-scious thoughts, attitudes, judgments, feelings, and the like, concerning any aspect of a social cognitive enterprise an individual is engaged in. I hypothesize that both metacognitive knowledge and metacognitive expe-riences can have very important influences on the formation, pursuit, and achievement of social cognitive goals. I also believe that the developmen-tal study of this sort of monitoring may prove to be a fruitful new line of inquiry within the field of social cognitive development. Speculations about some of the possibilities that might develop in this area were pre-sented in the final section of the chapter.

Notes

1 Much of social cognition is itself metacognitive in nature, of course. For example, if I know that you (or I) know X, the first "know" clearly refers to knowledge about cognition, and hence is an instance of metacognition. In this chapter, however, I shall be concerned primarily with the monitoring and regulating functions of metacognition (metacognitive knowledge and experiences) *about* social cognition, not with social cogni-tion *as* metacognition.

2 In previous writings (Flavell, 1977, 1978a, in press; Flavell & Wellman, 1977) this sort of sensitivity was classified as a separate category of metacognitive knowledge, distinct from knowledge about person, task, and strategy variables. I now believe it logically belongs in this subcategory of task knowledge.

References

Brown, A. L. Knowing when, where, and how to remember: A problem of metacognition. In R. Glaser (Ed.), *Advances in instructional psychology.* New York: Halsted Press, 1978.

Damon, W. *The social world of the child.* San Francisco: Jossey-Bass, 1977.

Elkind, D. Egocentrism in adolescence. *Child Development,* 1967, *38,* 1025–34.

Flavell, J. H. *Cognitive development.* Englewood Cliffs, N.J.: Prentice-Hall, 1977.

Metacognitive development. In J. M. Scandura & C. J. Brainerd (Eds.), *Structural/process theories of complex human behavior.* Alphen a. d. Rijn, The Netherlands: Sijthoff and Noordhoff, 1978. (a)

Metacognition. In E. Langer (Chair), *Current perspectives on awareness and cognitive processes.* Symposium presented at the meeting of the American Psychological Association, Toronto, 1978. (b)

Metacognition and cognitive monitoring: A new area of psychological inquiry. *American Psychologist,* 1979, *34,* 906–11.

Cognitive monitoring. In W. P. Dickson (Ed.), *Children's oral communication skills.* New York: Academic Press, in press.

Flavell, J. H., & Wellman H. M. Metamemory. In R. V. Kail & J. W. Hagen (Eds.), *Perspectives on the development of memory and cognition.* Hillsdale, N.J.: Lawrence Erlbaum Associates, 1977.

Langer, E. J. Rethinking the role of thought in social interaction. In J. H. Harvey, W. J. Ickes, & R. F. Kidd (Eds.), *New directions in attribution research* (Vol. 2). Hillsdale, N.J.: Lawrence Erlbaum Associates, 1978.

Markman, E. M. Comprehension monitoring. In W. P. Dickson (Ed.), *Children's oral communication skills.* New York: Academic Press, in press.

Schank, R., & Abelson, R. *Scripts, plans, goals and understanding: An inquiry into human knowledge structures.* Hillsdale, N.J.: Lawrence Erlbaum Associates, 1977.

Wellman, H. M. Knowledge of the interaction of memory variables: A developmental study of metamemory. *Developmental Psychology,* 1978, *14,* 24–9.

12   The moral intuitions of the child

Richard A. Shweder, Elliot Turiel, and Nancy C. Much

Young children are intuitive moralists. Although four- to six-year-olds have little reflective understanding of their moral knowledge, they nevertheless have an intuitive moral competence that displays itself in the way they answer questions about moral rules and in the way they excuse their transgressions and react to the transgressions of others. Recent research by Much and Shweder (1978), Nucci and Turiel (1978), Pool, Shweder, and Much (in press), and Turiel (in press), indicates that they have moral understandings that are distinguished from nonmoral forms of appraisal. In fact, at this relatively early age, four to six, children not only seem to distinguish and identify moral versus conventional versus prudential rules using the same formal principles (e.g., obligatoriness, importance, generalizability) employed by adults; they also seem to agree with the adults of their society about the moral versus conventional versus prudential status of particular substantive events (e.g., throwing paint in another child's face versus wearing the same clothes to school every day).

These recent findings are in sharp contrast with many accounts of the development of social thought in which it is asserted that young children lack moral understanding per se and that they confuse moral and nonmoral forms of appraisal. In analyses of both the evolution of social systems (Gellner, 1973; Horton, 1968; Hobhouse, 1906) and the ontogenesis of children's moral judgments (Kohlberg, 1963, 1969, 1971; Piaget, 1932) it has been proposed that development entails the differentiation of domains of appraisal. In this view, children's judgments are dominated by nonmoral appraisals and true moral understanding only comes about after a gradual process of separating nonmoral judgments from moral ones. For example, Piaget (1932) and Kohlberg (1963, 1969, 1971) view social cognitive development as a process of differentiation and replacement in which moral understandings come to be distinguished from prudential and conventional understandings and then supersede them. This process of differentiation and replacement takes place at what are considered to be the most advanced developmental levels; indeed, by Kohlberg's account all young children and most adults in all cultures never display pure moral understandings.

Studies showing that young children have moral understandings do not imply that substantive moral development ceases at an early age. Rather, those findings suggest that it is necessary to distinguish intuitive abilities from reflective abilities. It appears that some (e.g., Piaget and Kohlberg) have traced the ontogenesis of reflective understanding and the ability to *articulate* the formal principles that define morality. In contrast, Much and Shweder (1978), Nucci and Turiel (1978), Pool, Shweder, and Much (in press), and Turiel (in press) have examined these same formal principles, but from the point of view of intuitive understanding.

In the first part of this chapter we argue that the young child is an "intuitive moralist"; the intuitive moralist knows a good deal more about morality, convention, and utility than he or she can deliberately formulate (see Nisbett & Wilson, 1977, on "knowing more than one can tell"; also Searle, 1969, p. 41). On the assumption that young children do possess intuitive moral knowledge, we then turn to the developmental question, "where do the moral intuitions of the young come from and how are those intuitions of childhood related to the moral order of the adult?" One of the best-suited methods for answering this question is cross-cultural developmental research. Accordingly, the second part of the chapter analyzes the development of intuitive moral knowledge as related to philosophical assumptions regarding moral universalism and relativism.

What is a moral issue?

Before one can speak of the moral intuitions of children one must define morality and identify moral issues. The meaning of "morality" is something discovered, not stipulated. Adults normally employ a vocabulary of moral appraisal exemplified by such terms as "immoral," "unfair," "unethical," a vocabulary that can be distinguished from nonmoral vocabularies of appraisal exemplified by such terms as "rude," "discourteous," "inappropriate," "inefficient," "impractical," "short-sighted," "illogical," and "unauthorized." A vocabulary of appraisal, whether moral or nonmoral, is applied when certain implicit or explicit prescriptions for conduct ("one should not steal"; "one should return a greeting") are violated. One way to discover the meaning of morality is to identify the formal criteria or principles that characterize and distinguish moral from nonmoral prescriptions.

The formal criteria or principles that define "morality" are relatively few in number. Gewirth (1978, p. 1) describes the core meaning as follows:

A morality is a set of categorically obligatory requirements for action that are addressed at least in part to every actual or prospective agent, and that are concerned with furthering the interests, especially the most important interests, of persons or recipients other than or in addition to the agent or the speaker. The requirements are categorically obligatory in that compliance with them is mandatory for the conduct of every person to whom they are addressed regardless of whether he wants to accept them or their results, and regardless also of the requirements of any other institutions such as law or etiquette, whose obligatoriness may itself be doubtful or variable. Thus, although one moral requirement may be overridden by another, it may not be overridden by any non-moral requirement, nor can its normative bindingness be escaped by shifting one's inclinations, opinions, or ideals.

According to this definition a transgression (e.g., a promise is broken) should elicit moral terms of appraisal (e.g., "wrong," "unfair," "immoral") if its governing prescription is perceived to satisfy certain formal criteria. Prescriptions will be classified as moral if they are (1) *obligatory,* that is, duties are invoked that do not depend on what anyone happens to want to do, (2) *generalizable or just,* that is, what is right or wrong for one is right or wrong for any similar person in similar circumstances, and (3) *important,* that is, the moral has precedence. If we subdivide "obligation" into some of its components, moral prescriptions are also perceived as (4) *impersonal or external,* that is, what is right or wrong is right or wrong regardless of whether people recognize it as such, (5) *unalterable,* that is, what is right or wrong cannot be changed by consensus or legislation, and (6) *ahistorical,* that is, although its recognition may be historical, there is no point in time at which the validity of what is right or wrong changes. (See Whiting & Whiting (1960), Hart (1961), Black (1962), Kohlberg (1971), Much & Shweder (1978), Nucci & Turiel (1978), and Turiel (1979), and Pool, Shweder, and Much (in press) for overlapping formal definitions of morality.)

Moral prescriptions are perceived as obligatory (impersonal, unalterable, ahistorical), generalizable, and important, at least by adults. The question arises, do children identify and distinguish moral prescriptions by means of the same formal criteria? Two independent lines of research suggest that they do.

The child as an intuitive moralist

Much and Shweder (1978) conducted a sociolinguistic analysis of naturally occurring excuses and justifications elicited by accusations of wrongdoing in a kindergarten setting. Three hundred twelve transgressions committed by five- and six-year-old children were classified as either breaches of morality, convention, law (school rules), belief, or "know-how" (pragmatic instructions) using adult formal criteria derived from Black (1962). The formal criteria included alterability and historicity as previously discussed. The 312 transgressions were reliably classified by two adults. What follows is an example of a transgression classified as a moral breach:

> Sally: That was my chair, Diane, get out of it.
> Diane: You can get another one, see?
> Sally: I don't have enough room. You stealed my chair.
> Diane: Nobody was in it and I sat in it.
> Sally: I'm sitting here first. I was sitting here first!

Much and Shweder discovered that for kindergarten children the things talked about and some of the ways of talking in transgression situations varied by type of breach (moral, conventional, prudential, etc.), as classified by adults using formal criteria (alterability, historicity, etc.). An analysis of the excuses and justifications of kindergarten children suggested that five- and six-year-olds distinguish among breach types in much the same way adults do, and adjust their speech behavior accordingly.

As Much and Shweder point out, breaches of conventions (e.g., "Thou shalt not stare at someone while they undress") and school rules (e.g., "Children are expected to be in school every day") elicit a legalistic orientation rich in explicit references to rules. Breaches of these kinds are explained with reference to myriad circumstantial or contextual conditions. Much and Shweder also found that breaches of pragmatic instructions (e.g., "Don't take freshly painted articles home in the rain") elicit "knowledge talk" and references to what one is trying to accomplish, his or her goals, wants, preferences. Moral breaches, in contrast, elicit negotiations over what it is that was done and who did it. Reference to the nature of the untoward act occurs most typically in connection with breaches of this type. Children either deny the act of which they have been accused, or that the accused did it, or they redefine the act to make it appear innocent instead of blameworthy. In the previous example, Diane, accused of "stealing" Sandra's chair, notes that because the chair was empty, she didn't steal it, she "sat in it." This verbal strategy ("redefine in order to avoid blame") is consistent with the view that children (like adults) perceive moral prescriptions as unalterable, obligatory, and general. Special circumstances do not excuse them. When, on occasion, a child does proffer what he or she believes to be a justification for a moral breach, it is justification of a special type: The child explains his act as punishment or retribution for someone else's wrongdoing ("Why did you pinch Tammy?" "She wouldn't let Alice play.") The research suggests that young children distinguish the moral versus conventional versus prudential status of a prescription and modulate their speech accordingly.

Research by Nucci and Turiel (1978) and Turiel (1979) and Weston and Turiel (1979) provides us with even more direct evidence that young children possess intuitive knowledge of the formal criteria that define "morality" and distinguish it from other types of prescriptions. In the Nucci and Turiel study, preschool children and adults were asked to classify seventy-two observed transgressions of moral and conventional prescriptions in terms of obligatoriness, alterability, and generalizability as measured by responses to the question: "What if there weren't a rule in the school about [the observed act], would it be right to do it then? "The preschoolers and adults agreed 83 percent of the time. In addition, preschoolers were observed to display different reaction patterns to actual rule violations, which paralleled their formal classification of the violation as either moral or conventional.

In the Turiel study subjects ranging from six to seventeen years of age were questioned about a series of rules selected to represent the distinction between moral and conventional prescriptions. The prescriptions pertained to such matters as stealing, dress codes, use of titles in school, games, and so on. Queries were posed concerning the importance of the various moral and conventional prescriptions, their perceived alterability ("Can the rule be changed?") and perceived generalizability ("Suppose there is another country in which no families have that rule. Is that all right?"). At *all* ages, subjects were discriminating in their responses and tended to agree with each other about which prescriptions were important, which could or could not be altered, and which did or did not generalize. Similar results have been obtained by Nucci (1977).

In the study by Weston and Turiel (1979) subjects from five to eleven years of age were questioned about hypothetical stories describing (1) a school in which children are allowed to hit each other (i.e., no rule exists regarding a moral prescription), and (2) a school in which children are allowed to be without any clothes (i.e., no rule exists regarding a convention). In each story the children evaluated the school policy (that permitted the act) and a child who had engaged in the permitted act. At all ages the majority of children stated a school should not permit hitting, but that a school could allow children to be undressed (even though the children, in the absence of information about school policy, had stated that one should not go around undressed). The following example of a five-year-old boy's responses is typical:

David (five years old): (This is a story about Park School. In Park School the children are allowed to hit and push others if they want. It's okay to hit and push others. Do you think it is alright for Park School to say children can hit and push others if they want to?)

No, it is not okay. (Why not?) Because that is like making other people unhappy. You can hurt them that way. It hurts other people, hurting is not good. (Mark goes to Park School. Today in school he wants to swing but he finds that all the swings are being used by other children. So he decides to hit one of the children and take the swing. Is it okay for Mark to do that?) No. Because he is hurting someone else. . . .

[Prior to specifying the school rule David was told about a boy who took his clothes off because he was warm from running around and asked if that was alright.] No, because it's a school and other people don't like to see you without your clothes on. It looks silly. (I know about another school in a different city. It's called Grove School. . . . At Grove School the children are allowed to take their clothes off if they want to. Is it okay or not okay for Grove School to say children can take their clothes off if they want to?) Yes. Because that is the rule. (Why can they have that rule?) If that's what the boss wants to do, he can do that. (How come?) Because he's the boss, he is in charge of the school. (Bob goes to Grove School. This is a warm day at Grove School. He has been running in the play area outside and he is hot so he decides to take off his clothes. Is it okay for Bob to do that?) Yes, if he wants to he can because it is the rule.

As noted earlier, the results of all these studies serve to question the commonly held view that young children do not differentiate moral and nonmoral forms of understanding. Moreover, the evidence of pure moral understandings in such young children serves to highlight the importance of distinguishing between *intuitive* and *reflective* understanding. It may be the failure to make such a distinction that has led to the belief that children confuse morality, convention, and prudence. Consider a concrete example. It is frequently thought that children confuse morality with prudence, believing that right and wrong is defined by reward and punishment; as in a child who responds to the question "Why is it wrong to steal?" with "because you will be punished for it." However, the results of the studies just reviewed suggest that such responses are a consequence of the child's difficulty in articulating justifications for their moral prescriptions. When initially asked for a justification children do indeed sometimes express themselves in the idiom of reward and punishment. However, the child does not seem to define rightness or wrongness by punishment. Rather, the resulting punishment for transgression is seen as a demonstration of its wrongness. In other words, the child is not stating that because you will be punished it is wrong, but instead is stating you will be punished because it is wrong. In fact, when the issue is pressed a little further and children are asked a question like "what if there were no punishment" for the transgression, they maintain that the act would still be wrong.

This point can be clarified through an analogy with grammatical intuitions. The young intuitive grammarian can distinguish a grammatical utterance from an ungrammatical utterance. Whatever its origin, this early competence emerges independently of either the ability to describe grammatical principles or the inclination to speak grammatically. Grammatical competence, grammatical theorizing, and speech performance undergo separate courses of development that must be explained in somewhat different terms. Similarly, it is necessary to distinguish moral intuition from moral reflection. Young children possess knowledge of the formal criteria that define "morality," but their knowledge does not involve deliberate reflection and cannot necessarily be articulated.

There are two versions of the analogy with grammar that have somewhat different implications for moral development. In the "strong" version, it would be asserted that evidence of an early intuitive ability of children to distinguish moral versus nonmoral forms of appraisal means that reflective moral *articulation* is analogous to writing the grammar of one's language. For both the intuitive grammarian and the intuitive moralist, reflective understanding is an intellectual pastime that has little bearing on either the development of grammatical or moral competence, or on the inclination to engage in appropriate behavior, either linguistic or moral. According to the "strong" version of the analogy most young children have moral intuitions. None are moral philosophers, and only a few are paragons of virtue. In the "weak" version of the analogy, however, it would be maintained that moral reflection is different from grammatical reflection in certain crucial respects. Whereas reflection upon grammatical principles does not necessarily alter one's grammatical intuitions or speech performance, reflection upon the moral reasoning of the self or others may very well result in substantive transformations in moral judgments and/or moral conduct. That is, reflection upon morality may be an intellectual activity that has a significant bearing on the development of moral competence and the regulation of behavior.

There are, then, three issues regarding the child's orientation to rules that need to be kept separate. Rules, to the extent they are *legitimately*, not whimsically or arbitrarily, enjoined, are designed to influence conduct by appealing to what is reasonable. Thus, one issue deals with the existence (or nonexistence) of an intuitive *grasp* of the requirements set by reason and an appreciation of the difference between moral and nonmoral forms of appraisal. That is the issue that concerns us in this chapter. The second issue deals with the development of skills of moral reflection, *articulation*, and reasoned argumentation. The third issue is about the fit (or lack of fit) of moral conduct and moral reason. This last issue might be viewed affectively as a problem in the development of a *respect* for the requirements set by reason (i.e., superego formation), or cognitively as a problem in the *coordination* of two subsystems, judgment and behavior. Each of these problems is compelling in its own right. When accused of wrongdoing, young intuitive moralists often fail to articulate adequate reasons for their apparent transgression, and they are not always inclined to convince themselves or others that the appearance that they have behaved in an arbitrary and unjustifiable way is merely an appearance. Both the concern with justifying oneself to oneself (and others), and the intellectual tools for doing so may or may not yet be or ever get acquired. Finally, it must be asked whether or not either intuitive or reflective understanding has a bearing on moral conduct. Nevertheless, to distinguish moral intuitions from moral articulation is an important first step in the examination of a five-year-old's orientation to rules. The second step is to penetrate more deeply into the nature of intuitive understanding.

Intuitive knowledge: perceptible, elementary, innate or merely – tacit?

As we have said, intuitive knowledge is knowledge possessed without deliberate reflection. There are several different ways that the early appearance of intuitive knowledge can be interpreted.

1. Knowledge may be intuitive in that it is "there for all to see." Such intuitions are immediate, perceptible, simple, given (so to speak) directly from the world to the senses. For example, ". . . if you cut your finger deeply with a knife, it bleeds."

2. Knowledge may be intuitive in that it involves "elementary logical deductions" that are difficult to intelligibly doubt. Although it may be said that knowledge appearing by four or five years of age appears early, it is also the case that children at that age have had four or five years of interaction with the environment for their logical schemata to develop. By age five the mind of the child is sufficiently developed so as to make elementary deductions routinely. For example, "a whole is greater than any of its parts."

3. Knowledge may be intuitive in that "nature wired us that way." Such intuitions have been given in the evolutionary past of one's species, genetically transmitted, "prepared" to emerge with minimal assistance from the environment. For example, "nothing can be perceived as red and green all over."

4. Knowledge may be intuitive in that it has been "tacitly conveyed." Such intuitions are given by one's symbolic community; they are the unconscious, acquired, unstated messages, implicit in the ongoing prac-

tices of a group. For example, "the uses of the prefix un- to reverse the meaning of an English verb coincides with the centripetal enclosing, covering and surface attaching meaning of the verb. We say, uncover, uncoil, undress, unfasten, unfold, unlock, unroll, untangle, untie, unwind, 'but not' unbreak, undry, unhang, unheat, unlift, unmelt . . ." (Whorf, 1956, p. 71, paraphrased). Whorf referred to such intuitions as "crypotypes."

Which of the four interpretations (if any) of the early appearance of intuitive knowledge best explains the development of the moral understandings of the young? The currently available data come from studies of American children. The American five-year-old does have an intuitive grasp of both the form and substance (content) of adult moral codes. By a "formal" grasp we mean that the young intuitive moralist understands the principles of obligatoriness, generalizability, importance, and so forth, that distinguish moral prescriptions from nonmoral prescriptions. By a "substantive" grasp we mean that the five-year-old understands which of his prescriptions are moral (e.g., promises should be kept), which are conventional (e.g., greetings should be returned), and which are prudential (e.g., sharp objects should be handled carefully). It could be argued that the evidence of the early appearance of unarticulated moral knowledge is compatible with all four of the interpretations. Knowledge that is "there for all of us to see," easily deduced, already available in the genes, or tacitly (if repetitively) conveyed need not take long to appear. Therefore, all four approaches to intuitive knowledge might conceivably predict that five-year-old children know much about morality and know more than they can tell. The different interpretations also have implications for later moral development. For instance, if moral intuitions are genetically transmitted, it would not be surprising if all moral competence had emerged by the age of five. However, if moral intuitions are deduced, it is likely that further age-related changes will occur.

To choose among the different interpretations of intuitive knowledge other types of evidence are required, especially evidence on the degree and nature of cross-cultural variability in the moral codes of children and adults. For example, if moral knowledge is "there for all to see" or is easily deduced then it should not be acquired by children in only some cultures but not others, unless there are peculiar mitigating circumstances (e.g., differential "blindness" or "feeble-mindedness"). That is, such explanations are most compatible with *universality*. Cross-cultural variability in childhood moral codes is more easily explained by the notion of "tacit communication." If moral knowledge is "tacitly conveyed," then children should not endorse moral rules at variance with adult practices recognized as legitimate and consistent in their own symbolic community (unless they have not been exposed to these practices). Parallel evidence of a universal childhood moral code and a cross-culturally variable adult moral code would be inconsistent with the proposition that moral knowledge stems from tacit communications received by children. The idea that morality is tacitly conveyed is most compatible with *relativism*.

The required evidence on variability in moral codes is presently unavailable. There are many historical and ethnographic accounts of other people's customs and manners, but very few of these studies, if any, examine the rule understandings of children. And it is the rare study, indeed, that provides the type of interview protocol necessary to answer the question "do such and such people perceive such and such rule as moral, or do they perceive it as conventional, or prudential, and why?" Because relevant evidence on the cross-cultural variability of childhood moral codes is not yet available we cannot review it. Instead we shall discuss the implications of certain hypothetical patterns of cross-cultural evidence for the two major philosophical approaches to the development of moral codes, namely, universalism and relativism. How does each approach interpret the moral intuitions of the child? What does each approach have to say about the relationship of the child's moral intuitions to the moral order of adults?

Intuitive knowledge: moral universalism and moral relativism

Moral universalists differ from moral relativists in their answer to the question: Is the relationship between the formal criteria of a moral code (the various criteria discussed earlier) and the content of a moral code (e.g., promises should not be broken) ultimately arbitrary? The relationship between the form and content of a moral code is *not* arbitrary to the extent that some law of nature enables you to induce, or some canon of logic enables you to deduce the content of a moral code from formal principles such as obligatoriness, generalizability, and importance. Moral universalists are typically involved in a search for some canon of logic or universal generalization that will help specify a content for a moral code that all peoples should endorse. For relativists, in contrast, the individual's moral codes are derived from premises concerning matters of fact, importance, and value (e.g. all persons are created equal) that may vary from culture to culture. Therefore, for a relativist, the content of a moral code has no determinate relation to the formal criteria that define morality.

Universalism

In the universalist view there are a number of ways to link the formal criteria and content of a moral code in a determinate relationship. Deductive universalists (e.g., Kohlberg, 1971; Gewirth, 1978) argue that formal principles such as generalizability (justice) enable you to logically deduce the content that ought to be part of any moral code (e.g., respect for another's physical and psychological well being). Notably, universalists of this type do not make clear-cut predictions about the cross-cultural or developmental *content* of extant moral codes. What they do maintain is that proper deductive reasoning from undeniable premises, combined with a willingness to accept the requirements set by reason would lead to unanimity about how one is obligated to behave, although because people often commit logical errors or hold false or contradictory beliefs, the deductive universalist would not be surprised by evidence that what is thought to be moral on one side of the Red Sea is not thought to be moral on the other side. However, they would expect cross-cultural commonalities in the developmental sequences of reasoning about what are considered moral contents.

Inductive universalists, in contrast, do expect extant moral rules (i.e., rules that are perceived as obligatory, impersonal, unalterable, ahistorical, generalizable, and important) to in fact concentrate on a predictable and universal content, such as the value of life, physical and psychological harm to others, truthfulness, and so on. First, certain species-wide goals (e.g., survival) are attributed to the child. Furthermore, inductive universalists maintain that interpersonal actions are the basis for the formation of prescriptive judgments in childhood. Morality entails judgments (initially intuitive) and judgments are generated out of experiences. Although moral judgments stem from experiences, they are not directly given in the experiences: Inferences about events and about relations between events result in moral prescriptions. In conjunction with the goal of survival the perceived consequences of, for example, attacks on persons, property, and promises constitute the experiences that stimulate the development of a moral orientation. Therefore, moral development stems from the child's interpretations of events experienced, rather than from the social transmission of rules, values or instructions as to how to behave. Certain social events (e.g., those entailing the infliction of harm by one person upon another) are likely to be perceived as nonarbitrary, whereas other events (e.g., a uniformity in mode of dress) will be perceived as arbitrary. It is events perceived as nonarbitrary that lead to the construction of moral prescriptions, whereas it is events perceived as arbitrary, insofar as they are subject to social regulation, that lead to conventional appraisals.

Given the proposition that inferences about the consequences of social interactions are the source of a moral orientation, inductive universalists claim that in all cultures a limited number of content areas (e.g., violence to persons, properties, or promises) will be viewed in moral terms. However, inductive universalists may differ as to whether or not those are the only content areas treated as moral. Those who may be referred to as *maximal* inductive universalists would claim that moral rules will focus *exclusively* on a limited number of content areas. In contrast, those who may be referred to as *minimal* inductive universalists would claim that all people view the same *few* content areas in moral terms, but they may differ about other content areas. This is a more restricted claim because it leaves many other content areas (sexuality, dress code, dietary customs, marriage rules, etc.) free to vary in their moral versus nonmoral status from society to society. *Maximal* inductive universalists would, thus, look skeptically upon reports that, for example, female dress codes are a moral issue for Iranian Moslems and dietary codes a moral issue for Brahmanic Hindus. In contrast, *minimal* inductive universalists do not deny the moral status of a veiled face in the Middle East or a beef-free diet in South Asia. They will insist, however, that such issues as the protection of persons, property, and promises have a moral status across cultures.

The position taken by inductive universalists has implications for cross-cultural developmental research. From this viewpoint, cross-cultural research must do more than catalogue cultural uniformities or practices. In cross-cultural research it is necessary to do in-depth study of individuals' reasoning about specific rules and thereby assess the formal criteria used by them. Moreover, it is necessary to compare the formal criteria used for different rules. The inductive universalist would expect to find that in certain equivalent content areas rules will be viewed and treated as important, obligatory, impersonal, unalterable, ahistorical, and generalizable for all peoples. However, rules in other content areas will be viewed and treated as (1) important and obligatory for members of the group, and (2) alterable, historical, and not necessarily obligatory for members outside the group (nongeneralizable across groups).

The prediction is that moral forms of appraisal are nonarbitrarily linked to certain content areas that are, across cultures, distinguished from conventional forms of appraisal that are recognized as specific to their own culture. Moreover, it is claimed that the evidence is not in yet, in spite of frequent social scientific assertions to the contrary. This is because what may actually be conventional forms of appraisal by peoples in other lands may be misinterpreted by social scientists as moral forms of appraisal. Only cross-cultural research that makes in-depth study of individuals' orientations to a variety of specific rules can begin to answer these questions.

Such cross-cultural research must also be developmental, focusing on the experiences that stimulate moral development and the types of moral judgments made by young children. In that way it would be possible to determine how the moral judgments of children in various cultures compare with each other and how children's moral judgments within a culture compare with those of adults. The prediction most consistent with the interepretation of inductive universalism is that children around the world will agree with each other about what is and what is not a moral issue regardless of the content of adult moral codes in the child's own society. The prediction that children around the world subscribe to similar moral codes, an intuitive code derived directly from experience and reason, must be reconciled with the apparent correspondence between *American* children and *adults* of their culture in what is and what is not regarded as a moral issue.

Two interpretive possibilities can explain transgenerational consensus. Maximal inductive universalists would maintain that the moral codes of adults in all cultures is an amplification of universal childhood intuitions. That is, the child's moral intuitions form the basis for subsequent transformations into reflective moral judgments evident among adults in all cultures. Minimal inductive universalists might maintain that (1) in all cultures there would be substantial correspondence between childhood and adult moral codes for a limited number of content areas, and (2) within some cultures other content areas are treated by adults as moral but not by children.

Relativism

According to universalists moral judgments arise out of intuitive responses to the consequences of certain types of human social interactions in relationship to certain universal human goals. Therefore, the basis of morality does not stem from cultural consensus. In contrast, according to relativists, moral codes do arise from direct and indirect cultural transmission: The moral intuitions of the child are tacit, culturally conveyed understandings and the content of moral intuitions will vary from culture to culture. Relativists grant that for any person or people moral codes may be supported by reasons, considerations, and so on, but they insist that, for any person or people, reasons and considerations ultimately give out. Ultimately, a relativist will argue, moral codes rest upon declarations of what is of importance, value, and significance, declarations that cannot themselves be justified and are matters of preference that have neither an inductive nor a deductive warrant (see Perelman, 1963).

Relativism is associated with the view that the formal principles that define morality do not contribute any content to a moral code. As examples consider, first, the formal principle of importance and then the principle of generalizability (or justice). Briefly, relativists argue that judgments about what is morally important are cross-culturally variable, potentially charged with symbolic value, and typically disproportionate to the substance of the valued conduct. From not worshipping idols to not coveting thy neighbor's wife to not spending money on luxuries to not remarrying if one's husband dies to veiling one's face, what are matters of importance on one side of the globe are not matters of importance on the other. The collection of practices thought to be morally important by one people or other at one time or other is a diverse and unpredictable set, or so the relativist would argue.

The same relativist argument (the formal criteria and content of a moral code are unrelated) can be applied to the principle of generalizability or justice. The principle of justice states, "What is right (or wrong) for one is right (or wrong) for any similar person in similar circumstances" (Singer, 1963, p. 19), "persons who belong to the same essential category ought to be treated in the same way" (Perelman, 1963, p. 29), "treat like cases alike and different cases differently" (Hart, 1961, p. 155). Relativists will point out, along with Hart, that justice

cannot afford any determinate guide to conduct. . . "Treat like cases alike and different cases differently" is the central element in the idea of justice [but] it is by itself incomplete. . . This is so because any set of human beings will resemble each other in some respects and differ from each other in others and, until it is established what resemblances and differences are relevant, "treat like cases alike" must remain an empty form (Hart, 1961, p. 155).

Thus, for example, given our culture's belief that there are relevant differences between an adolescent and an adult in the capacity for responsible judgment, there is nothing unjust or unfair about denying a thirteen-year-old the right to vote or enter into a contract. To be just, fair, equitable, or impartial is not necessarily to treat all sentient beings in identical fashion. Quite the contrary. It is out of respect for the principle of justice that relevant differences between people must make a difference for how they are treated. As relativists see it, the principle of justice is compatible with all sorts of nonidentical treatment and diverse (but only "apparently" inequitable) social classifications. Many peoples, the relativist will argue, perceive the difference between a woman and a man, a slave and a master, a "black" and a "white," an animal and a person to be as significant as the difference between a thirteen-year-old and an adult appears to us.

As the relativist sees it, the principle of justice (treat like cases alike and different cases differently) not only fails to specify who it is that is to be treated in like or different fashion; it also fails to specify in what particular way those treated in like fashion are to be treated. Thus, in our culture, it might be unjust, as Hart notes (1961, p. 155), if a father "arbitrarily selected one of his children for severer punishment than that given to others guilty of the same fault." However, if all children guilty of the same fault are treated in like fashion, it is no less just to spank each of them than to reason with each of them, or psychologically torment them by withdrawing love. Again, the formal principle of justice contributes little to the content of a moral code; the content derives instead from historically specific and culturally relative premises about the nature of the person, society, and social relationships.

Relativists radically separate the formal criteria of a moral code from its content. This radical separation makes it possible for relativists to admit the possibility that the formal principles (obligatoriness, generalizability, importance) underlying moral (versus nonmoral) appraisal are universal while arguing at the same time that the content of moral codes is cross-culturally variable. Thus, relativists are amenable to the idea that any single content area (e.g., sexuality, possession of property) can be covered by rules of more than one type (e.g., moral prescriptions against certain "animal-like" postures, prudential rules for maximizing pleasure, conventions governing who does what when); a relativist will argue that for any person or people matters such as how to do it, what to do, when not to do it, and who not to do it with may or may not be viewed as moral, conventional, or prudential issues. It all depends upon the importance, value, and significance assigned to the practice. A rule prescribing vegetarianism (or proscribing the eating of beef) might be viewed by one people as a moral injunction against the killing of animals (or the murder of "sacred cows"), whereas for another people it might be viewed as a prudential rule for achieving good health.

Although within any given culture certain content areas may be treated as moral in a formal sense, relativists maintain that individuals come by their morality via conversational routines and the incidental learning of ongoing practices. Therefore, the moral intuitions of the American five-year-old are regarded as tacit-covert understandings, achieved primarily from having lived for a half a decade in a distinctive cultural environment packed with implicit messages about what is of importance, what is of value, which differences between people should be overlooked, which should be emphasized, and so on. Because, from a relativistic viewpoint, the form of a moral code does not determine its content, the young intuitive moralist has no other way to achieve a substantive moral understanding except by making sense of, and with, the values and beliefs that are part of his peculiar cultural inheritance. If moral codes are historically and cross-culturally variable, then they are not "there for all to see," (unless some people are blind), nor are they likely to be innate (unless biological evolution occurs in historical timeframes and unless there are "racial" differences in moral sensibilities) or self-evident (unless some peoples are feebleminded). Relativists do not deny that the intuitive moral understandings of the child may *seem* directly apprehended to the child, but, a relativist will argue that some of the obviousness is the product of overlearning a tacit code that one has never had the opportunity to question or doubt.

Relativists make two strong predictions about what cross-cultural developmental evidence on moral codes will reveal: (1) the formal principles of obligatoriness (impersonality, unalterability, ahistoricity), generalizability, and importance will not enable you to determine the content of adult moral codes; that is, what is perceived as obligatory, impersonal, unalterable, ahistorical, just, and important in one land will not correspond to what is perceived in that way in other lands; (2) to the extent that children are exposed to adult practices, the substantive moral intuitions of children in different lands will correspond more closely to the moral codes of adults in their own culture than to the moral intuitions of children in different cultures. In other words, the content of moral codes will vary for both children and adults across time and culture. Furthermore, relativists emphasize the symbolic character of social interactions, and predict that children everywhere learn to interpret the meaning of a social event by applying, misapplying and reapplying extant adult moral codes.

Summary

In the foregoing pages our aim has been to identify some questions worth asking in the investigation of moral development. As an essay in conceptual clarification we have (1) distinguished between intuitive moral understanding and reflective moral understanding; (2) outlined four possible interpretations for the existence of an intuitive moral competence in American five-year-olds; and (3) examined the problem of "arbitrariness" in moral codes.

The interpretive options currently available to moral development re-

searchers are rich, spanning the full philosophical spectrum from universalism to relativism. A major conclusion of our chapter is that a reduction
in the degrees of theoretical freedom is desirable and can be best
achieved by means of relevant cross-cultural developmental research.

References

Black, M. The analysis of rules. In M. Black, *Models and metaphors*. Ithacs, N.Y.: Cornell
    University Press, 1962.
Gellner, E. The savage and the modern mind. In R. Horton and R. Finnegan (Eds.),
    Modes of Thought. London: Faber and Faber, 1973.
Gewirth, A. *Reason and morality*. Chicago: University of Chicago Press, 1978.
Hart, H. L. A. *The concept of law*. London: Oxford University Press, 1961.
Hobhouse, L. T. *Morals in Evolution*. London: Chapman and Hall, 1906.
Horton, R. Neo-Tylorianism: Sound sense or sinister prejudice? *Man*, 1968, *3*, 625–34.
Kohlberg, L. The development of children's orientation toward a moral order. 1. Sequence
    in the development of moral thought. *Vita Humana*, 1963, *6*, 11–33.
    Stage and sequence: The cognitive developmental approach to socialization. In D. A.
    Goslin (Ed.), *Handbook of socialization theory and research*. New York: Rand
    McNally, 1969.
    From is to ought: How to commit the naturalistic fallacy and get away with it in the study
    of moral development. In T. Mischel (Ed.), *Cognitive development and epistemology*.
    New York: Academic Press, 1971.
Much, N., & Shweder, R. A. Speaking of rules: The analysis of culture in breach. In W.
    Damon (Ed.), *New directions for child development, Vol. 2: Moral development*. San
    Francisco: Jossey-Bass, 1978.
Nisbett, R. E. and Wilson, T. D. Telling more than we can know: Verbal reports on mental
    processes. *Psychological Review*, 1977, *84*, 231–59.
Nucci, L. *Social development: Personal, conventional and moral concepts*. Unpublished
    doctoral dissertation, University of California, Santa Cruz, 1977.
Nucci, L. P., & Turiel, E. Social interactions and the development of social concepts in
    preschool children. *Child Development*, 1978, *49*, 400–7.
Perelman, C. *The idea of justice and the problem of argument*. New York: Humanities
    Press, 1963.
Piaget, J. *The moral judgment of the child* (1932). New York: Free Press, 1965.
Pool, D. L., Shweder, R. A., and Much, N. C. Culture as a cognitive system: Differenti-
    ated rule understandings in children and other savages. In E. T. Higgins, D. N. Ruble,
    & W. W. Hartup (Eds.), *Social Cognition and Social Behavior: Developmental Perspec-
    tives*. In preparation, 1980.
Searle, J. R. *Speech Acts*. Cambridge: Cambridge University Press, 1969.
Singer, M. G. *Generalization in ethics*. London: Eyre & Spottiswoode, 1963.
Turiel, E. Distinct conceptual and developmental domains: Social-convention and morality.
    In C. B. Keasy (Ed.) *Nebraska Symposium on Motivation, 1977*, (Vol. 25). Lincoln:
    University of Nebraska Press, 1979.
    Domains and categories in social cognitive development. In W. Overton (Ed.), *The
    Relationship Between Social and Cognitive Development*. Hillsdale, N.J.: Lawrence Erl-
    baum Associates, in press.
Weston, D. and Turiel, E. *Act-rule relations: Children's concepts of social rules*. Unpub-
    lished manuscript, University of California, Berkeley, 1979.

Whiting, J. W. M., & Whiting, B. B. Contributions of anthropology to the methods of studying child rearing. In P. H. Mussen (Ed.), *Handbook of research methods in child psychology*. New York: Wiley, 1960.

Whorf, B. L. *Language, Thought and Reality*. Cambridge, Mass.: MIT Press, 1956.

13   Concluding remarks

John H. Flavell and Lee Ross

Two related beliefs have been instrumental in stimulating both this volume and the Social Science Research Council conferences that preceded it. The first belief was that the topic of social cognitive development should be viewed less as a discrete area within developmental psychology than as an important point of contact between developmental psychology and several other disciplines, notably social anthropology, social psychology, and cognitive psychology. The second, and consequent belief was that leading practitioners in these other disciplines would have some interesting things to say to and learn from those who study social cognitive development. Our concluding essay speaks more explicitly to the basis for these beliefs by outlining some important differences between developmental and nondevelopmental approaches and exploring the strategic advantages of recognizing and exploiting such differences. It also attempts both to underscore some recurrent themes sounded by our various contributors and to identify a pair of research topics relating to social cognition that seem particularly ripe for developmental consideration.

Developmental versus nondevelopmental approaches

Developmentalists often deplore the apparent obliviousness to developmental concerns that is characteristically shown by investigators of adult social and nonsocial cognition. Such obliviousness, we suspect, may cost the nondevelopmentalist dearly – in terms of the phenomena selected for study, the hypotheses entertained, the methodology employed, and perhaps even the conclusions reached. Paradoxically, however, we also suspect that developmentalists might do well to adopt, or at least be able to better appreciate, that stance in their own efforts to understand the nature and growth of the child's social understanding and behavior. This is the case with respect to two related features that distinguish developmentalist from "nondevelopmentalist" orientations: (1) the assumption of

306

universality versus nonuniversality in underlying processes; and (2) the relative emphasis on adult competence versus shortcomings.

The assumption of universality

Investigators of adult cognitive processes make the working assumption that the essential features of such processes are universal and invariable within the species. They assume they are studying the way that the class of organisms called "people" comprehend, remember, make social inferences, and act or inhibit action accordingly. Moreover, the class members who are most "available" for them as subjects, and most apt to be treated as "representative," are college students. Thus, phenomena and functional relationships discovered in research with these subjects are assumed (more tacitly than explicitly) to apply to adults of other ages, ability levels, life histories, and cultures. Similarly, although few researchers would deny the existence of age-related differences in sophistication, knowledge, experience, and skill, children are nevertheless assumed to be governed by the same basic psychological principles and processes that are discovered in research with young adults.

It is true that juvenile members of the species are sometimes used as experimental subjects by the researchers in question. However, this is often done simply to demonstrate that "children" – a subset of the species that is rarely further differentiated – do indeed act in a "person"-like fashion and, more importantly, that their behavior can be understood in terms of the same theories or principles that apply to the whole class of people. By such demonstrations, of course, the investigator seeks to validate not only the robustness of the relevant theories or principles but also the legitimacy of the underlying assumption of invariance in the cognitive makeup of the human species. Such studies demonstrate that, for example, children *too* show constructive processes in comprehension of complex social and nonsocial events.

Lest the reader feel compelled at this point to defend his or her nondevelopmentalist colleagues against our oversimplified caricature, let us emphasize from the outset that we do not intend to criticize this aspect of the nondevelopmental perspective. Quite the contrary, we shall argue that it constitutes a kind of "null hypothesis" that developmentalists in the area of social cognition would do well to consider more carefully and reject more cautiously.

Developmentalists (not excluding the senior author of this essay) tend to look at a segment of adult social cognition and almost reflexively wonder how it evolved during childhood into its present form. Their working hypothesis is apt to be that the segment must not have existed at all during the earliest months or years of childhood but then may have assumed a succession of qualitatively different forms during subsequent childhood periods. This general "schema" for developmental theorizing seems particularly applicable in the social domain, perhaps because the social domain is one in which age-related differences in the nature and overall quality of observed performance seem particularly obvious. Developmentalists, in short, are "set" to look for rich and complex developmental stories behind segments of adult social cognition. The hypothesis that a given segment of adult social cognition may have a relatively impoverished (and thus an "uninteresting") ontogenetic history, or essentially no history at all, is not a highly available alternative. Moreover, any evidence that such a hypothesis may be warranted with respect to a given class of phenomena may make the developmentalist reluctant to pursue such phenomena further.

The nondevelopmentalist stance we have described, by contrast, would neither expect nor search for significant age-related changes in performance or in the processes that are reflected in performance. It views the child as most interesting and worthy of detailed investigation when that child's behavior seems very similar to the adult's, or better still when it seems to offer a particularly clear illustration of some principle or process that is somehow obscured by subtle and complex influences in the adult. Hence the attractiveness of using children to study modeling effects in aggression, or to illustrate the capacity of extrinsic rewards to undermine intrinsic interests. Purported evidence of fundamental changes in cognitive structures or processes, or of discontinuities over the lifespan in the functional relationships embodied in psychological principles or laws, are apt to be either regarded with skepticism or dismissed as isolated and particularistic. Most important, the nondevelopmentalist is prepared to argue that age-related differences in observed performance are less profound in their implications concerning underlying processes than might be assumed from the magnitude of such differences. When they can plausibly do so, nondevelopmentalists attribute discontinuities between the performances of younger and older individuals simply to "additional learning and experience" or, less simply, to "the older subjects' superior mastery of the goals and rules that characterize experimenter–subject interactions." And where such explanations seem least plausible or least satisfying, the nondevelopmentalist becomes least interested in using the young as experimental subjects.

For the field of psychology as a whole, these alternative stances we have caricatured constitute two dangerous extremes to be avoided. But for practitioners who find that either caricature describes themselves a little too accurately for comfort, a willingness to adopt or at least role play the "mind set" of the opposing camp can pay important intellectual dividends. We will not pause here to defend and elaborate the proposition that students of adult social cognition may benefit from entertaining a more developmental perspective – such a defense, we suspect, would be a gratuitous exercise given the disposition of most of our readers. However we will try to emphasize the importance for the developmentalist to at least periodically entertain a nondevelopmental mind set – one that assumes minimal changes in basic cognitive capacities or processes until evidence demands a contrary interpretation, and one that regards the absence of marked age-related changes in performance as no less interesting than the presence of such changes. Even Piaget, the quintessential developmentalist, was careful from the beginning to distinguish those things that do not change with ontogenesis (such as the "functional invariants" of assimilation and accommodation) from those that do.

Several essays in this volume profitably adopted some version of this universalistic, nondevelopmental mind set in considering social cognitive development, and there are at least hints of it in others. Some essays have spoken particularly forcefully about specific domains where youthful understanding and performance seem surprisingly sophisticated (e.g., Hoffman; Mischel; Shweder, Turiel, & Much). Others have described sources of age differences that seem related much less to basic cognitive capacities than to the mastery of specific theories, scripts, or other bodies of knowledge (e.g., Berndt; Damon; Flavell; Gelman & Spelke; Higgins; Kosslyn & Kagan; and Nelson) or even to the availability of adequate firsthand or secondhand "data samples" from which to draw social inferences (e.g., Bandura; Ross). In several of these essays, analyses dealing with age-related changes in "perspective taking" or "role playing" or "empathic abilities" were particularly notable in this regard, as were discussions of the various factors that made mastery of social knowledge and performance both easier and more difficult than nonsocial knowledge for the young.

The recognition and investigation of adult shortcomings

We turn now to a second, but closely related feature distinguishing developmental from nondevelopmental mind sets – one that likewise offers important intellectual dividends for the investigator willing to seriously entertain the perspectives of the opposing camp. Nondevelopmentalists, we have claimed, are wont to think of the creatures they study as "people" or "subjects," not as "outcomes of cognitive growth." As a consequence, they are less likely than the developmentalist to accept as an article of faith the notion that these creatures are always and everywhere highly rational, logical, and effective thinkers. Developmentalists cannot help comparing mature intellectual performance with that of the infants or young children that they see in their daily research. For them, adults are former infants and children who have "grown up" – with considerable emphasis on the "up." It is extremely tempting for most developmentalists to see the passage from birth to adulthood as a Horatio Alger-like increase in cognitive fortune, whereby growing older means growing wiser, more competent, and less prone to the follies of youth.

For the nondevelopmentalist, by contrast, adults are not consequences of a grand and inexorable perfecting process. Adult subjects are simply "people" – the kind of people who misunderstand the point of one's argument, vote for the wrong candidate, and hand in illogical and incoherent essay exams. Indeed, if invidious comparisons are made, they are apt to be between the layperson and the scientist (see Ross, 1977; Nisbett & Ross, 1980) or the novice and the expert in some domain (Simon & Simon, 1978).

Thus, where cognitive developmentalists look for sophisticated formal-operational level thought, nondevelopmentalists find an ever-growing list of intellectual shortcomings. Adults' social inferences are frequently the products of judgmental heuristics or scripts, schemas, and other knowledge structures that may be ill-suited for the purpose to which they are put. Far from the essentially rational paragon seen emerging by the contemporary cognitive developmentalist, the adult is viewed as a creature whose most impressive intellectual triumphs are matched by equally impressive failures. The failures, moreover, are not simply regressions to childish modes of inference; indeed, many are part and parcel of the same adult strategies and priorities that have been "developing" and becoming more pervasive over the life span (see Ross's essay in this volume; also Shaklee, 1979). (Interestingly, it appears that developmental psychologists who are not cognitive developmentalists are also less likely to conceive of ontogenesis as unswerving progress toward the good and positive. For example, developmental psychologists who study socialization effects may try to find out why some children grow up to be antisocial, intellectually inactive, prejudiced, etc.).

Nondevelopmentalists continually dispute the diagnosis of the various performance deficiencies that have been demonstrated, and some question whether they are really dysfunction or even are really clear violations of normative principles of inference. Currently, such disputes seem to be raging quite heatedly (see Cohen, 1980), but there is little dispute about the fact that adult capacities are indeed imperfect and limited. All contemporary information-processing models stress how attention, coding, storage, and retrieval of information compromise the quality and complexity of adult thinking. And even the most sympathetic review of human inference would agree that there exist particular inferential domains (e.g., appreciating regression phenomena, or updating hypotheses in light of new data) in which adult performances leave much to be desired.

Undoubtedly, nondevelopmentalists might be led to a more charitable, and perhaps more balanced view of human intellectual performance by recognizing how far the adult has "advanced." But the opposite advantage of perspective-switching also merits considerable emphasis. The developmentalists' tendency to focus on cognitive shortcomings that are largely overcome by the end of adolescence has understandably led them to be overly impressed with adult capacities and insufficiently concerned with adult deficiencies. Furthermore, by recognizing this fact a new and unusual scientific task for developmentalists now becomes more imaginable – studying the ontogenesis of our intellectual warts. What sorts of developmental histories might they have? Some, of course, may undergo essentially no developmental changes at all. They may simply testify to the continuity between the child's and the adult's modes of thinking. These differences may reflect, and thus may help us to discover and understand, "hard-wired" properties of every human intellect, that is, structurally dictated ways that all people think as soon as they become able to think at all. Other shortcomings, as Chapter 1 suggests, may actually develop with age. They may develop as a consequence of exposure to culturally shared ideas or to uniquely distorted sources of data, or to ever-increasing cognitive demands to do more, to do it more quickly, or to do it more "thoughtlessly." The development of such shortcomings may be a straightforward and nonstagelike increase in the relevant tendency, or it might consist of a succession of qualitatively different-looking steps. Still other shortcomings, although still clearly present in adult cognitive functioning, may become less pronounced in the course of ontogenesis. In such cases, domain-specific insights, gathered from one's individual experience or the collective experience of one's tribe, one's profession, or the "experts" in one's culture, may hold the relevant differences in check and curb their influence. Clearly, cross-cultural studies (developmental and nondevelopmental alike) would go a long way in speaking to the issues of universality and developmental malleability that are raised by these speculations. They might also lead to some qualification or regrouping of, and almost certainly make some interesting additions to, the presently still modest list of shortcomings that has been drawn up by students of adult cognition.

Attention to the possibility of studying the developmental history of our species' inferential shortcomings alerts the developmentalist to another set of research possibilities. Consider the familiar psycholinguistic distinction between competence and performance. A segment of linguistic or cognitive competence is of course assumed to be a positive, desirable thing. We *want* it to find expression in performance. The opposite, however, is true in the case of our cognitive shortcomings (one is tempted to call them *in*competences). In all likelihood we could not expunge them from our cognitive repertoires; and even if we could it is doubtful that we would be well served by an indiscriminate abandoning of inferential strategies that are undeniably efficient, and perhaps even "cost effective," for many types of everyday problems (see Ross, in this volume; also Nisbett & Ross, 1980). What the cognitively maturing individual must learn to do, therefore, is to become more aware of his or her inferential strategies, of the respect in which they may violate particular normative dictates, and of the tasks or inferential domains in which such violations are too likely or too costly to bear. People, in a sense, are forced to learn how to block or attenuate the passage of their "incompetences" into performance. The development in question thus seems to be of the metacognition, monitoring, and regulation variety described in Flavell's essay. Bandura's and Mischel's essays similarly whet one's appetite for research that focuses more specifically on the child's developing awareness of the relationship between his or her own capacities and limitations and the performance demands of everyday cognitive and social tasks.

We do not know the extent to which adults may have developed an awareness of some of their social cognitive strategies and shortcomings (see also Nisbett & Wilson, 1977). Nor do we know the extent to which they may have developed the inclination and ability to blunt the effects of those they have identified. We have little doubt, however, that the search for these sorts of metacognitive knowledge and skills will be an important future task for social cognitive developmentalists.

Frontiers and possible futures: on action, affect, and cognition

The contributors to this volume have already suggested an abundance of frontiers and future possibilities for exploration. Nevertheless, we wish to conclude essay and volume by calling attention to a few additional possibilities.

From Heider's early work on attribution theory to Kahneman and Tversky's recent work on judgmental heuristics and Abelson's on scripts, research on adult social cognition has always helped to define targets for developmental consideration. However, the almost exclusively cognitive orientation of contemporary social psychology, and indeed of almost all experimental psychology, presents a risk for the developmentalist. Specifically, developmentalists may find themselves aping a similarly one-dimensional approach at exactly the time when some nondevelopmentalists are beginning to rediscover the other two components of the traditional cognitive-conative-affective (or thinking-acting-feeling) trinity.

Action and cognition

With regard to the problem of "action," we shall say little beyond reiterating the folly of portraying human beings as creatures who, like Tolman's rat, seem doomed to remain "lost in thought" – attending, evaluating, comprehending, and remembering, but not actually *doing* anything. Psychology as a whole obviously needs to know a great deal more about when judgments, inferences, or other cognitive events lead first to behavioral intentions, and then to behavior itself. When is behavior "thoughtful" and when is it "thoughtless" (Langer, 1978), or the consequence of "top of the head" (Taylor & Fiske, 1978) processes?

Developmentally, many key issues invite exploration. How, when, and at what level of awareness do children learn strategies or decision rules for taking or inhibiting actions consistent with their various impressions, beliefs, and impulses? Similarly, when, and how, and why, do particular classes of overt behavior – and perhaps the inferential or judgmental processes that underlie them – become either more automatic or less so, that is, either more or less subject to conscious consideration of alternatives, priorities, and decision rules? In this volume, Berndt's essay with its particular adaptation of Fishbein and Ajzen's work on the specificity of attitude–behavior linkages, suggested one fruitful path to be followed in the developmental study of symmetries and asymmetries between cognition and behavior. Mischel's essay took an intriguing new look at the classic "behavioral" problem of impulse control or delay of gratification. Bandura's social learning analysis of the problem of self-efficacy offered yet another path toward the integration of research on social (and self) cognition with that on social behavior. Flavell likewise alluded to the metacognitive aspects involved in the self-control of behavior and the selection of appropriate social strategies. Finally, Shweder, Turiel, and Much reminded us of the cognition versus action question that is as old as speculative philosophy itself – the relationship between moral knowledge and moral behavior. Nevertheless systematic study of the links between the child's growing cognitive competencies and the evolving relationship between contemplation, intention, and action remains almost virgin terrain for the developmentalist.

Affect and cognition

The portrait of the adult human as an information-processing computer or analytic scientist preoccupied with interpreting stimuli and event sequences and with updating generic knowledge undeniably has been useful in formulating questions for psychological research. But it is a portrait that cannot easily be reconciled with an ongoing phenomenological experience that is apt to be highly affective and evaluative.

As Zajonc (1980) argues, in an essay that is bound to be both influential and controversial, the contemporary cognitive emphasis in psychology has failed to recognize both the pervasiveness and the immediateness of our positive or negative responses to stimuli. In encountering many types of stimuli (such as sounds, shapes, or even the human face) affective or evaluative responses seem to *precede*, rather than follow from, more "cognitive" processes such as feature analysis, interpretation, or even recognition. Zajonc goes so far as to speculate about the existence of two relatively autonomous processing systems that independently mediate these two types of responses.

If Zajonc's speculations bear fruit, the developmental implications will be important and obvious. The early onset of affective responding and the early existence of visual and other sensory preferences in the very young have been well documented, and have generally been regarded as evidence of the dawning of the *cognitive* capacities of the neonate. If Zajonc is right, we may be obliged to rethink the relationship among the infant's earliest responses to its environment. But even if Zajonc's radical suggestions about independent systems and processes prove to be unfounded, there is little doubt that the role of affective response will receive increased attention in the decade ahead. We will be forced to portray a creature who feels, as well as analyses, and who must therefore try to reconcile any discrepancies between affective and "intellectual" responses.

With an increasingly affective (or at least "hotter" cognitive) emphasis in psychology as a whole, the opportunities for research on affective development and its relationship to social cognitive development should become even more obvious. For example, one could search for regular sequences and timetables in children's initial experience and expression of different feelings, and in their sensitivity to the occurrence of these feelings in others. In so doing the need to relate affective and cognitive developments becomes apparent. Thus, longing for a specific person and other attachment-related feelings obviously presuppose some level of development of Piagetian object permanence. Various levels of shame and self-consciousness must depend upon corresponding levels of self-awareness and the concept of self. Feelings of personal efficacy or inefficacy (recall Bandura's essay in this volume) presuppose some acquired conceptions about abilities, performance norms and standards, task difficulty, and so forth. And we know essentially nothing about the development and possible cognitive underpinnings of more mature sounding feelings – feeling foolish, humiliated, penitent, moved to tears, regretful over what might have been, and the like.

Similarly, we could explore the development of children's theoretical (à la Mischel) knowledge concerning the nature, expression, and control of various kinds of affect. When and how do children come to understand that some kinds of emotions tend to be more transient and situation-bound than others, that a person can experience affective blends or ambivalences (mixtures of love and hate, joy and sadness, etc.), that people may not always really feel the way they appear to feel, and so on? There must also be interesting developmental stories concerning the prediction and control of emotions. People may develop the tendency to try to prepare themselves for strong feelings they believe are upcoming, in hopes of controlling the expression of these feelings and their effect on the self or others. They may have learned that it is sometimes easier to manage the desired expression and impact of an emotion if one prepares in advance. When about to undergo a turbulent airplane flight, for example, a parent may brace himself to control both the experience and the expression of fear; for example, try not to let his child see that he is frightened. Adults could also have learned that one may be able to prevent the occurrence of some unwanted affects in self or others by taking appropriate planful action, such as changing the topic of thought or conversation (see Chapter 10). Similarly, many people have acquired the ability to postpone affective experience until a later, more "convenient" time. Examples are delaying your emotional collapse until after the crisis is over and containing your exuberance until you actually get written notification of your Nobel prize. Do we really know *anything* about these important-seeming forms of "affect management" knowledge and ability? Affects are notoriously difficult to manage but they are not wholly unmanageable, and there simply has to be a great deal for the child to develop here. Mapping the what, when, and how of development in this area seems an important scientific task.

We will resist the temptation to expand our list of things affective or affective/cognitive that develop. We will similarly resist the temptation to speculate about new and promising methodologies for such investigations (but see again the essays by Bandura, Berndt, Damon, and Kossyln & Kagan). Instead we will close by renewing our plea for closer and more sympathetic contact between developmentalists and nondevelopmentalists who, sometimes inadvertently and sometimes deliberately, blaze exciting trails for one another to follow.

References

Cohen, L. J. On the psychology of prediction: Whose is the fallacy? *Cognition*, 1979, *7*, 385–407.

Langer, E. J. Rethinking the role of thought in social interaction. In J. H. Harvey, W. J. Ickes, & R. F. Kidd (Eds.), *New directions in attribution research*, (Vol. 2). Hillsdale, N.J.: Lawrence Erlbaum Associates, 1978.

Nisbett, R., & Ross, L. *Human inference: Strategies and shortcomings of social judgment.* Englewood Cliffs, N.J.: Prentice-Hall, 1980.

Nisbett, R. E., & Wilson, T. D. Telling more than we can know: Verbal reports on mental processes. *Psychological Review, 1977, 84,* 231–59.

Ross, L. The intuitive psychologist and his shortcomings. In L. Berkowitz (Ed.), *Advances in experimental social psychology,* (Vol. 10). New York: Academic Press, 1977.

Shaklee, H. Bounded rationality and cognitive development: Upper limits on growth? *Cognitive Psychology*, 1979, *11,* 327–45.

Simon, D. P., & Simon, H. A. Individual differences in solving physics problems. In R. S. Siegler (Ed.) *Children's thinking: What develops?* Hillsdale, N.J.: Lawrence Erlbaum Associates, 1978.

Taylor, S. E., & Fiske, S. T. Salience, attention and attribution: Top of the head phenomena. In L. Berkowitz (Ed.), *Advances in experimental social psychology,* (Vol. 11). New York: Academic Press, 1978.

Zajonc, R. B. Feeling and thinking: Preferences need no inferences. *American Psychologist,* 1980, *35,* 151–75.

Index

Abelson, R. P., 101, 103, 105, 107, 116, 313
Abrahams, B., 54
abstracting from script representations, 113–16
abstraction level, schema, 99
accommodation of theory to subsequent experience, 11
accomplishments, and self-efficacy, 203
acquisition: of knowledge content, 18–20; of script, 105–8
action(s): animate and inanimate objects as recipients of, 46–7; child's understanding of, 52–4; and cognition, 313–14; defined, 273; and metacognitive experiences, 281–3; and outcomes, role-biased, 25–8; and observers, attribution, 20–2
Adolescence, transitional experiences, and growth of self-efficacy, 215
Adulthood: origins of shortcomings, 17–18; recognition and investigation of shortcomings, 309–12; self-efficacy concerns, 215–16
affect: and cognition, 314–16; and empathy, 75–6; and information processing, 93–4
age: and discovery of attitudes and beliefs, 90–2; and reappraisals of self-efficacy, 216–18; and representation, 88–90; and social behavior, 188–92; and susceptibility to fundamental attribution error, intuitive scientist, 28–32
Ajzen, I., 186, 187, 188, 190, 193, 313
altruism, and role taking, 145
animate and inanimate objects, 43–4; and causal reasoning, 61–3; and child's developing system of knowledge, 54–6; child's understanding of properties of, 48–51; development of distinction between, 47–8; as different natural kinds, 45; and object permanence and attachment, 57–60; as objects of perception, 46, child's understanding of, 49, 51–2; as recipient of action, 46–7, child's understanding of, 52–4; and social and nonsocial cognition,

57–63; systems of knowledge about, 47; *see also* people vs. things; social cognition
application, of scripts, 108–13
Aristotle, 176–7
arousal, emotional, and self-efficacy, 204
arousal information, cognitive processing, and self-efficacy, 208–10
articulation, and orientation to rules, 294
Asch, S., 2, 241
assessment: causal, and prediction, 10–11; covariation, 9–10
assimilation: biased, 13; of data, 11
association, and friendship, 178
attachment, and object permanence, 57–60
attention, and self-control, 251–2
attention to outcomes, and waiting behavior, 246–9
attitudes: and age, 90–2; and social behavior, 186
attributes, of friends, 178
attribution: of actors and observers, 20–2; vs. bias, 3–4; false consensus or egocentric bias, 22–5; intuitive scientist's age-related susceptibility to fundamental error, 28–32; and prediction, 5–7; social, and causal reasoning, 61–3
attribution theory, to intuitive psychology from, 2–7
availability heuristic, and intuitive scientist, 15–16

Bacon, Francis, 11
Bailey, D. E., 139
Baker, N., 259
Baldwin, J. M., 159
Bandura, A., 241, 312, 313
Bartlett, F. C., 100
Bates, E., 53
Beck, A. T., 229
behavior: control, and self-efficacy, 228–9; and social cognition, 185–95; waiting, and attention to outcomes, 246–9

beliefs: and age, 90–2; perseverance of, 11–12
Bem, D. J., 2, 27
Bem, S., 27
Berlyne, D. E., 255
Berndt, T. J., 125, 313
bias: vs. attribution, 3–4; inferential, 20–8
biased assimilation, 13
Black, M., 291
Borgida, E., 6
Borke, H., 73, 130, 137
Botvin, G. J., 164
brain, child's understanding of, 49
Brainerd, C. J., 182
Brown, I. Jr., 207
Bruner, J. S., 13, 158, 163
Bullock, M., 50, 62
Byrne, D. F., 122, 130

Campos, J. J., 69
capabilities, and self-efficacy, 215–16
Carey, S., 48–9
causal assessment, and prediction, 10–11
causality, and cognition, 69–71
causal judgment, and attribution, 2
causal reasoning, development of, 61–3
Chandler, M. J., 121, 162
Chapin, M., 224
classical conditioning, and empathy, 75
Clement, D. C., 115
cognition: and action, 313–14; and affect, 314–16; and assessing inner states, 71–2; and causality, 69–71; and permanence, 68–9; *see also* social cognition
cognitive control, and self-efficacy, 229–30
cognitive development: nonsocial, 182–3; and social interaction, 165–7
cognitive distraction, and delay, 249–54
cognitive modeling, and self-efficacy, 224
cognitive operations to transform stimulus, and delay, 257–62
cognitive self-efficacy, and school, 214–15
Coie, J. D., 132
Collins, W. A., 125
comparison judgments, 129–30
competence-contingency incentives, and growth of interest and self-efficacy, 232–3
conflict, and social cognition, 183–5
congruity effect, and imagery, 87
conservation: and nonsocial cognition, 180; and role taking, 145
conservation training, and social interaction, 164
control: behavioral, and fear arousal, 228–9; cognitive, and self-efficacy, 229–30; *see also* self-control
coordinated intentions, and social interaction, 158–9

coordinated social exchanges, 159–61
coordination, and respect for rules, 295
corrective modeling, and self-efficacy, 224
Costanzo, P. R., 132
covariant principle, and attribution, 3
covariation, assessment, 9–10
Croft, K., 49
Cronbach, L. J., 3

Damon, W., 187, 272
datum, characterizing, 8
Davis, K. E., 2
death, child's understanding of, 48
decentration, and role taking, 131
deductive inference: and role taking, 139; and social reference, 141
delay: child's knowledge of rules, 262–6; and cognitive distraction, 249–54; and cognitive operations to transform stimulus, 257–62; and growth of self-control competencies, 266–7; origins of, 245–6; and symbolically presented rewards, 254–7
developmental vs. nondevelopmental approaches to social cognition, 306–12
Devin, J., 136
DeVries, R., 130
didactic treatment, and self-efficacy, 224
discounting principle, and atttribution, 3
distraction, cognitive, and delay, 249–54
Doise, Willem, 164–6, 168
dreaming, child's understanding of, 49–50
Dyck, D. G., 224

effectance motivation, and self-efficacy, 226–7
egocentric attribution bias, 22–5
egocentrism: and metacognitive knowledge, 275; and role taking, 131; vs. self-reference, 141–4
emotional arousal, and self-efficacy, 204
empathy, and social cognition, 74–8
enactive information, cognitive processing, and self-efficacy, 205–6
environment, and social cognition, 182
equilibration, and social cognition, 163–4
Estes, W. K., 255
evaluation, of role-biased actions and outcomes, 25–8
event, representation of, 101–5
exchanges, coordinated, 159–60
experience, vicarious, and self-efficacy, 203–4
experimental techniques, in studying development of social cognition, 86–8

facilitators of social cognition, 72–8
fairness, and peer influence, 169–71

faithfulness, and friendship, 179
false consensus, attribution bias, 22–5
family, and self-efficacy, 212–13
Farnill, D., 132
fear arousal, and self-efficacy, 228–31
feelings, child's understanding of, 50
Feffer, M., 123, 137
Fein, D. A., 69, 70
Feldman, N.S., 123, 137
Fishbein, M., 186, 187, 188, 190, 193, 313
Fisher, K. W., 69
Flavell, E.R., 49
Flavell, J. H., 49, 120, 121, 122, 127, 128, 134, 135, 162, 169, 183, 312, 313
Freud, S., 245, 254, 257, 264
friendship, conception of, 176–80
fundamental attribution error, and age, intuitive scientist, 28–32

Gelman, R., 50, 62, 67, 136, 265
generalizing from sample, 9
Gewirth, A., 290
Glick, J., 67
Glucksberg, S., 127, 129
goals: defined, 273; and metacognitive experiences, 281–3
Golinkoff, R. M., 48
gratification, *see* delay
Grim, P. F., 251
growth, children's understanding of, 48
Gruendel, J. M., 116
Grumet, J. F., 132

Halliday, M. A. K., 97
Harding, C. G., 48
Hart, H. L. A., 301, 302
Hartshorne, H., 251
heart attack, and self-efficacy, 217
Heider, F., 2, 313
Hess, V. L., 125
heuristics, judgmental, and intuitive scientist, 14–15
Higgins, E. T., 137, 139, 140, 142, 143
Huttenlocher, J., 128

Icheiser, G., 2
illness, and self-efficacy, 217
imagery: and representation, 88–90; research program, 82–6; and social cognition, 86–92
incentives, and development of interest, 231–3
individual role taking, 127–8, 129–31
inductive inference, and role taking, 139
inferred similarity vs. egocentrism, 141–4
information on efficacy, cognitive processing of, 204–10
information processing, and affect, 93–4

Inhelder, B., 168
inner states, assessing, 71–2
Inouye, D. K., 207
intentions, coordinated, in social interaction, 158–9
interaction: and cognition, 155–8; and cognitive development, 165–7; and conservation training, 164; coordinated intentions in, 158–9; and culture, 164; model, 169–71; participatory, 106
interest, intrinsic, and self-efficacy, 231–4
intimacy, and friendship, 179
intrinsic interest, and self-efficacy, 231–4
intuitive knowledge: interpretations, 195–7; and universalism vs. relativism, 297–303
intuitive moralist, child as, 290–5
intuitive psychologist, child as, 240–5

Jackson, E., 69
James, William, 251
Johnson, C. N., 49
Jones, E. E., 2, 20–1, 22
judgment: self-efficacy, 201–2, 223; *see also* role taking
judgmental heuristics, and intuitive scientist, 14–16
justice reasoning, and peer influence, 169–71

Kahneman, Daniel, 5, 14, 17, 93, 313
Karniol, R., 124, 264
Keil, F., 50, 51
Kelley, H. H., 2
Kelly G., 2
Kessel, F. S., 121
Klosson, E. C., 123
knowledge: about animate and inanimate objects, 47; content, acquisition of, 18–20; of delay rules, 262–6; intuitive, 295–303; and schema, 98–9; social cognition and acquisition of, 162–7; and social judgment, 146–7; *see also* metacognitive knowledge
knowledge structures, and intuitive scientist, 13–14
knowledge systems, child's developing, 54–6
Kohlberg, L., 183, 188, 189–90, 191, 288
Kosslyn, S. M., 83, 87, 89, 93
Krauss, R. M., 127, 129
Kun, A., 62, 125

Laird, J. D., 76
Langer, E. J., 276
language acquisition, and self-efficacy, 213
Lempers, J. D., 49
Lepper, M., 12
level of efficiency judgments, 223

Lockhart, K. L., 54
loyalty, and friendship, 179
Lyons, J., 114

Macmurray, J., 158
Markham, E., 141
maximal inductive universalists, 299
May, M. A., 251
Mead, G. H., 130, 159
mediating mechanism, self-efficacy as, 230–1
Meichenbaum, D., 229
memory capacity, and representation, 89
mental image scanning, 86
metacognition, *See* delay; metacognitive experience; metacognitive knowledge
metacognitive experience, 278–81; defined, 273; effect on goals, metacognitive knowledge, and actions, 281–3
metacognitive knowledge: defined, 273; and metacognitive experiences, 281–3; and monitoring of social cognitive enterprises, 277–8; person variables, 274–6; strategy variables, 277; task variables, 276–7; *see also* knowledge
metacognitive psychology, and cognitive content, 20
microanalytic efficacy methodology, 222–5
Miller, D. T., 264
Miller, P. H., 121, 122
mind, child's understanding of, 50–1
minimal inductive universalists, 299
Mischel, H. N., 191
Mischel, W., 191, 254, 258, 259, 260, 263, 264, 265, 312, 313
monitoring of social cognitive enterprises, 272–3
Moore, B., 254, 258, 260
moral intuition: and child as intuitive moralist, 290–5; and intuitive knowledge, 295–303
moral issue, defined, 289–90
moral judgments, and role taking, 123–4
moral reasoning, and role taking, 190
moral relativism, 297, 300–3
Morris, W. N., 220
motivation, effectance, and self-efficacy, 226–7
motivation to comply, and self-efficacy, 226–7
Much, N. C., 288, 289, 290, 291, 313
Murray, F. B., 164
musculature, somatic, and empathy, 76
mutuality, and social interaction, 159
mutual role taking, 122–3

Nemcek, D., 220
Nisbett, R. E., 6, 20–1, 22, 198

nonsocial cognition: development of, 57–63; and social cognition, 180–5; *see also* animate and inanimate objects; people vs. things; social cognition; social cognitive enterprises
normative beliefs, and social behavior, 187
Nucci, L. P., 288, 289, 292

object permanence, and attachment, 57–60
observers and actors, attribution, 20–2
occupation, and self efficacy, 215
Oppenheimer, L., 71
origins of adult shortcomings, 17–18
Ortony, A., 99
Osherson, D. N., 54
outcomes: and actions, role-biased, 25–8; waiting behavior and attention to, 246–9

Paige, Satchel, 217
parsimony, and causal assessment, 11
Parsons, J. E., 123, 125
Pascual-Leone, J., 126
Pavlov, I., 241, 244
peers: influence, and fairness, 169–71; and validation of self-efficacy, 213–14
people vs. things: assessing inner states, 71–2; causality, 69–71; development of distinction between, 47–56; and empathy, 74; interactional context, 73–4; permanence, 68–9; and similarities among people, 74; and social and nonsocial cognition, 68–72; understanding, 67–68; *see also* animate and inanimate objects
perceived efficacy, beginnings, 211
perception, and animate and inanimate objects as objects of, 46; child's understanding of, 49, 51–2
performance: and role taking, 135–44; and self-efficacy, 203
permanence, and cognition, 68–9
perseverance of beliefs, 11–12
personal normative beliefs, and social behavior, 187
personal relations, and intentions, 158–9
personal variables, metacognitive knowledge, 174–6
persuasion, verbal, and self-efficacy, 204
persuasory information, cognitive processing, and self-efficacy, 208
physical cognition vs. social cognition, 157–61
physical mechanisms, and causal reasoning, 61–3
Piaget, Jean, 48, 50, 53, 57, 59, 61, 67, 70, 71, 100, 120, 126, 163, 182, 288, 309
play, and friendship, 178
Pool, D. L., 288, 289

prediction: and attribution, 5–7; and causal assessment, 10–11
Premack, D., 51
Presson, C. C., 128
prosocial behavior, and friendship, 178
proximal self-motivation, and growth of interest and self-efficacy, 233–4
psychology, intuitive, from attribution theory to, 2–7

reasoning, causal, development of, 61–3
reciprocity, child's understanding of, 53–4
relativism, moral, and intuitive knowledge, 297, 300–3
representation: development over age, 88–90; of event, 101–5; script, abstracting from, 113–16
representativeness, and social reference, 140–1
representativeness heuristic, and intuitive scientist, 15–16
reproduction, children's understanding of, 48
respect, and orientation to rules, 295
retroactive self-reference vs. egocentrism, 143
rewards: and development of interest, 231–2; symbolically presented, and delay, 254–7
Rholes, W. S., 123
role-biased actions and outcomes, 25–8
role taking: and content of judgments, 120–2; and controlling self, 126–31; dimensions underlying development of, 119–20; independence from stimulus input, 120; integrated perspective on development of, 131–5; and interrelating multiple events, 122–6; and moral reasoning, 190; and performance, 135–44; situational vs. individual, 127–31; social reference and social deduction, as alternative processes, 139–41
Rosch, E., 139
Ross, L., 25, 26, 124, 162, 169
Ruble, D. N., 123, 125, 137
Rumelhart, D. E., 99

Sachs, J., 136
sample: characterizing, 8; generalizing from, 9
Sarason, I. G., 229
Sarbin, T.R., 120, 139
scanning, mental image, 86
schachter, S., 2
Schank, R. C., 101, 103, 105, 107, 116
schema: features, 99; and intuitive scientist, 14; theories, 98–100
school, and cognitive self-efficacy, 214–15

Schunk, D. H., 223
script: abstracting from representations, 113–16; acquisition, 105–8; event representation, 101–5
self-appraisal, skills development, 219–22
self-as-object judgments, 130–1
self-concept, and self-efficacy, 225
self-control: and attention, 251–2; and delay, 266–7; and social judgments, 126–31
self-discovery, 182–3; and social cognition, 185
self-motivation, proximal, and growth of interest and self-efficacy, 233–4
self-reference vs. egocentrism, in role taking, 141–4
self-reflective role taking, 122, 130
Selman, R. L., 122, 127, 130
sexes: and friendship conceptions, 181–2; and self-efficacy, 218
Shatz, M., 50, 136, 141, 143
Shipstead, S. G., 49
Shwartz, S. P., 89
Shweder, R. A., 288, 289, 290, 291, 313
similarity: and friendship, 177; inferred, vs. egocentrism, 141–4
Singer, J. E., 2
situational role taking, 127–9
Skinner, B. F., 241
social attribution, and causal reasoning, 61–3
social behavior, and social cognition, 185–95
social conflict, and social cognition, 183–5
social deduction, and role taking, 139–41
social exchanges, coordinated, 159–61
social inference, and attribution, 2
social interaction, *see* interaction
social judgments, *see* role taking
social normative beliefs, and social behavior, 186–7
social reference, and role taking, 139–41
social relations, as coordinated exchanges, 159–61
somatic musculature, and empathy, 76
speech, style, and age of listener, 136–7
Spelke, E., 67
stimulus, cognitive operations to transform, and delay, 257–62
stimulus input, and role taking, 120
strategy variables, metacognitive knowledge, 277
strength, of efficacy judgments, 223
subjective role taking, 122, 130
Sullivan, H. S., 183
symbolically presented rewards, and delay, 254–7

Taft, R., 139
target-only judgments, 129–30

task variables, metacognitive knowledge,
  276–7
theories: schema, 98–100; testing and revising, 11–13
things vs. people, *see* animate and inanimate
  objects; people vs. things
thought, child's understanding of, 49–50
time-binding, and delay, 245, 251
Trevarthen, C., 97
trust, and friendship, 179
Turiel, E., 54, 187, 288, 289, 292, 313
tutorial methods, and cognitive development, 182–3
Tversky, Amos, 5, 14, 17, 93, 313

understanding: intuitive vs. reflective, 293;
  of people vs. things, *see* people vs. things
universalism, moral, and intuitive knowledge, 297–300
universality: and intuitive knowledge, 296;
  social cognition and assumption of, 307–9

validation of self-efficacy, peers and, 213–14
Van der Lee, H., 71

Variables: person, 274–6; schema, 99;
  strategy, 277; task, 276–7
verbal persuasion, and self-efficacy, 204
vicarious experience, and self-efficacy,
  203–4
vicarious information, cognitive processing,
  and self-efficacy, 206–8
visual contact, and attachment, 58–9
Vygotsky, L., 163

waiting behavior, and attention to outcomes,
  246–9
Wellman, H. M., 49
Weston, D., 292
White, R. W., 226, 227
Whorf, B. L., 296
Wilson, T. D., 194
Wine, J., 229
Woodruff, G., 51

Yates, B. T., 264, 265

Zajonc, R. B., 79, 314
Zeiss, A., 260